350 best vegan recipes

350 best vegan recipes

Deb Roussou

Robert ROSE

350 Best Vegan Recipes
Text copyright © 2012 Deb Roussou
Photographs copyright © 2012 Robert Rose Inc. (except as listed below)
Cover and text design copyright © 2012 Robert Rose Inc.

For complete cataloguing information, see page 384.

Disclaimer
The recipes in this book have been carefully tested by our kitchen and our tasters. To the best of our knowledge, they are safe and nutritious for ordinary use and users. For those people with food or other allergies, or who have special food requirements or health issues, please read the suggested contents of each recipe carefully and determine whether or not they may create a problem for you. All recipes are used at the risk of the consumer.

We cannot be responsible for any hazards, loss or damage that may occur as a result of any recipe use.

For those with special needs, allergies, requirements or health problems, in the event of any doubt, please contact your medical adviser prior to the use of any recipe.

Design and production: Daniella Zanchetta/PageWave Graphics Inc.
Editor: Carol Sherman
Recipe editor: Jennifer MacKenzie
Copy editor: Karen Campbell-Sheviak
Photographer: Colin Erricson
Associate photographer: Matt Johannsson
Food stylist: Kathryn Robertson
Prop stylist: Charlene Erricson

Cover image: Sautéed Slivered Brussels Sprouts over Wild Rice Cakes (page 132)

Additional photographs: Soy Milk © iStock/Sze Fei Wong; Creamy Mayonnaise © iStock/Lilyana Vynogradova; Caramel Sauce © iStock/Giuseppe Parisi; Greek Herbed Soy Feta in Olive Oil © iStock/Lilyana Vynogradova; Basil Lemon Gremolata Pesto © iStock/Viktorija Kuprijanova; Ranch Dressing © iStock/Lauri Patterson; Bouquet Garni © iStock/Maria Gerasimenko; Cajun Spice © iStock/Kelly Cline.

We acknowledge the financial support of the Government of Canada through the Book Publishing Industry Development Program (BPIDP) for our publishing activities.

Published by Robert Rose Inc.
120 Eglinton Avenue East, Suite 800, Toronto, Ontario, Canada M4P 1E2
Tel: (416) 322-6552 Fax: (416) 322-6936
www.robertrose.ca

Printed and bound in Canada

1 2 3 4 5 6 7 8 9 TG | LBF 20 19 18 17 16 15 14 13 12

Contents

Acknowledgments

Many thanks to everyone who contributed knowledge, inspiration, support and snacks to this project. Endless thanks to Diane Durrett for getting this party started. A colossal thanks to Melinda Van Doren for being so very literal and incredibly good at everything she does. To Kathleen Pedulla for her limitless knowledge of all things baked, given so generously. Thanks to Lynda Scheben for the nutritional bounty, to Suzanne Perkins for her universal savvy and to Linda Meeks for the old-school schooling.

A massive thanks to Sally Ekus and the Lisa Ekus Group for putting this project together. To Bob Dees and his team at Robert Rose for all their hard work, most particularly Carol Sherman, Marian Jarkovich and Martine Quibell. And to Daniella Zanchetta and the staff at PageWave Graphics for wrapping it all up in a beautiful book.

Introduction

❈—❈—❈—❈—❈—❈—❈—❈—❈—❈—❈—❈—❈

Good food is good food no matter what the label and this cookbook is a celebration of just that! These vegan recipes will guide you while making edibles for every occasion and for all in attendance. This is gorgeous food, simple food, party food and healthy food you will enjoy cooking and sharing with your family and friends. And that is what really great vegan food is about!

The recipes in this cookbook are vast and varied from regional favorites to worldly bites like Northwest Passage Cedar-Planked Tofu, County Fair Corn Chip Pie, Greek Herbed Soy Feta in Olive Oil and Tempeh Mango Lettuce Cups with Chile-Garlic Dipping Sauce. Get your party started with the absolutely fabulous McGillicuddy's Irish Cream or a Mexican Velvet Elvis cocktail. Find recipes for luminous lunches such as Roasted Beet Tacos with Marinated Shredded Kale and lazy weekend French Herbed Strata brunches. From artisan breads to fresh summertime grills, this cookbook offers 350 great recipes to choose from and I feel certain you will find just the right ones. You can always start with the cocktails.

The recipes in the Vegan from Scratch chapter are affordable and healthy alternatives to many hard to find and or expensive vegan ingredients such as heavy cream, sweetened condensed milk, creamy mayonnaise and seitan. These recipes use readily available ingredients generally present in a vegan pantry or refrigerator.

The first chapters offer tips on ingredients and tools. The Vegan Pantry suggests food items that are practical to have on hand. Most you will already have, a few ingredients may be new to you. Purchase one or two at a time and use liberally to get a feel for how they act. Tools and Equipment suggests kitchen tools helpful to have but by no means required. A blender can make your life easier but many times a glass jar with a tight-fitting lid will do the job.

Beyond the recipes, Suggested Menus is helpful for planning almost any occasion, from a Southwestern Brunch to a Super Bowl Sunday bash or a New Year's Eve Cocktail Party.

The key to kitchen bliss is innovation with tools and ingredients. Don't be afraid to adjust recipes to celebrate seasonal vegetables, try a new spice or use up ingredients you have on hand. Many memorable successes were born of improvisation. And remember; have fun, it's all good!

– Deb Roussou

Tools and Equipment

X—X—X—X—X—X—X—X—X—X—X—X—X—X

For many, money is the deciding factor in the number of kitchen tools that end up gathering dust in drawers, purchasing as many as the budget will allow. This contributes to the clutter in your brain, in your kitchen and on the planet. The more we buy, the more is made, the more is thrown away and the cycle continues.

Before buying, think about how you cook. What tools do you really use? Do you spend your weekend crafting the perfect loaf of bread or chocolate fudge? If so a stand mixer, cooling rack or candy thermometer might enhance your kitchen time. If you tend a garden or have earned your own parking space at the weekly farmer's market, your money might be better spent on a few good knives, a chinois strainer and canning kit. So clean out those drawers, get real about what you need and spread those tools around. Tools that haven't seen the light of day in years may find a starring role in a friend's kitchen; one person's garlic press is another's paperweight. That said, it is fun to broaden your cooking repertoire. If you feel a julienne peeler may open up a world of culinary possibilities, try one. If you find you do not use it, pass it along to a friend. For years I resisted purchasing a zester, instead cutting strips and mincing. Who knew a zester could bring such joy?

With this in mind, I offer a few suggestions for tools that make my life easier and kitchen time more fun. This does not include the obvious knives, measuring cups and spoons, mixing bowls, rolling pin, wooden spoons, whisks, slotted spoons, ladles, rubber spatulas, cooling racks, cutting board, can and wine openers, large and small glass or metal baking dishes, a variety of saucepans and nonstick and cast-iron skillets. For seasoning and cleaning cast-iron skillets, see page 101.

Dutch oven

OK, it is a bit of a splurge, but if you can swing it you will be happy you did. The enameled cast iron will disperse heat evenly and is perfect for a long slow simmer. Dutch ovens are superior for stove top browning and oven completion of a dish. The enamel makes for easy cleanup.

Food processor

If I had to choose between a blender and a food processor, I would choose the food processor every time. Select one with a powerful motor, nesting bowls and adjustable slicing and shredding attachments. For smooth tofu or vegetable purées, for quickly shredding potatoes or onions or for perfect ground seitan, nothing beats a food processor.

Glass jars with tight-fitting lids

You can never have too many jars as they are wonderful for storing food in the pantry, refrigerator or freezer. And they are a great way to combine ingredients such as salad dressings or marinades.

Immersion blender

Perfect for blending small amounts (use a deep jar or bowl) and of course, in-pan, stove-top blending. They are actually quite reasonable and will save you time and cleanup.

Kitchen scissors

Often overlooked, this tool will really make your life easier — from opening the paper towel package to trimming herbs.

Stock pot

A large 8- to 10-quart (8 to 10 L) stock pot comes in handy for making pasta, boiling potatoes or corn, steaming large amounts of vegetables, making a nice pot of soup or chili and, of course, making stock.

Strainer

A fine-wire mesh strainer and cheesecloth really come in handy in a vegan kitchen. Essential for straining fine grit from reconstituted mushrooms and essential when making soy or nut milks.

Tongs

You will find yourself reaching for them over and over and wondering why you waited until now to buy them.

Vegetable peeler

Such a simple and inexpensive solution to a potentially aggravating task.

Zester

Yes, you can cut strips of citrus and finely mince or shred your fingertips along with the ginger on the tiny protruding metal shards of a grater, but why?

Vegan Pantry

Just a few additions to a basic well-stocked pantry will accommodate a vegan diet. Here are a few suggested ingredients and a little about each to guide you while purchasing. It is not necessary to purchase every item listed. A large variety of pantry ingredients will increase spur-of-the-moment options, but lesser-used items often find their way to a back corner and lose freshness. When possible, purchase lesser-used items from bulk bins, choosing only the amount needed for your recipe. And of course, only buy what you like. The recipes in this book are easily adaptable to personal taste.

When food shopping, it is important to read labels as animal products appear in the strangest places. Research trusted online sites to gain knowledge and information that may not be available on a product label. For instance, many liquors use animal products in the filtration process, but this fact is not stated on the label.

Vegan store-bought products can be expensive and a "vegan" label does not automatically equate to the healthiest choice. Many are high in sodium with trans-fats, stabilizers and preservatives. Some of the items listed are used in the Vegan from Scratch chapter, which offers recipes for typically purchased items. These cost-effective recipes come with the added bonus of knowing exactly what is in your food.

For additional information on the ingredients listed below, look to your local library or a trusted online source.

Agar

A natural gelatin used as a thickener made from algae. Agar is available in both flake and powder form. It is dissolved in water and thickens at room temperature or at a boil. Agar is available online or in most natural food and Asian food stores.

Agave nectar

A sweetener from the sap of the agave plant. Agave has a mild yet sweet flavor and is lower on the glycemic index than refined sugar.

Baking powder

Baking powder is often made with aluminum. Look for labels that specify non-aluminum baking powder.

Browning sauce

A seasoning or browning sauce made from roasted vegetables adds a hearty base and depth to many recipes such as stews, chilis and casseroles. I use the product made by Kitchen Bouquet.

Brown rice syrup

An absolutely delicious sweetener, smooth as glass with a very subtle hint of molasses. Made from brown rice, the rich amber syrup is a healthy alternative to sugar, great in recipes or drizzled on waffles.

Coconut oil

I use coconut oil in this book for many of the recipes. It adds a very faint, if any, taste of coconut to the finished product.

Confectioner's (icing) sugar

This sugar is made with cornstarch. Check the label for genetically modified (GMO) information.

Cornstarch

Cornstarch is often made with corn that is genetically modified for a variety of reasons that include resistance to pesticides. Read labels to ensure cornstarch is GMO free. Soy beans, corn, canola crops, rice and cotton seed are among plants that are modified. There is a multitude of information available on this subject online and at your local library.

Egg replacer

If necessary, I use commercial egg replacer only when absolutely nothing else will do, mostly in place of whipped egg whites. I like the product from Ener-G. As a substitute thickener, for each egg use ¼ cup (60 mL) puréed tofu or 1 tbsp (15 mL) chickpea flour mixed with 2 tbsp (30 mL) water. Chickpea flour added directly to a mixture such as bean burgers is a great binder. For baking, for each egg substitute ¼ cup (60 mL) applesauce, mashed banana or pumpkin, or mix 1 tbsp (15 mL) flax seeds with 2 tbsp (30 mL) water and let stand for 10 minutes.

Evaporated cane sugar

Refined granulated white sugar is processed using bone char. Substitute evaporated cane juice sugar, which is also made from sugar cane but is not refined. Brown sugar is made from white sugar with molasses added for color. Substitute muscovado, a raw and unrefined sugar with a molasses flavor. These good but pricey substitutes are available in most natural food stores.

Flour

I generally use unbleached all-purpose flour in most of my recipes. I also use buckwheat flour, chickpea or garbanzo bean flour, hard winter wheat flour, rye flour, semolina flour, tapioca flour, vital wheat gluten flour, whole wheat flour and whole wheat pastry flour. Look for these flours in health food stores or well-stocked grocery stores.

Fruits and vegetables

Fruits and vegetables are always better local and organic when available. If it is not possible to purchase organic, just be aware that apples, cherries, grapes, nectarines, peaches, pears, raspberries, strawberries, bell peppers, celery, potatoes and spinach are referred to as the "Dirty Dozen" due to their higher concentration of pesticides. Recipes do not call for organic or local but it is highly recommended.

Liquid amino acids

A non-GMO liquid protein concentrate containing 16 essential and non-essential amino acids. It is a delicious substitute for tamari or soy, adding depth and flavor to soups, stews and many of the recipes in this cookbook. Bragg Liquid Amino is a product I like and is available in many grocery stores and most natural food stores.

Liquid smoke

A product that is created by collecting smoke and combining it with water. It adds a distinctive smoky flavor and is used in seasoning many food products.

Margarine

When vegan margarine is called for in recipes, I suggest Earth Balance, available in hard sticks or whipped. The hard sticks are best for baking and the whipped has a delightful flavor and is fabulous on toast or pancakes.

Mayonnaise

Vegan mayonnaise is included as a tofu-based recipe in Vegan from Scratch (see Creamy Mayonnaise, page 19). If a fat-based mayonnaise is required, as in a few recipes in this cookbook, I far prefer to purchase Vegenaise.

Molasses

Molasses is made from the juice extracted from sugar cane and processed into three grades, each a little less sweet and darker. Sulphur dioxide is used to process young sugar cane. Molasses from mature cane is unsulphured. The first concentration of cane juice is called light (fancy) or Barbados. The second processing or concentration is dark (cooking) molasses and the third is blackstrap. Look for unsulphured molasses in your grocery or natural food store.

New Mexico ground red chile powder

A superior product with a deep rich flavor. It is called for in many recipes in this book and well worth seeking out. It is available in mild, medium and hot. Find it in your local grocery store or online.

Nutritional yeast

A deactivated yeast with a nutty and somewhat cheesy flavor. It has the look of cornmeal and is popular as an additive to recipes or sprinkled on dishes such as pasta or popcorn. It may be found in most natural food stores.

Seitan

A protein made from wheat gluten. I have included two recipes in this cookbook for making seitan from scratch, one from hard winter wheat (see Old-School Seitan, page 28) and the other from vital wheat gluten flour (see Quick Basic Seitan, page 29). Both are simmered in a broth to create a protein with a chewy texture and hearty flavor. Seitan is wonderful added to casseroles or soups, ground and added to sauces and burgers or sliced and sautéed.

Prepared seitan is available in many grocery or natural food stores.

Hard winter wheat has a higher protein gluten content and less starch than other wheat. This is ideal for making seitan from scratch as more gluten is retained during the washing process. Look for the words "hard winter wheat" on flour labels.

Vital wheat gluten is the natural protein gluten found in wheat and contributes to the elasticity in bread dough. It is used in this cookbook as a main ingredient in making quick seitan. It is available in most natural food stores or online.

Tempeh

A fantastic tasty and versatile soy product with a nutty flavor and hearty texture that is high in protein and low in fat. Cooked and fermented soy beans are formed and packaged into blocks or patties that can be sliced or crumbled and sautéed or added to recipes. Added grains, flavoring and spices create a variety of products to choose from. Tempeh is readily available in many grocery and natural food stores.

Textured vegetable protein (TVP)

Often referred to as textured soy protein (TSP), this product is made from defatted soy flour and sometimes fillers such as wheat or oats. It is available in granules or flakes and takes on the flavors of the re-constructing liquid. It must be noted that there is concern as much of the TVP available is made with soy that has been genetically modified.

Tofu

A versatile soy product that is produced in both a silken and regular form.

Silken tofu is packaged in a shelf-stable container and has a custard-like consistency. It is available in soft, firm and extra-firm, however, the firm and extra-firm are so close in texture they are interchangeable in the recipes in this book. When processed in a blender or food processor, silken tofu is an excellent substitute for heavy cream.

Regular tofu is packaged in water and found in the refrigerator section of the grocery store. It is delicious in dips, crumbled for scrambles, tossed in stir-fries or pressed, marinated then baked or grilled.

To press tofu: Drain well and wrap in a kitchen towel or a few layers of paper towels. Set wrapped tofu on a plate, cover with another plate and place a heavy object, such as a 28-oz (796 mL) can of tomatoes on top. Transfer to the refrigerator and let stand for about 1 hour. Unwrap and cut into desired pieces.

To steam tofu: Steaming tofu extracts excess water, as does pressing tofu. The process takes less time and produces a tofu that is firm yet moist. Cut tofu into pieces about 1-inch (2.5 cm) thick and gently simmer directly in water or in a basket over water for 12 minutes. Carefully transfer tofu to a colander and drain.

To freeze tofu: When drained and pressed tofu is frozen, bits of moisture freeze and produce tiny pockets when thawed, creating a hearty texture. Freeze tofu in a resealable freezer bag for at least 12 hours. Thaw completely and use as desired.

Vegetables. See Fruits and vegetables

Menu Suggestions

Recipes from this cookbook are grouped to build balanced and beautiful menus for a variety of occasions. There are fun menus and formal menus, indoor menus and outdoor menus; switch them up to your liking.

Springtime Sunday Brunch
Raspberry Streusel Muffins (page 69)
French Herbed Strata (page 94)
Pan-Fried Onion and Potato Hash Browns (page 104)
Maple Bourbon Tempehacon (page 27)
Mimosas
Freshly squeezed orange juice
Freshly brewed coffee

Southwestern Sunday Brunch
Baja Fruit Skewers with Lime and Pico de Gallo (page 34)
Texas Tofu Migas (page 99)
Stuffed Sopapillas (page 199)
New Mexican Home-Fried Potatoes (page 103)
Blue Cornmeal Green Chile Scones (page 70)
Year-Round Blender Tomato Salsa (page 300)
Blazing Mary (page 323)
Freshly brewed coffee

Summertime Patio Picnic
White Bean Hummus with Spiced Baked Pita Chips (page 64)
Classic Tempehacon Avocado Burger (page 176)
Cuban-Spiced Corn on the Cob (page 145)
Sweet Mini Peppers and Broccoli Slaw (page 164)
Warm Rainbow Potato Salad (page 166)
Yellow Tomato and Three-Melon Salad (page 171)
Rustic Open-Faced Peach Pie (page 365)
Fresh Ginger Lemonade (page 329)
Cold beer

Fiesta Mixed Grill
Guacamole with Blue Corn Chips (page 50)
White tortilla chips
Stone-Fruit Salsa (page 289)
Year-Round Blender Tomato Salsa (page 300)
Orange Tequila Sizzlin' Fajitas (page 182)
Cilantro Black Bean Burgers (page 220)
Fiesta Pasta Salad (page 160)
Black Bean, White Corn and Nectarine Salad (page 157)
Blended Top-Shelf Margarita (page 325)
Tomatillo-Lime Sorbet (page 373)
Upside-Down Berry Cornmeal Cake (page 340)

Al Fresco Dinner Party
French Lentil Dip with Herbed Crostini (page 48)
Chesapeake Bay Cakes (page 37)
Roasted Garlic with Crusty Baguette (page 53)
Northwest Passage Cedar-Planked Tofu (page 214)
Grilled Artichokes with Jalapeño Mignonette Sauce (page 142)
Shallot and Strawberry Risotto (page 254)
Iceberg Wedge with Ranch Dressing (page 162)
Blackberry Mint Sorbet (page 370)
Balsamic Roasted Figs in Phyllo Cups (page 369)

New Year's Eve Cocktail Party

Pick and choose recipes from this suggested menu list to suit your taste and need, or enlist a few friends and go for broke.

Sake Martini with Fresh Pomegranate and Ginger (page 318)
Golden Autumn Holiday (page 320)
The Famous and Fabulous St. Germain Cocktail (page 324)
Coconut Russian (page 326)
Spicy, Sweet and Tart Roasted Chickpeas (page 58)
Crudités Piped with Vodka and Lemon Cream Cheese (page 44)
Garden Party Vegetable Platter (page 45)
Shanghai Shiitake Pâté (page 57)
Scattered-Seed Crackers (page 128)
Big Island Nori Rolls (page 38)
Toasted Tofu with Onion Miso Jam (page 61)
Tempeh Mango Lettuce Cups with Chile-Garlic Dipping Sauce (page 60)
Green Papaya Salad (page 170)
Crystallized Ginger Cookies (page 346)
Decadent Chocolate Truffles (page 370)
Mocha Cupcakes with Almond Icing (page 342)

Celebration Buffet

French Lentil Dip with Herbed Crostini (page 48)
Cremini and Kalamata Olivada (page 43)
Layered Pesto and Macadamia Nut Cream Cheese Torte (page 62)
Manicotti Florentine (page 243)
Roasted Potatoes and Tofu (page 207) with Caper and Pine Nut Vinaigrette (page 302)
Braised Baby Artichokes with Wine and Herbs (page 143)
Hearts of Palm and Mushroom Salad with Lemon Parsley Vinaigrette (page 161)
Apricot Brownies (page 357)
Jade Green Tea Pound Cake (page 334)

Super Bowl Sunday

Avocado Cilantro Dip (page 291)
Roasted Red Pepper and Chipotle Dip (page 292)
Roasted Root Vegetable Chips (page 56)
Boy Howdy Texas Chili and Beans (page 279)
Serrano and Roasted Pepper Cornbread (page 117)
Carolina Barbecued Seitan Sandwich with Vinegar Cole Slaw (page 206)
County Fair Corn Chip Pie (page 211)
Warm Rainbow Potato Salad (page 166)
Chocolate Cherry Brownies (page 358)
Chocolate Espresso Cowgirl Cookies (page 344)
Pistachio Brittle (page 359)

Winter Holiday Dinner

Holiday Nut Nog (page 321)
Nouveau Beaujolais
Dry white wine
Winter micro-brewed beer
White Bean Hummus with Spiced Baked Pita Chips (page 64)
Baked Green Chile Artichoke Dip (page 35) with garlic crostini
Olive, celery and carrot sticks with Basic Soy and Nut Smear (page 20)
Savory Porcini Lasagna (page 244)
Balsamic Asparagus with Walnuts (page 138)
Smashed Russets and Garnet Yams (page 147)
Chestnut and Cranberry Holiday Non-Stuffed Stuffing (page 140)
Mushroom gravy
Saffron Squash Rolls (page 124)
Pistachio Biscotti (page 347)
Plymouth Rock Pie (page 366)
Figgy Pudding with Brandy Hard Sauce (page 348)
McGillicuddy's Irish Cream over ice (page 317)

Vegan from Scratch

❌—❌—❌—❌—❌—❌—❌—❌—❌—❌—❌—❌

Almond crème fraîche

Spoon this fabulous thick and perfectly sweetened topping over fresh fruit, pound cake, granola, or baked goods that benefit from a little dab of cream and wait for the rave reviews.

❖ Variation

For an autumn topping, substitute maple syrup for agave nectar and add ¼ tsp (1 mL) maple extract, ¼ tsp (1 mL) ground cinnamon and a sprinkle of nutmeg.

❖ Blender

1	package (12.3 oz/350 g) firm or extra-firm silken tofu	1
1 cup	Almond Milk (page 19) or plain store-bought	250 mL
2½ tbsp	coconut oil, liquefied	37 mL
2½ tbsp	agave nectar	37 mL
½ tsp	vanilla extract	2 mL
¼ tsp	almond extract	1 mL
⅛ tsp	salt	0.5 mL

1. In blender, pulse tofu and almond milk until smooth and well combined. Add coconut oil, agave, vanilla and almond extracts and salt and blend until very smooth and creamy. Mixture will be frothy and is ready to use or let settle and thicken overnight in refrigerator. Refrigerate crème fraîche in an airtight container for up to 5 days. Stir well before using.

Silken crème fraîche

Even the name sounds rich and luscious. Traditionally made with products high in fat, this lovely vegan version is not only delicious but also much healthier. Use as a creamy topping for dishes such as Root Vegetable Latkes with Crème Fraîche and Chives (page 150) or in recipes calling for crème fraîche.

❖ Blender

1	package (12.3 oz/350 g) firm or extra-firm silken tofu	1
1 cup	plain hemp milk	250 mL
2 tbsp	coconut oil, liquefied	30 mL
2 tbsp	agave nectar	30 mL
1 tbsp	freshly squeezed lemon juice	15 mL
⅛ tsp	salt	0.5 mL

1. In blender, pulse tofu and hemp milk until smooth and well combined. Add coconut oil, agave, lemon juice and salt and blend until very smooth and creamy. Mixture will be frothy and is ready to use or let settle and thicken overnight in refrigerator. Refrigerate crème fraîche in an airtight container for up to 5 days. Stir well before using.

Toasted okara

Okara is the ivory-colored fibrous soy pulp left behind when making soy milk. It has very little flavor but is high in nutrients. Oven drying at a low temperature creates a nutty, crisp granule. Add to baked goods, cereals or savory dishes for a healthy crunch. Add it to Sprinkle (page 30), a homemade alternative to finely grated cheeses.

✖ **Preheat oven to 225°F (110°C)**
✖ **Baking sheet, lined with parchment paper**

²/₃ cup	okara reserved from Soy Milk recipe (page 18)	150 mL

1. Scatter okara on prepared baking sheet as thinly as possible. Bake in preheated oven, stirring, respreading and breaking up any clumps every 15 minutes, until dry and lightly toasted, about 1 hour.

2. Let cool completely. Ground toasted okara in a spice or coffee grinder for a finer granule, if desired. Transfer to an airtight container and store in a cool, dry place for up to 1 month.

Sweetened condensed milk

Thick and sweet, just like the original. Use this luscious sauce as a dip for fruit, in dessert recipes, as a sweetener for breakfast cereals or add a spoonful to a beverage for a rich spot of decadence.

✖ **Tip**

This recipe may be doubled if more is needed.

³/₄ cup	granulated sugar	175 mL
½ cup	boiling water	125 mL
3 tbsp	vegan hard margarine, melted	45 mL
³/₄ cup	powdered non-dairy milk, such as soy, hemp or nut	175 mL

1. In a small heavy-bottomed saucepan, combine sugar, water and margarine. Bring to a low boil over medium heat and cook, swirling pan gently, until sugar is melted. Remove from heat and gradually whisk in powdered milk.

2. Return mixture to medium heat and bring to a gentle boil. Adjust heat as necessary to keep mixture gently boiling with small bubbles breaking the surface consistently, whisking frequently, until slightly thickened and blended, 2 to 3 minutes. Remove from heat and let cool (the mixture will thicken as it cools). Use immediately or refrigerate in an airtight container for up to 2 days.

Soy milk

A few good reasons to make your own soy milk include the incredible fresh taste not found in store-bought, the low cost and, of course, the bragging rights.

Tips

The soy pulp left behind after the puréed soy beans are strained is called okara. Reserve this nutritious pulp and make Toasted Okara (page 17) or freeze for later use.

A fine-mesh nut bag, available in most kitchen or natural food stores, makes straining nut or soy pulp easy.

* Blender
* Wire mesh strainer and mesh nut bag or double layer of cheesecloth (see Tips, left)

1 cup	dried soy beans, picked through and rinsed	250 mL
	Water	

1. Place soy beans in a bowl and add water to cover by 3 inches (7.5 cm). Cover bowl and let soak for 10 to 12 hours.

2. Drain beans and rinse well. Place half of the beans and 1⅓ cups (325 mL) warm water into blender and blend into a thin smooth paste, 3 to 4 minutes. Transfer mixture to a bowl. Add remaining beans to blender, add 1⅓ cups (325 mL) warm water and repeat process.

3. In a heavy-bottomed saucepan, bring 1 cup (250 mL) water to a boil over high heat. Stir in puréed mixture and bring to a boil, stirring frequently, watching constantly as mixture will quickly froth over. Remove from heat and let cool slightly.

4. Place nut bag into a large wire mesh strainer over a large bowl and pour soy mixture into bag. Close bag and use the bottom of a measuring cup or mug to gently press liquid from soy pulp. When pulp appears dry, pour 1 cup (250 mL) warm water into nut bag and press again. Discard soy pulp or reserve, if desired, to make Toasted Okara (page 17).

5. Pour soy milk from bowl into a clean saucepan and bring to a boil over medium heat. Reduce heat and simmer, stirring occasionally, until bitterness has cooked out, 10 to 20 minutes. Let cool completely and transfer to a glass airtight container and refrigerate for up to 5 days.

Variations

Add 2 tbsp (30 mL) or more to taste of a sweetener such as agave nectar, brown rice syrup or pure maple syrup, or flavorings such as vanilla extract, almond extract or Divine Chocolate Sauce (page 22) to taste.

Almond milk

Nut milks are simple to make. Use purified water and organic raw nuts and know that you are treating yourself to the finest milk for drinking, baking and cooking.

✖ Tip
Soaking nuts is essential for optimal digestion and makes blending easier.

✖ Blender
✖ Wire-mesh strainer or double layer of cheesecloth (see Tips, page 18)

1 cup	raw almonds (see Tips, left)	250 mL
	Water	

1. Place almonds in a bowl and add water to cover by 3 inches (7.5 cm). Cover bowl and let soak for at least 8 hours or overnight.

2. Drain nuts and rinse well. In blender, combine nuts and 2 cups (500 mL) water for 1 minute. Add 2 cups (500 mL) water and blend again at high speed until nuts are pulverized and almost smooth, about 1 minute. Pour nut milk mixture through cheesecloth-lined strainer into a large bowl to remove solids from milk. Strain again if necessary. Refrigerate Almond Milk in an airtight container for up to 4 days.

Creamy mayonnaise

This creamy and absolutely delicious spread has the consistency and taste of mayonnaise and uses dry mustard powder to give it a little snap. It is excellent on sandwiches. Easily infused with roasted garlic, chopped herbs, curry or a multitude of flavorings, it is equally at home in a macaroni, grain or potato salad. Thin with water, wine or juice for a quick dressing or sauce.

✖ Immersion blender or small food processor

4 oz	firm or extra-firm silken tofu	125 g
2 oz	extra-firm tofu, drained	60 g
4¾ tsp	freshly squeezed lemon juice	23 mL
4 tsp	olive oil	20 mL
¼ tsp	Dijon mustard	1 mL
⅛ tsp	salt, approx.	0.5 mL
⅛ tsp	dry mustard (approx.)	0.5 mL

1. In a small deep bowl, combine silken and extra-firm tofu, lemon juice, oil, Dijon mustard, salt and dry mustard. Use an immersion blender to thoroughly blend ingredients into a very creamy, smooth mixture with the texture of mayonnaise, 2 to 3 minutes. Taste and adjust seasoning, adding a pinch each of dry mustard and salt, if desired. Store mayonnaise in an airtight container in the refrigerator for up to 1 week.

Basic nut smear

The base recipe provides a luscious nut smear with a spreading consistency of cream cheese and stores well in the refrigerator. Delicious as is, this spread also shines with the addition of fresh herbs, spices or sweeteners. Spread on toasted bagels with roasted red pepper and arugula, or thin slightly to create a dip for crackers and crudités.

❖ Food processor or blender

3 cups	raw cashews	750 mL
3 tbsp	freshly squeezed lemon juice	45 mL
2¹/₂ tsp	white wine vinegar	12 mL
2 tsp	nutritional yeast	10 mL
1¹/₂ tsp	salt	7 mL

1. Place cashews in a bowl and add water to cover by 3 inches (7.5 cm). Cover bowl and let soak for 4 to 5 hours.

2. Drain and place nuts in food processor. Add ¹/₂ cup (125 mL) water and pulse until coarsely chopped. Add lemon juice and vinegar and pulse into a rough paste, adding more water as necessary, 1 tbsp (15 mL) at a time. Scrape sides, add nutritional yeast and salt and process until smooth and creamy, 4 to 5 minutes.

3. Transfer to an airtight container and refrigerate for at least 6 hours or overnight, until set. Smear keeps, covered and refrigerated, for up to 10 days.

Basic soy and nut smear

This spread makes a great appetizer served with seeded crackers. Add a few spoonfuls of chipotle jelly for a lively twist.

❖ Variation

Add flavorings such as 2 tbsp (30 mL) mango ginger chutney and ¹/₂ seeded and chopped jalapeño in Step 2.

❖ Food processor or blender

³/₄ cup	macadamia nuts	175 mL
1 tsp	white wine vinegar	5 mL
2 tsp	freshly squeezed lemon juice	10 mL
³/₄ tsp	nutritional yeast	3 mL
¹/₄ tsp	salt	1 mL
8 oz	firm or extra-firm silken tofu	250 g

1. In a food processor, combine macadamia nuts, 2 tbsp (30 mL) water, vinegar and lemon juice and process nuts to a rough paste, adding more water as necessary, 1 tbsp (15 mL) at a time.

2. Scrape down sides, add nutritional yeast, salt and tofu and process until smooth and creamy, 4 to 5 minutes. Transfer to an airtight container and refrigerate for at least 6 hours or overnight, until set. Smear keeps, covered and refrigerated, for up to 4 days.

Basic ricotta

Whip up this basic ricotta in a snap. It is neither sweet nor savory, thus perfectly suited as a base for recipes, and is called for in many recipes in this book.

✜ Immersion blender

16 oz	extra-firm tofu, in water, drained	500 g
8 oz	firm or extra-firm silken tofu, drained	250 g
1 tsp	granulated sugar	5 mL
1 tsp	freshly squeezed lemon juice	5 mL
2 tsp	grapeseed oil	10 mL
¾ tsp	salt	3 mL

1. In a large bowl, combine extra-firm and silken tofus and using a potato masher, mash into small crumbs. In a small bowl, combine sugar, lemon juice, oil and salt. Add to tofu mixture. Use an immersion blender, pulsing on and off until mixture is semi-smooth but still very grainy. (If immersion blender is not available, continue with potato masher.) Refrigerate in an airtight container for up to 10 days.

Basic sour cream

With a creamy texture and a slight tart flavor, this basic sour cream alternative is sensational as a base for dips, sauces and toppings. Spoon a dollop or two on a baked potato or tostada.

✜ Tips

Extra-firm silken tofu is so similar in texture to firm silken tofu that either may be used in a recipe calling for one or the other.

Transfer to an airtight container and refrigerate for up to 1 week. Stir well before using.

✜ Food processor

1	package (12.3 oz/350 g) firm or extra-firm silken tofu (see Tips, left)	1
1½ tbsp	safflower or canola oil	22 mL
2 tbsp	freshly squeezed lemon juice	30 mL
2 tsp	white wine vinegar	10 mL
¾ tsp	granulated sugar	3 mL
½ tsp	salt	2 mL

1. In food processor, process tofu, oil, lemon juice, vinegar, sugar and salt until thoroughly smooth. Adjust flavors, adding more lemon juice, sugar or salt to taste and pulse to incorporate. Best if chilled before using.

✜ Variation

Creamy Dip: Mix 1 cup (250 mL) Basic Sour Cream with ¼ cup (60 mL) Creamy Mayonnaise (page 19) for a fabulous base for dips. Simply stir in your favorite flavorings, refrigerate for at least 2 hours or overnight, until set, and serve.

Crunchy tempehacon bits

These crispy bits are the perfect little crunch in every bite of a salad or tofu scramble. Great as a tasty topping for vegetables, on baked potatoes or tossed into pasta or grain dishes.

1/4 cup	soy sauce	60 mL
2 tbsp	pure maple syrup	30 mL
1 tsp	liquid smoke	5 mL
8 oz	tempeh, well crumbled	250 g
2 tbsp	grapeseed oil	30 mL

1. In a small shallow container, whisk together soy sauce, maple syrup and liquid smoke until well combined. Add tempeh crumbles and toss to coat. Cover and refrigerate, stirring occasionally, for at least 4 hours or up to overnight.

2. Spread marinated crumbles on a plate and let air dry for 10 minutes.

3. Place a large skillet over medium–high heat and let pan get hot. Add oil and tip pan to coat. Transfer crumbles to skillet, reduce heat to medium and cook, stirring frequently, until bits are very crisp and browned, 4 to 6 minutes.

Divine chocolate sauce

This recipe whips together in no time to create a delicious syrup. Refrigerate the syrup overnight to thicken into a luscious fudgy chocolate sauce that elevates even store-bought desserts to new heights.

1 cup	unsweetened non-dairy cocoa powder, sifted	250 mL
3/4 cup	natural cane sugar	175 mL
1/2 cup	corn syrup	125 mL
1 cup	Soy Milk (page 18) or store-bought	250 mL
1/2 tsp	vanilla extract	2 mL

1. In a heavy-bottomed saucepan, whisk together cocoa powder, sugar and corn syrup. Whisk in soy milk, a little at a time, until mixture comes together to form a smooth sauce and bring to a boil over medium heat.

2. Reduce heat to low and simmer, stirring constantly, for 1 minute. Remove from heat, stir in vanilla and let cool completely. Transfer to a glass airtight container and refrigerate until thickened, for at least 4 hours. Store, covered and refrigerated, for up to 2 weeks.

✖ Tip

For hot chocolate, blend 2 tbsp (30 mL) Chocolate Sauce with 1 cup (250 mL) of unsweetened vanilla nut milk or coconut milk and microwave until steaming, about 1 1/2 minutes.

✖ Variation
Substitute almond extract for vanilla.

Caramel sauce

A luscious caramel sauce that is easy to make, scrumptious to eat and dairy-free; what more could you ask for? It's a decadent dip for apples and pears, a delirious drizzle for frozen desserts and a special treat spooned into hot almond milk.

:: Tips

When using corn syrup, I prefer to use non-GMO corn syrup such as Wholesome Sweeteners Organic Light Corn Syrup, available at health food stores, well-stocked supermarkets in the natural food section and online.

Use a heavy-bottomed pan to prevent sugar from quickly burning. Even in a heavy-bottomed pot, boiling sugar turns from pale yellow to golden fairly quickly. Once past this stage, it turns from gold, to amber, to burnt in a matter of seconds. Watch closely.

Resist the temptation to stir the sugar while it is boiling. A simple swirl of the pan every now and then is all that is needed.

2 cups	granulated sugar	500 mL
$\frac{1}{4}$ cup	corn syrup (see Tips, left)	60 mL
$\frac{3}{4}$ cup	vegan hard margarine	175 mL
1 cup	Heavy Cream (page 26) or store-bought vegan cream alternative	250 mL

1. In a heavy-bottomed saucepan, combine sugar and corn syrup. (Mixture will be lumpy.) Bring to a low boil over medium-high heat, stirring constantly until sugar is melted. Boil, without stirring, until sugar turns golden, 5 to 6 minutes, keeping a very close watch as sugar will advance in color quickly.

2. Immediately remove from heat, whisk in margarine and gradually add heavy cream, whisking until smooth, 2 to 3 minutes. Set aside and let cool completely to thicken.

3. Refrigerate in an airtight glass container for up to 1 month. If refrigerated, bring sauce to room temperature or warm before using to thin slightly, if desired.

:: Variation

Chocolate Caramel Sauce: Add $1\frac{1}{2}$ oz (45 g) coarsely chopped dairy-free dark chocolate along with the margarine.

Greek herbed soy feta in olive oil

Salty soy feta cubes swirl in rich olive oil with intense red and green jewels of flavor. Choose a lovely jar to complete the stunning presentation. A gorgeous addition to an appetizer platter, these spicy, salty little pillows are scrumptious on crackers or grilled slices of Three-Olive Focaccia (page 108).

✖ Tip

Vary the salty flavor of the soy feta by increasing or decreasing the salt brine soaking time.

4 oz	extra-firm tofu	125 g
¼ cup	kosher salt	60 mL
1 tbsp	white wine vinegar	15 mL
2 cups	water	500 mL
1 cup	olive oil	250 mL
1 tbsp	drained oil-packed sun-dried tomato strips	15 mL
1	large clove garlic, slivered	1
1	bay leaf, crumbled	1
1 ½ tsp	drained capers	7 mL
½ tsp	mixed whole black and red peppercorns	2 mL
¼ tsp	hot pepper flakes	1 mL
¼ tsp	dried oregano	1 mL

1. Drain tofu, wrap in a clean thick kitchen towel or paper towels and place on a dinner plate. Place a second dinner plate on top, place a heavy can on top and set aside for 1 hour. Transfer to a resealable freezer bag and freeze for at least 12 hours.

2. Let frozen tofu thaw at room temperature and cut into 1-inch (2.5 cm) cubes. In a bowl, combine salt, vinegar and water. Add tofu cubes and immerse in liquid. Cover and refrigerate for 4 to 6 hours (see Tip, left). Remove tofu from brine and carefully pat dry. Discard brine.

3. In a glass jar with a tight-fitting lid, combine oil, sun-dried tomatoes, garlic, bay leaf, capers, peppercorns, hot pepper flakes and oregano. Add tofu and gently stir to distribute ingredients. Store in refrigerator for up to 1 week. Before serving let mixture stand at room temperature for 30 minutes to allow oil to re-liquefy.

Hearty savory baked tofu

Makes 4 pieces

This simple dish is a satisfying and flavorful addition to stir-fries, casseroles, salads or sandwiches. Try it sliced into savory strips for snacking. Bake up a double batch and refrigerate the unused portion to have on hand for up to a week.

✖ Tip

To steam tofu: Steaming tofu extracts excess water, as does pressing tofu. The process takes less time and produces a tofu that is firm yet moist. Cut tofu into pieces about 1-inch (2.5 cm) thick and gently simmer directly in water or in basket over water for 12 minutes. Carefully transfer tofu to a colander and drain.

✖ **Baking sheet, lined with lightly oiled foil or silicone liner**

16 oz	extra-firm tofu (see Tip, left)	500 g
6 tbsp	whiskey	90 mL
1/4 cup	water	60 mL
2 tbsp	balsamic vinegar	30 mL
1 1/2 tsp	onion powder	7 mL
1/2 tsp	garlic powder	2 mL
1/4 tsp	freshly ground black pepper	1 mL

1. Drain tofu, wrap in a clean thick kitchen towel or paper towels and place on a dinner plate. Place a second dinner plate on top, place a heavy can on top and set aside for 1 hour.

2. In a glass pie plate, whisk together whiskey, water, vinegar, onion powder, garlic powder and pepper until well incorporated. Cut tofu, crosswise into 4 pieces and place in pie plate and turn to coat. Cover and refrigerate for 1 hour or up to overnight, turning at least once.

3. Preheat oven to 375°F (190°C). Place tofu on prepared baking sheet and bake in preheated oven for 15 minutes. Flip tofu and bake for 10 minutes for moist tofu or 15 to 20 minutes for more dense and chewy tofu.

> ## ✖ Variation
> To create a very chewy crust, just before flipping, brush top of tofu with oil, flip and brush again.

Light savory baked tofu

Makes 4 pieces

A wine-based marinade infuses this tofu with a light yet savory flavor, creating a baked tofu, perfect for dishes requiring a protein that blends rather than dominates other ingredients.

Tip

To create a very chewy crust, just before flipping, brush top of tofu with oil, flip and brush again.

Baking sheet, lined with lightly oiled foil or silicone liner

1 cup	water	250 mL
1/2 cup	white wine	125 mL
1 tsp	Homemade Vegetable Bouillon (page 32) or store-bought powdered or cubed	5 mL
1 tsp	dried parsley	5 mL
1/2 tsp	Sage Seasoning Blend (page 314) or store-bought sage-based seasoning blend	2 mL
16 oz	extra-firm tofu, drained and pressed (see page 12)	500 g

1. In a glass pie plate, whisk together water, wine, bouillon, parsley and seasoning blend until well incorporated. Cut tofu, crosswise into 4 pieces, place in pie plate and turn to coat. Cover and refrigerate for 1 hour or up to overnight, turning at least once.
2. Preheat oven to 375°F (190°C). Place tofu on prepared baking sheet. Bake in preheated oven for 15 minutes. Flip tofu and bake for 10 minutes for moist tofu or 15 to 20 minutes for dense and chewy tofu.

Heavy cream

Makes about 2 1/2 cups (625 mL)

Thick and pourable, this simple combination is fantastic whenever heavy cream is called for. The cream is unflavored and therefore suitable in both sweet and savory dishes.

Food processor or blender

1	package (12.3 oz/350 g) firm or extra-firm silken tofu	1
1 cup + 2 tbsp	plain hemp milk	280 mL
2 tsp	agave nectar	10 mL

1. In a food processor, blend tofu, hemp milk and agave nectar until very smooth and creamy. Mixture will be frothy and can be used as is but is best covered and refrigerated for 2 hours to thicken slightly. Stir well before using. Refrigerate in an airtight container for up to 5 days.

Maple bourbon tempehacon

Makes 24 slices

When feeling the need for some love, just whip up a batch of crispy, maple-flavored, smoky tempehacon. So good, it is just the thing to make a plate of pancakes sing.

Tips

If splatter screen is unavailable, loosely cover with foil.

For added flavor, drizzle a few drops of marinade on cooking slices after flipping.

- **13- by 9-inch (33 by 23 cm) glass baking dish**
- **Splatter screen (see Tips, left)**

1/4 cup	tamari	60 mL
1 tbsp	pure maple syrup	15 mL
2 3/4 tsp	brown rice syrup	13 mL
2 tsp	bourbon whiskey	10 mL
1 tsp	liquid smoke	5 mL
8 oz	soy and grain tempeh	250 g
2 to 4 tbsp	grapeseed oil	30 to 60 mL

1. In a small saucepan, combine tamari, maple syrup, brown rice syrup, whiskey and liquid smoke. Place pan over medium heat and bring to a boil, stirring occasionally. Remove from heat and set aside to cool.
2. Using a sharp thin knife, cut block of tempeh in half horizontally. Cut each half lengthwise into thin 1/8-inch (3 mm) slices. Pour cooled marinade into baking dish, arrange tempeh slices in a single layer and carefully turn to coat. Cover dish and refrigerate for at least 4 hours or up to overnight, flipping tempeh at least once.
3. Place a large skillet over medium-high heat until hot. Add 2 tbsp (30 mL) oil and tip pan to coat. Remove pan from heat and quickly arrange 12 slices of tempehacon in pan in a single layer. Work quickly so oil does not cool. Return pan to heat, cover with splatter screen and fry, carefully flipping once, until browned and crisp, 30 seconds to 1 minute per side. Transfer cooked tempehacon to a plate.
4. Let pan cool slightly, wipe oil and any crisp or burnt residue from pan with paper towels, return to heat and repeat process. Serve immediately.

Old-school seitan

This recipe uses the harder winter wheat, which retains more gluten than soft spring and summer wheat, usually sold as Durham wheat. Although the total time required may seem lengthy, the actual preparation time is well under an hour and is definitely worth the effort. Seitan is a versatile protein substitute and may be used in many ways. It is excellent pulsed in a food processor to the consistency of ground protein, for use in chili, tacos, burgers or pasta sauce. Cube seitan for a hearty addition to stir-fries, slice and sauté for sandwiches or serve roasted and sliced with potatoes and gravy for a satisfying meal.

✖ Tip

It is important to use winter wheat flour as soft wheat will wash away, since there is very little gluten.

Gluten

8 cups	hard winter wheat flour, divided (see Tip, left)	2 L
2 tbsp	Homemade Vegetable Bouillon (page 32) or store-bought powdered or cubed	30 mL

1. *Gluten:* Place 7 cups (1.75 L) of the flour in a large bowl. Add 3½ cups (875 mL) water and mix to combine. While still in the bowl, knead mixture until dough ball forms and starts to become elastic, about 5 to 7 minutes, gradually adding enough reserved flour to create a dough ball that is easy to work with and does not stick to your hands. Add cold water to cover dough. Cover bowl and refrigerate for at least 4 hours or up to overnight.

2. Transfer bowl to sink and under running water, knead dough until water in bowl runs almost clear, 6 to 10 minutes (this rinses milky starch from gluten). Transfer gluten ball to a wire mesh strainer set over a bowl or in the sink and let rest, allowing gluten strands to bind, about 10 minutes.

3. In a large stockpot, bring 6 cups (1.5 L) water to a boil over high heat. Stir in bouillon. Tear 2- to 3-inch (5 to 7.5 cm) chunks from gluten ball, stretching each slightly and carefully drop into broth. Partially cover pot, reduce heat and gently simmer, turning occasionally, until cooked through and slightly firm, about 1 hour. Let seitan cool in broth. Use immediately or transfer to an airtight container with about 3 tbsp (45 mL) of cooking broth and refrigerate for up to 1 week or freeze for up to 2 months.

✖ Variation

Seitan Roast: Instead of breaking gluten ball into chunks, form it into a roast shape, then wrap in a double layer of cheesecloth and tie with kitchen twine. Place in simmering broth and cook, turning roast every 15 minutes, for 1 hour. Remove from broth and let cool. Unwrap roast and slice to serve.

Quick basic seitan

Makes about 1 lb (500 g)

Unlike Old-School Seitan, which relies on a simmering broth to add flavor, this quick seitan is infused by flavoring the dry and/or wet recipe components before blending, adding complexity to your finished dish. This recipe is a very basic savory seitan suitable for roasting, broiling, braising or simmering. Flavors may be added to complement the dish in which it will be used — the possibilities are endless. See Variations (right) for suggestions.

✕ Tip

It is important to use fresh vital wheat gluten flour because older flour can add a bitter taste to seitan. You can find vital wheat gluten flour at health food stores and well-stocked supermarkets in the natural foods section.

Gluten

1 cup	vital wheat gluten flour (see Tip, left)	250 mL
1 tsp	onion powder	5 mL
1 tsp	garlic powder	5 mL
3/4 cup + 1 tbsp	boiling water	190 mL
7 tsp	Homemade Vegetable Bouillon (page 32) or store-bought powdered or cubed, divided	35 mL

1. *Gluten:* In a bowl, whisk together wheat gluten and onion and garlic powders. In a small bowl, combine boiling water and 1 tsp (5 mL) vegetable bouillon. Stir liquid mixture into dry ingredients, mixing well to combine. When liquid is incorporated, leave mixture in bowl and knead gluten dough until elastic strands begin to form, 2 to 3 minutes. Let dough rest for 10 minutes to let gluten bind.

2. In a large stockpot, bring 6 cups (1.5 L) water to a boil and stir in 2 tbsp (30 mL) bouillon. Tear 2- to 3-inch (5 to 7.5 cm) chunks from gluten ball, stretching each slightly and carefully drop into broth. Partially cover pot, reduce heat and simmer, turning occasionally, until cooked through and slightly firm, about 1 hour. Let seitan cool in broth and use immediately or transfer to an airtight container with about 3 tbsp (45 mL) of cooking broth and refrigerate for up to 1 week or freeze for up to 2 months.

✕ Variations

Add ethnic flavorings to seitan by adding 1/4 to 1 tsp (1 to 5 mL) curry powder, chile powder, herbes de Provence, ras el hanout, mango powder or oregano to dry mixture. Add 1 tsp (5 mL) to 1 tbsp (15 mL) grated fresh gingerroot, chopped garlic, minced shallot, bottled hot sauce, tamari, sesame oil, miso, flavored vinegars or wine to liquid mixture.

Sprinkle

Makes $1/4$ cup (60 mL)

A finely ground combo with a subtle onion flavor will add just the right kick when sprinkled onto steamed vegetables or grain, bean and pasta dishes. Fantastic sprinkled on popcorn. The recipe makes use of pantry staples but does not keep long, so grind up a fresh batch and use liberally.

Tip

Toasted Okara is made from dried soy pulp left behind when straining soy milk from ground soy beans. It is full of nutrients and adds a fiber and nutty crunch to this recipe. It is available in Asian grocery stores as Dry Okara and it is also sometimes called Unohana Dorai. If you can't find it and haven't made your own, simply omit it.

Spice or coffee grinder

3 tbsp	ground almonds (almond meal)	45 mL
2 tbsp	sesame seeds	30 mL
1 tbsp	Toasted Okara (page 17) or store-bought, optional (see Tip, left)	15 mL
$1/2$ tsp	dried onion flakes	2 mL
$1/8$ tsp	salt	0.5 mL

1. In spice or coffee grinder, combine almond meal, sesame seeds, okara, onion flakes and salt and pulse 6 times. Scrape bottom edges and pulse until sesame seeds are finely ground but not powdered, 6 to 8 times. Transfer to a small airtight container, scraping bottom edges. Mix well to blend. Use immediately or refrigerate for up to 3 days.

Crunch

Whip up a batch of Crunch to have on hand for when you need a little, well, crunch. The flavor is light and a perfect crispy complement to savory creamy casseroles. Try it on roasting vegetables, create a crispy crust for chickpea or vegetable fries, or use it to encrust your favorite oven-baked protein.

❖ **Preheat oven to 250°F (120°C)**
❖ **Rimmed baking sheet**

3 tbsp	water	45 mL
1 tsp	nutritional yeast	5 mL
1 tbsp	Homemade Vegetable Bouillon (page 32) or store-bought powdered or cubed	15 mL
1 cup	panko bread crumbs	250 mL
2 tbsp	ground almonds (almond meal)	30 mL
1 tbsp	dried parsley	15 mL

1. In a small cup, combine water and nutritional yeast, stirring well to dissolve. Stir in bouillon and let stand for 10 minutes.

2. In a small bowl, stir together bread crumbs, almond meal and parsley until well combined.

3. Add bouillon mixture to bread crumb mixture and use fingers to gently but firmly crumble mixture to incorporate wet into dry.

4. Spread mixture on baking sheet in a thin layer and bake in preheated oven for 12 to 15 minutes. Let cool on baking sheet until crisp. Store cooled Crunch in an airtight container in a cool, dry place for up to 3 weeks.

Vegetable broth

Certainly one of the most valuable resources in a kitchen is homemade vegetable broth, and creating it instantly from homemade vegetable bouillon is a revelation!

1 cup	hot water	250 mL
1 tsp	Homemade Vegetable Bouillon (page 32)	5 mL

1. In a small bowl, combine hot water and bouillon. Let steep for 30 seconds to 1 minute. Use in a recipe or serve as a delicious drink.

❖ **Variation**
Vary strength and flavor to taste, adding more bouillon and less water as necessary. Take into consideration that bouillon is salted, so the salt flavor increases proportionally.

Homemade vegetable bouillon

This clever recipe makes use of salt grains to prevent a simple root vegetable paste from freezing into a solid block. Stored in the freezer, the granulated bouillon is loose and easily spooned out in the desired amount. Inspired by Pam Corbin's *Preserves: River Cottage Handbook,* this versatile recipe works like a charm with most herbs and root vegetables, but for a well rounded flavor base be sure to include the classic French combination of aromatics: carrots, celery root or celery and onion, referred to as a mirepoix.

⁑ Tips

If using organic produce there is no need to peel carrots. Simply scrub well and enjoy the extra nutrients.

Pint (500 mL) canning jars with tight-fitting two-piece lids make great storage containers for this beautiful blend.

Add by the spoonful to soups, stews, rice or grain cooking liquid or enjoy as a warm beverage.

⁑ Food processor

1	small bulb fennel, trimmed	1
2	large carrots, peeled	2
1	celery root, peeled (about 8 oz/250 g)	1
10	small green onions, white and light green parts only	10
4	medium shallots	4
1	bunch parsley, tough ends trimmed	1
3	cloves garlic	3
2/3 cup	thyme leaves	150 mL
1 tbsp	tomato paste	15 mL
2/3 cup	salt	150 mL

1. Chop fennel, carrots, celery root, green onions, shallots and parsley into about 1-inch (2.5 cm) pieces and combine in a large bowl. Stir in garlic and thyme.

2. In a food processor, pulse about one-third of the mixture until reduced in volume, 10 to 15 times. Scrape sides and bottom, coaxing the less chopped vegetables into a better position. Add half of the remaining vegetables and repeat process until all the chopped vegetables are processed.

3. Add tomato paste and salt and pulse until incorporated, about 6 times. Process mixture for 5 to 10 seconds to form a finely chopped scoopable blend. Do not overblend mixture into a smooth paste.

4. Use immediately or transfer to an airtight container and store in freezer for up to 3 months.

5. To use: Ratio is approximately 1 tsp (5 mL) bouillon to 1 cup (250 mL) hot water, adding more or less according to taste.

Small Plate Starters

Baja fruit skewers with lime and pico de gallo

In Mexico many street vendors sell refreshing fruit skewers drizzled with lime juice and sprinkled with the spicy and tart pico de gallo powder.

✖ Tip

Pico de gallo is a Mexican spice mixture of red chile, spices and lime powder and can be found in the ethnic section of most grocery stores, your local Mexican grocery store or purchased online. It is referred to as pico de gallo as well as pico de gallo con limon. Pico de gallo is Spanish for "rooster's beak."

✖ 12-inch (30 cm) bamboo skewers

4	large limes	4
2	mangos, cubed	2
1/2	medium pineapple, cored and cubed	1/2
1/2	small watermelon, seeded and cubed (about 4 cups/1 L)	1/2
1	small jicama, peeled and cubed	1
2	seedless cucumbers, peeled and cubed	2
	Pico de gallo con limon powder (see Tip, left)	

1. Juice three of the limes and cut the fourth one into wedges.

2. Thread mangos, pineapple, watermelon, jicama and cucumbers on skewers, alternating to create a colorful arrangement. Place skewers on a platter.

3. Drizzle with lime juice and sprinkle with powdered pico de gallo. Serve fruit skewers and pass bowls of lime wedges and powdered pico de gallo.

> ## ✖ Variations
> Add or substitute nectarines, plums, grapefruit, oranges, apples, pears or your favorite in-season fruit.

Baked green chile artichoke dip

Serves 6 to 8

Because this creamy dip is baked and served in the same vessel, it is fun to use a decorative ceramic baking dish that matches the theme of your party. Or bake in 6 (4 oz/125 g) ramekins, place on a nice platter and surround with crostini or crackers.

✖ Tips

If artichoke hearts are unavailable, you can substitute artichoke crowns in water.

Look for an oil-based mayonnaise, such as Vegenaise, rather than a tofu-based one. This recipe benefits from the extra richness provided by the oil.

Most canned green chile is mild so if using, increase hot pepper flakes for additional heat.

✖ Preheat oven to 350°F (180°C)
✖ Food processor or blender
✖ 8-inch (20 cm) square glass baking dish

2	cans (each 14 oz/398 mL) artichoke hearts in water, drained, divided (see Tips, left)	2
½ cup	vegan oil-based mayonnaise (see Tips, left)	125 mL
½ cup	canned roasted diced mild or medium green chile peppers (or one 4 oz/127 mL can)	125 mL
2	cloves garlic, minced	2
½ tsp	salt	2 mL
¼ tsp	hot pepper flakes	1 mL
1	red bell pepper, halved	1
4 oz	firm or extra-firm silken tofu	125 g
2 tbsp	olive oil	30 mL

1. Chop half of the artichokes and place in a large bowl. Set remaining aside. Add mayonnaise, green chile, garlic, salt and hot pepper flakes to bowl. Chop half the bell pepper into a medium dice, add to bowl and stir to combine. Thinly slice remaining red bell pepper and set aside.

2. In food processor, pulse tofu and reserved artichokes into a thick and slightly chunky purée, stopping a few times to scrape sides. Add to vegetables in bowl and stir well to incorporate.

3. Spread mixture evenly in baking dish and brush top liberally with oil. Arrange bell pepper slices on top and bake until heated through and bubbly, 40 to 45 minutes. Set oven to broil and broil until top is golden, 5 to 10 minutes. Let cool slightly before serving.

Basil lemon gremolata dip

Makes about 1 ½ cups (375 mL)

Try this very simple yet distinctly different dip with kettle chips, crudités or spread on crostini.

Tip

You could also use store-bought vegan basil pesto with 1 tbsp (15 mL) lemon zest added.

1 cup	Basic Sour Cream (page 21) or vegan store-bought	250 mL
¼ cup	Creamy Mayonnaise (page 19) or vegan store-bought	60 mL
6 tbsp	Basil Lemon Gremolata Pesto (page 285)	90 mL

1. In a small bowl, combine sour cream, mayonnaise and pesto until well blended. Serve immediately or refrigerate in an airtight container for 2 days.

Variation

This ratio of sour cream and mayonnaise produces an excellent base for dips. Add 3 to 6 tbsp (45 to 90 mL) vegan olive tapenade, finely chopped sun-dried tomatoes or chopped drained marinated artichoke hearts in place of pesto.

Caprese salad with tomatoes, basil and avocado

Serves 4

A fresh play on a classic Caprese, perfectly ripe avocado is a creamy stand in for buffalo mozzarella. Ripe tomatoes are essential to making this refreshing summer salad. Serve with a loaf of crusty bread to sop up the treasured juices.

4	large ripe tomatoes, sliced ¼ inch (0.5 cm) thick	4
½ cup	fresh basil leaves	125 mL
2	large ripe avocados, sliced ½ inch (1 cm) thick	2
3 tbsp	good-quality olive oil	45 mL
	Salt and freshly ground black pepper	

1. On a large platter or 4 individual plates, arrange in an overlapping pattern placing slices of tomato between basil and avocado in the following order: tomato, basil, tomato, avocado, tomato, basil, etc. Drizzle with oil and sprinkle with salt and pepper to taste. Serve immediately.

Variation

If basil is unavailable, use arugula, mâche or baby spinach.

Chesapeake bay cakes

Makes 10 to 12

These delicate cakes are the perfect starter for a dinner party or a satisfying main course served with grilled vegetables.

✖ Tip

Use a food processor to make quick work of chopping the vegetables and crumbling the tofu with just a few pulses.

✖ Preheat oven to 400°F (200°C)
✖ 2 baking sheets, lined with parchment, each brushed with 2 tbsp (30 mL) olive oil

1 tbsp	olive oil, divided	15 mL
1/4 cup	finely chopped red bell pepper	60 mL
1/4 cup	finely chopped onion	60 mL
1/4 cup	finely chopped celery	60 mL
2 1/2 cups	panko bread crumbs, divided	625 mL
1 lb	firm tofu, drained, crumbled	500 g
1/2 cup	Creamy Mayonnaise (page 19) or store-bought vegan alternative	125 mL
1/4 cup	minced fresh parsley	60 mL
1 tbsp	Old Bay Seasoning	15 mL
2 tsp	hot pepper sauce	10 mL
1 tsp	Nori Sesame Salt (page 313) or salt	5 mL
1/2 tsp	freshly ground black pepper	2 mL
	Cocktail sauce	
	Vegan tartar sauce	
	Lemon wedges	

1. Place a skillet over medium heat and let pan get hot. Add oil and tip pan to coat. Add bell pepper, onion and celery and cook, stirring occasionally, until softened, 3 to 5 minutes. Transfer to a large bowl.

2. Add 1 1/2 cups (375 mL) of the panko, tofu, mayonnaise, parsley, seasoning, hot pepper sauce, salt and pepper to vegetables in bowl. Using hands, mix to combine well.

3. Place remaining panko in a pie plate. Form tofu mixture into 3- by 1/2-inch (7.5 by 1 cm) patties and gently press into crumbs, coating lightly on both sides, and place on prepared baking sheet, at least 1 inch (2.5 cm) apart.

4. Bake in preheated oven for 12 minutes. Gently flip patties over, rotate pans and bake until crispy and golden, about 12 minutes. Serve immediately with your favorite cocktail or tartar sauce and lemon wedges.

Big island nori rolls

A sushi-style roll filled with Hawaiian macadamia nuts, sweet onion, jalapeño, avocado and cucumber has something for everyone. Don't forget the wasabi and tamari for dipping, which some feel is the best part.

⚒ Tip

Fill a small bowl with water and 2 tbsp (30 mL) rice vinegar and use to wet fingertips to prevent sticking while rolling the rolls.

⚒ Food processor
⚒ Bamboo sushi rolling mat

¹⁄₂ cup	walnut halves	125 mL
2 tbsp	tamari	30 mL

Rice

2 cups	sushi or short-grain rice, rinsed	500 mL
2 cups	water	500 mL
3 tbsp	rice vinegar	45 mL
7 tsp	granulated sugar	35 mL
2 tsp	salt	10 mL

Filling

3 tbsp	freshly squeezed lime juice	45 mL
3 to 4 tbsp	walnut or olive oil	45 to 60 mL
2 tbsp	toasted sesame seeds	30 mL
1 tsp	Hawaiian salt or sea salt	5 mL
1	sweet onion, cut into 1-inch (2.5 cm) pieces	1
1 cup	macadamia nuts	250 mL
1	jalapeño, seeded and quartered	1
3 tbsp	chopped fresh cilantro	45 mL
4	sheets nori, toasted (see Tip, right)	4
1	avocado, thinly sliced	1
1	seedless cucumber, cut into matchsticks	1
2 tbsp	rice wine vinegar	30 mL
	Tamari	
	Wasabi	

1. In a small bowl, combine tamari and walnuts and set aside to soak for 2 hours.

2. *Rice:* Place rice in a medium saucepan, add water and bring to a boil over high heat. Cover, reduce heat to low and cook for 15 minutes. Remove pan from heat and let stand, covered, without stirring or lifting lid, for 10 minutes.

3. Meanwhile, in a small microwave-safe bowl, combine vinegar, sugar and salt. Microwave for 10 seconds and let cool.

✖ Tip

To toast nori: Turn heat to medium-high on stovetop. Hold nori with metal tongs and toast about 4 inches (10 cm) above heat until darkened and crisp, 3 to 5 seconds per side. Let cool completely before using.

4. Fluff rice with a fork or paddle and transfer to a large bowl. Sprinkle vinegar mixture over rice while gently folding to combine and completely coat. Fan rice while fluffing until just warm.

5. *Filling:* In another small bowl, whisk together lime juice, 3 tbsp (45 mL) of the oil, sesame seeds and salt.

6. Drain walnuts. In food processor, pulse onion, macadamia nuts, walnuts, jalapeño and cilantro until finely chopped, 10 to 12 times. Add 1 tbsp (15 mL) of the lime juice mixture and pulse, adding additional juice mixture, 1 tbsp (15 mL) at a time, until mixture holds together.

7. Place bamboo rolling mat on work surface with bamboo strips running crosswise. Place a sheet of nori, shiny side down, lined up with mat edge closest to you. Cover nori sheet with about one-quarter of the rice, pressing and spreading until it is $\frac{1}{4}$ inch (0.5 cm) thick and leaving a $1\frac{1}{2}$ inch (4 cm) border along edge farthest away from you.

8. Place one-quarter of the filling in a line on rice crosswise about 1 inch (2.5 cm) from nearest edge. Lay rows of avocado and cucumber slices crosswise along upper edge of filling row. Starting at nearest edge, lift bamboo mat and fold nori sheet over ingredients, rolling with a light but steady pressure and peeling mat back as you roll. Use finger to moisten riceless nori border with vinegar and finish rolling. Use mat to press gently but firmly to close and seal roll.

9. Repeat process with remaining ingredients to make 3 more rolls. Cut roll crosswise into 6 or 8 slices. Serve with wasabi and tamari for dipping.

✖ Variation

Sweet onions are available from April through August. Look for varieties such as Maui, Walla Walla or Vidalia. If sweet onions are unavailable, substitute regular cooking onions, then rinse and drain onion and add 1 tsp (5 mL) granulated sugar while processing.

Caramelized leek and onion tart

This savory tart may be thinly sliced for appetizers or served in generous wedges as a light lunch with Sweet Mini Peppers and Broccoli Slaw (page 164).

✖ Tip

To clean leeks: Leeks are grown in sand and are sometimes difficult to clean. A good method of cleaning is to vertically slice through the white and light green leaves, leaving most of the dark green leaves intact. Grasp the leek by the dark green leaves, fan out the bottom white and light green portions, exposing much of the inside of the leek, and run under cold water.

✖ Food processor
✖ 9-inch (23 cm) tart pan

Crust

1⅛ cups	all-purpose flour	280 mL
2 tbsp	cornmeal	30 mL
¼ tsp	salt	1 mL
6 tbsp	vegetable shortening, chilled and cut into chunks	90 mL
3 to 4 tbsp	cold water	45 to 60 mL
½ tsp	fresh thyme leaves	2 mL

Filling

5 tbsp	olive oil, divided	75 mL
5 cups	sliced onions (about 4 medium)	1.25 L
1 tsp	salt, divided	5 mL
½ tsp	freshly ground black pepper, divided	2 mL
1 tsp	balsamic vinegar	5 mL
3	leeks, white part only (see Tip, left)	3
1½ tbsp	sun-dried tomatoes	22 mL
8 oz	firm or extra-firm silken tofu	250 g
1 tsp	fresh thyme leaves, divided	5 mL

1. *Crust:* In food processor, pulse flour, cornmeal and salt until blended. Add shortening and pulse until mixture resembles coarse meal. With motor running, add 3 tbsp (45 mL) cold water through the feed tube until incorporated. Pulse, adding 1 tbsp (15 mL) water at a time if mixture is too dry, just until dough starts to clump together. Add thyme and pulse to combine. Gather dough into a ball, press into a disk and wrap in plastic wrap and refrigerate for at least 30 minutes, until chilled, or for up to 24 hours.

2. On a lightly floured surface, roll dough into a circle slightly larger than tart pan. Fit dough into tart pan and trim edges. Refrigerate tart crust while preparing filling.

3. *Filling:* Place a large skillet over medium heat and let pan get hot. Add 2 tbsp (30 mL) of the olive oil and tip pan to coat. Add sliced onions, reduce heat to medium–low and cook, stirring frequently, until onions are very soft and beginning to take on a golden color, 40 minutes to 1 hour. Stir in $\frac{1}{2}$ tsp (2 mL) of the salt, $\frac{1}{4}$ tsp (1 mL) of the pepper and balsamic vinegar. Set aside.

4. Preheat oven to 425°F (220°C).

5. Slice leeks into $\frac{1}{8}$-inch (3 mm) slices and rinse carefully to remove any sand. Drain on clean kitchen towels and pat dry. Transfer to a bowl and toss with 1 tbsp (15 mL) of olive oil to coat. Set aside.

6. In clean food processor, pulse sun-dried tomatoes and remaining 2 tbsp (30 mL) of olive oil until coarsely chopped. Add tofu, $\frac{1}{2}$ tsp (2 mL) of the thyme, remaining $\frac{1}{2}$ tsp (2 mL) salt and $\frac{1}{4}$ tsp (1 mL) pepper and process until smooth. Spread mixture over prepared crust, smoothing top. Spread caramelized onions evenly over tofu mixture to cover completely. Place leek slices decoratively over onions, pressing down slightly.

7. Bake in preheated oven until crust is lightly browned, 40 to 45 minutes. Sprinkle remaining $\frac{1}{2}$ tsp (2 mL) thyme over top. Serve warm or at room temperature. Refrigerate any leftovers for up to 2 days.

Chile-dusted chickpea fries

With a crusty crunch, these tasty chickpea fries are nutty and satisfying to even the most discerning french fry connoisseur. Unlike when using potatoes, you can adjust the flavor to suit your whim.

:: Variations

Add flavorings, such as curry, ground ginger, parsley and thyme, olive tapenade, or garlic and lemon zest, to dry chickpea mixture before mixing with water. Flavors can also be added to the cornmeal, or vary the dipping flour; try blue cornmeal, rice flour or chickpea flour.

:: 9-inch (23 cm) square metal baking pan

1½ cups	chickpea flour, sifted	375 mL
1½ tsp	salt	7 mL
1½ tsp	freshly ground black pepper	7 mL
2 cups	water	500 mL
¼ cup	olive oil	50 mL
½ cup	cornmeal	125 mL
¾ tsp	New Mexico red chile powder	3 mL
	Canola oil	
	Salt and freshly ground black pepper	

1. Line square baking pan with a sheet of waxed paper with ends extending up beyond sides of pan. Set aside.

2. In a small bowl or large measuring cup, combine sifted chickpea flour, salt and pepper.

3. In a saucepan over medium-high heat, bring water to a simmer. Whisk in olive oil and remove from heat. Gradually add chickpea mixture, constantly whisking. Mixture will come together and pull away from sides of saucepan. Mix until well combined.

4. Transfer mixture to baking pan and top with another sheet of waxed paper. Use your hands to smooth and flatten the surface. Place in refrigerator to chill thoroughly, 4 hours to overnight. When mixture is set, peel off top sheet of waxed paper, place a cutting board over top of pan and invert to transfer mixture to cutting board. Peel off waxed paper. Cut mixture across center, then slice each half crosswise into ½-inch (1 cm) thick fries.

5. In a shallow dish, combine cornmeal and red chile powder. Place a heavy-bottomed skillet over medium heat and add 2 inches (5 cm) of canola oil. While oil is heating, gently roll a few fries in cornmeal mixture, taking care as fries break easily. When a pinch of cornmeal dropped into hot oil immediately bubbles up, carefully place fries in pan, in batches to avoid crowding, and fry, turning once, until golden brown, 2 to 4 minutes. Using a slotted spatula or tongs, transfer to a plate lined with paper towels to drain. Repeat with remaining fries, adjusting heat as necessary between batches. Sprinkle fries with salt and pepper to taste while hot and serve.

Cremini and kalamata olivada

Savory and pungent, this earthy dip adds balance to your appetizer menu. Spread it on crackers, sliced bread or fresh crudités. Serve in a decorative bowl dusted with paprika for a striking presentation.

⠿ Food processor

¼ cup	olive oil, divided	60 mL
8 oz	cremini mushrooms, sliced	250 g
1	shallot, sliced	1
¾ cup	pitted kalamata olives	175 mL
½ tsp	fennel seeds	2 mL
½ tsp	freshly ground black pepper	2 mL
¼ cup	packed Italian flat-leaf parsley	60 mL
1 tbsp	drained capers	15 mL

1. Place a skillet over medium heat and let pan get hot. Add 2 tbsp (30 mL) of the oil and tip pan to coat. Add mushrooms and shallot and cook, stirring occasionally, until softened and slightly browned, 5 to 6 minutes. Let cool.

2. In food processor, combine mushroom mixture, olives, fennel seeds, pepper and remaining oil and pulse until roughly chopped, about 10 times. Add parsley and capers and pulse again until coarsely chopped and incorporated, about 10 seconds. Taste and adjust seasonings and pulse to incorporate. Transfer to a serving bowl or refrigerate in an airtight container for up to 5 days.

Crudités piped with vodka and lemon cream cheese

This great make-ahead party dish easily adapts to your personal tastes or seasonal availability. Get creative with your garnishes, using toasted seeds, chopped nuts, hot pepper flakes or a few sprinkles of turmeric or smoky paprika.

✖ Tips

If you do not own a pastry bag, simply snip off a bottom corner of a large resealable plastic food storage bag.

Use the tender inside celery stalks for crudités and salads reserving outer stalks for cooking.

✖ **Pastry bag with medium plain or star tip (see Tips, left)**

1 1/2 cups	Basic Soy and Nut Smear (page 20) or store-bought vegan cream cheese	375 mL
1 1/2 tbsp	vodka (approx.)	22 mL
1 tsp	freshly squeezed lemon juice (approx.)	5 mL
1 tbsp	finely chopped fresh dill	15 mL
1/4 tsp	salt	1 mL
1	cucumber	1
6	radishes, trimmed	6
6	stalks celery (see Tips, left)	6
1	head Belgian endive, end trimmed, leaves separated	1
2 tbsp	chopped fresh chives	30 mL

1. In a small bowl, combine nut smear, vodka and lemon juice, mixing until well blended to a pipeable consistency, adding additional vodka or lemon juice as needed. Stir in dill and salt. Taste and adjust flavors with more dill or salt, if needed. Spoon mixture into pastry bag fitted with tip and refrigerate for 15 minutes.

2. Rake fork tines down the sides of the cucumber to create decorative ridges. Slice cucumber crosswise into 1/4-inch (0.5 cm) thick rounds. Slice radishes into 1/8-inch (3 mm) thick rounds. Cut each celery stalk into thirds.

3. Arrange cut vegetables on a platter along with endive leaves. Pipe cream cheese onto each piece and garnish with chopped chives.

> ## ✖ Variation
> Spice up your smear with a dash of hot pepper sauce or a dab of wasabi.

Garden party vegetable platter

Whether it is a party in the garden or a party in the house, this gorgeous platter of garden vegetables served with two colorful dips is sure to please your guests. Make good use of in-season produce when planning your platter because the vegetables will be at the height of their flavor and less expensive. Choose vegetables in a variety of colors to create a festive look.

✖ Tip

To save time, purchase pre-cut vegetables, trimming ends and refreshing with cold water. Arrange on your own platter and scoop purchased dips into prepared red bell pepper and purple cabbage. Your favorite vegan store-bought creamy salad dressings make instant dips.

1 lb	small red new potatoes	500 g
	Salt	
1 lb	green beans, ends trimmed	500 g
	Ice water	
1	red bell pepper	1
1	small head purple cabbage	1
2	heads broccoli, trimmed into florets	2
1 lb	cherry tomatoes	500 g
1	large yellow bell pepper, cored and cut into 1-inch (2.5 cm) strips	1
1	recipe Avocado Cilantro Dip (page 291)	1
1	recipe Roasted Red Pepper and Chipotle Dip (page 292)	1

1. Place potatoes in a large saucepan. Cover with water, add salt and bring to a boil over high heat. Reduce heat and boil gently until just tender, about 20 minutes. Transfer to a colander, drain and set aside to cool. When cool enough to handle, cut potatoes in half horizontally. Set aside.

2. Place a steamer basket into the same large saucepan. Add water, making sure it's well below the bottom of the basket and bring to a boil over high heat. Carefully add green beans, cover and steam until bright green and still crisp, 2 to 3 minutes. While beans are cooking, place a large bowl of ice water in the sink. Transfer beans to the ice bath and let stand until cold. Drain and pat dry.

3. Cut top from red bell pepper and carefully scoop out core and seeds. With a sharp paring knife, cut a hole through the top and down into the cabbage. Gradually cut away cabbage to create a small bowl–shaped space. Place bell pepper and cabbage on a platter and arrange potatoes, green beans, broccoli, tomatoes and yellow bell pepper around them. Carefully fill red bell pepper with Avocado Cilantro Dip and fill hollow in cabbage with Roasted Red Pepper and Chipotle Dip. Serve immediately or cover and refrigerate for up to 2 hours.

Eggplant fries with cucumber dipping sauce

Serves 4

Crispy and healthy, these delicious fries are terrific with the zesty dipping sauce. Serve with a large salad for a healthy and decidedly delectable dinner.

1 lb	eggplant, peeled and cut into strips	500 g
1/4 cup	kosher salt	60 mL

Cucumber Dipping Sauce

2 cups	plain soy yogurt	500 mL
1/4 cup	grated cucumber	60 mL
1/4 cup	finely chopped fresh parsley	60 mL
2	cloves garlic, minced	2
1 tbsp	grated lemon zest	15 mL
3 tbsp	freshly squeezed lemon juice	45 mL
1 tbsp	finely chopped fresh mint	15 mL
Pinch	each salt and freshly ground black pepper	Pinch
	Canola oil	
1 cup	all-purpose flour	250 mL
1 tbsp	garlic powder	15 mL
2 tsp	ground cumin	10 mL
1 tsp	smoked paprika	5 mL
1 tsp	salt	5 mL
1 tsp	freshly ground black pepper	5 mL
1/2 cup	dry white wine	125 mL

1. Place eggplant in a colander and toss with salt. Set colander over a plate and let stand for 1 hour.

2. *Cucumber Dipping Sauce:* Meanwhile, in a bowl, whisk together yogurt, cucumber, parsley, garlic, lemon zest, lemon juice, mint, salt and pepper. Transfer to an airtight container and refrigerate until needed.

3. Rinse eggplant under running water and drain well. Gently squeeze with a clean kitchen towel and pat dry.

4. Place large heavy-bottomed skillet over medium heat and add 2 inches (5 cm) of oil and heat oil until a pinch of flour dropped into hot oil immediately bubbles up.

5. In a shallow dish, whisk together flour, garlic powder, cumin, paprika, salt and pepper and set aside. Pour wine into a second shallow dish and set aside.

6. Working in batches, lightly toss eggplant strips in wine and dredge through flour mixture. Carefully place fries into oil and fry, turning once, until golden brown, 3 to 4 minutes. Transfer cooked fries to a plate lined with paper towels. Repeat with remaining eggplant, adjusting heat as necessary between batches. Serve immediately with dipping sauce.

✖ Variation

In place of the Cucumber Dipping sauce, a good store-bought jarred vegan spicy marinara sauce heated to a simmer makes a different and hearty dipping sauce.

French lentil dip with herbed crostini

Serves 4 to 6

With a little advanced preparation, you can throw this together after work for a quick and easy weeknight get-together. Making the dip in the morning before work gives the flavors time to blend. Toast the crostini just before guests arrive, add a bottle of dry white wine and enjoy the evening.

⚎ Food processor

French Lentil Dip

1 cup	dried French lentils (Puy lentils), picked through and rinsed	250 mL
1	small onion, finely chopped	1
1	bay leaf	1
2 cups	water	500 mL
1 tbsp	freshly squeezed lemon juice	15 mL
3 tbsp	olive oil, divided	45 mL
1 tbsp	chopped fresh tarragon	15 mL
1/2 tsp	fleur de sel or other sea salt	2 mL
1/2 tsp	freshly ground black pepper	2 mL
2 tbsp	chopped drained capers	30 mL
2 tbsp	toasted pine nuts	30 mL

Herbed Crostini

1 lb	loaf rustic baguette, sliced into 1/2-inch (1 cm) pieces (see Tips, right)	500 g
2 tbsp	olive oil	30 mL
2 tsp	herbes de Provence, crushed	10 mL

1. *French Lentil Dip:* In a saucepan, combine lentils, onion and bay leaf and cover with water. Bring to a boil over medium-high heat. Reduce heat and gently simmer, until lentils are just tender, 15 to 20 minutes. Let cool. Drain lentils, reserving cooking liquid. Discard bay leaf.

2. In food processor, combine lentils, lemon juice, 2 tbsp (30 mL) of the oil, tarragon and salt and pulse until rough and creamy but not yet smooth, adding a little reserved cooking liquid, if necessary. Taste and adjust seasoning with salt and pepper, if needed, and pulse to combine. If making ahead, cover and refrigerate for up to 5 days. When ready to serve, bring dip to room temperature, transfer to a serving bowl, drizzle with 1 tbsp (15 mL) of oil and garnish with capers and pine nuts.

✖ Tips

The average 1 lb (500 g) baguette will yield about 40 to 45 ½-inch (1 cm) slices.

Crostini can be prepared up to a week in advance. Store in a paper bag at room temperature and re-crisp on a baking sheet in a 350°F (180°C) oven for 3 to 4 minutes before serving.

3. Preheat oven to 350°F (180°C).

4. *Herbed Crostini:* Arrange baguette slices on a baking sheet. Brush each on both sides lightly with oil and sprinkle with a pinch of herbes de Provence. Bake in preheated oven, turning once, until lightly toasted, 4 to 6 minutes per side (watch closely as crostini will quickly burn).

5. To serve, place bowl of lentil dip in the center of a large platter and surround with herbed crostini.

Guacamole with blue corn chips

Perfect guacamole is one that uses few ingredients, celebrating simple fresh flavors. Quality ingredients, fresh and ripe, are paramount as each contributes heavily to the end result.

✄ Tips

Test oil readiness by dropping a small piece of tortilla into hot oil. If the tortilla instantly bubbles, the oil is ready.

A few paper bags torn open and doubled (inside up) are great for absorbing oil from chips.

Fry tortillas in small batches as large additions will lower oil temperature, resulting in oil-saturated chips.

3	large ripe avocados, halved and pitted	3
½ tsp	salt	2 mL
	Juice of 1 lime	
1	small serrano chile pepper, seeded and minced, divided	1
½	small onion, finely chopped, divided	½
1	tomato, chopped	1
12	6-inch (15 cm) blue, yellow or white corn tortillas, cut into large pieces	12
	Canola oil	

1. Scoop avocado pulp into a bowl and roughly mash with a fork. Mash in salt and lime juice. Stir in half of the minced chile and onion. Taste and add additional chile, salt and/or lime juice if needed. Gently fold in tomato. Cover bowl loosely and let stand for 30 minutes at room temperature to let flavors mingle.

2. In a deep saucepan, heat 2 inches (5 cm) of oil over medium–high heat (see Tips, left). When oil is hot, use tongs to carefully add tortillas in small batches and fry to desired crispness, 1 to 2 minutes. Transfer to a plate lined with paper towels to drain. Repeat with remaining tortillas, adjusting heat as necessary between batches.

3. Transfer chips to a large bowl or basket and serve while warm with guacamole.

Herbed golden tofu spread

Makes about 2¾ cups (675 mL)

This versatile golden spread flecked with fresh herbs is a rich addition to any menu. Serve with crackers or crudités for a light but filling midday snack or slather on crusty whole-grain bread piled with lettuce, tomatoes and red onion for a sumptuous lunch or dinnertime sandwich.

1 lb	firm tofu, drained	500 g
½ cup	Creamy Mayonnaise (page 19) or vegan store-bought mayonnaise	125 mL
2 tsp	Dijon mustard	10 mL
4 tsp	freshly squeezed lemon juice	20 mL
2 tbsp	finely chopped green onion, white part only	30 mL
1 tbsp	finely chopped fresh parsley	15 mL
1 tbsp	finely chopped fresh dill	15 mL
1½ tsp	ground turmeric	7 mL
½ tsp	garlic powder	2 mL
½ tsp	Nori Sesame Salt (page 313) or salt	2 mL
½ tsp	freshly ground black pepper	2 mL

1. In a bowl, using a potato masher, mash tofu into medium crumbs. Stir in mayonnaise, mustard, lemon juice, green onion, parsley, dill, turmeric, garlic powder, salt and pepper and mash to semi-smooth and slightly chunky mixture or desired consistency. Cover and refrigerate for at least 30 minutes or up to overnight. Taste and adjust seasonings, adding additional lemon juice, mustard, garlic powder, salt or pepper, if needed, before serving.

> ## Variation
> Finely shredded cabbage, grated carrot and minced celery are all great additions.

Ritzy roll-ups

Created by my friend
Suzanne Perkins, owner
of Cool Mint Café
near Austin, Texas,
these roll-ups are full
of intense flavors and
make a convenient
meal to take along on
a picnic or hike. Rings
of color shine through
when sliced for a
striking addition to
any appetizer table.

✕ Tip

If lavosh is hard, wet a
kitchen towel with hot
water. Wring out by hand,
leaving the towel very
damp with ample water.
Place lavosh in the towel,
fold to cover and let stand
for 20 minutes or until
lavosh will bend easily
without cracking.

1	soft lavosh bread, about 11- by 9-inches (28 by 23 cm) (see Tip, left)	1
1 cup	vegan roasted garlic hummus	250 mL
$\frac{1}{2}$ cup	chopped black olives	125 mL
$\frac{1}{2}$ cup	chopped red onion	125 mL
2 cups	baby spinach	500 mL
1	roasted red bell pepper, cut into long strips	1
2 tsp	olive oil	10 mL
1 tsp	balsamic vinegar	5 mL
	Salt and freshly ground black pepper	

1. Lay bread on a work surface and spread with hummus. Sprinkle chopped olives and red onion across bread half closest to you. Layer spinach across entire bread and place a wide row of pepper strips down the center, left to right. Sprinkle with oil and vinegar and season with salt and pepper to taste.

2. Starting at bottom closest to you, fold 1 inch (2.5 cm) of bread up over hummus. Roll bread, away from you, using light pressure to produce a tight roll without squeezing ingredients out at ends. Wrap tightly in plastic wrap. Refrigerate for at least 4 hours or for up to 6 hours.

3. Just before serving, unwrap and place roll on a cutting board. Slice roll on the diagonal into desired number of pieces.

✕ Variations

In place of hummus, use Basic Nut Smear (page 20) or store-bought vegan cream cheese and flavor with curry powder or blend with sun-dried tomatoes.

Substitute grated carrots and apples, arugula, sliced tomatoes and cucumber; or green bell peppers with kalamata olives.

Roasted garlic with crusty baguette

Roasting garlic softens its bite and creates a luscious garlicky spread that is guaranteed to become a favorite.

✖ Tip

The cut tops will contain small pieces of garlic, which can be roasted along with the large heads but will cook more quickly due to their size. Remove them from papery skins and use in dressings, garlic butter or as a flavor additive in everything from sauces to tempeh burgers.

✖ Preheat oven to 350°F (180°C)
✖ 8-cup (2 L) glass baking dish

4	large whole heads garlic (see Tip, left)	4
1/4 cup	olive oil	60 mL
2 tsp	finely chopped fresh thyme	10 mL
2 tsp	finely chopped fresh oregano	10 mL
1/2 tsp	salt	2 mL
1/2 tsp	freshly ground black pepper	2 mL
1 lb	crusty French baguette, sliced	500 g

1. Slice 1/2 inch (1 cm) off the top of garlic bulbs to expose individual cloves. Place garlic heads in baking dish and drizzle each with 1 tbsp (15 mL) oil and sprinkle with 1/2 tsp (2 mL) each thyme and oregano, and pinch of salt and black pepper. Cover loosely with foil, tucking outer edges down around garlic. Bake in preheated oven until garlic cloves are lightly browned and very tender, about 40 minutes.

2. To serve, place each head of garlic on a small plate surrounded by sliced baguette and accompanied by a small knife. Diners will scoop garlic from clove skin and spread on baguette slices.

> ## ✖ Variation
> Top garlic with a variety of herb combinations. Always include thyme to create a solid flavor base.

Rangoon vegetable samosas

Makes 12

A popular street food in South Asia, these jalapeño-spiked, curry-scented veggie turnovers will be a hit with everyone at your next appetizer party. Utopian with a cold beer! Serve with Mango Habanero Chutney (page 296) or Basil Lemon Gremolata Pesto (page 285).

- **Wok or deep skillet**
- **Food processor**
- **Candy/deep-fry thermometer with clip**

Filling

4	medium potatoes	4
5 tsp	salt, divided	25 mL
2 tsp	olive oil	10 mL
1/2 tsp	cumin seeds	2 mL
1 tbsp	grated gingerroot	15 mL
1	large carrot, diced and steamed (see Tip, right)	1
3/4 cup	steamed edamame or green peas (see Tip, right)	175 mL
1/4 cup	diced red bell pepper	60 mL
1	jalapeño pepper, seeded and diced	1
1 tsp	mango powder, optional	5 mL
1 tbsp	garam masala	15 mL
1/4 cup	water	60 mL
2 tbsp	chopped cilantro	30 mL

Dough

2 cups	all-purpose flour	500 mL
1/2 tsp	salt	2 mL
3 tbsp	vegetable oil	45 mL
1/2 cup	water	125 mL
	Canola oil	

1. *Filling:* Place potatoes in a large saucepan. Cover with water, add 3 tsp (15 mL) of the salt and bring to a boil over high heat. Reduce heat and boil gently until tender, 20 to 25 minutes. Let cool slightly. Peel and chop coarsely. Set aside. (Potatoes can be made ahead and refrigerated for up to 2 days.)
2. Place a large skillet over medium heat and let pan get hot. Add olive oil and tip pan to coat. Add cumin seeds and fry for a few seconds until fragrant, then add ginger. Stir in potatoes, carrot, edamame, bell pepper, jalapeño, mango powder, if using, and garam masala. Add 1/4 cup (60 mL) water, cover pan and reduce heat to low and cook, for 3 minutes. Remove from heat. Stir in cilantro and let stand, covered, for 6 minutes. Remove cover and set aside to cool while making dough.

To steam vegetables:
Steaming vegetables
retains nutrients and color.
Insert a steamer basket
into a saucepan and fill
with water about ½ inch
(1 cm) below basket. Add
vegetables and bring
water to a boil. Steam
carrots for 8 to 10 minutes
and edamame for 10 to
15 minutes, depending on
size, until softened but not
mushy.

3. *Dough:* In food processor, pulse flour and salt. Add oil. Through feed tube, gradually pulse in ½ cup (125 mL) water until dough forms. Transfer dough to floured work surface and knead until dough becomes smooth and soft, about 5 minutes. Divide dough into 12 balls. Roll each ball into approximately 5-inch (12.5 cm) circles. Cover circles with damp cloth to prevent dough drying out.

4. Place a small bowl of water next to work surface. Working with one piece of dough at time, fill with about 2 tbsp (30 mL) filling, being careful not to overstuff. Wet outside edge with finger then fold dough over to cover filling, pinching to seal edges tightly. Place under damp cloth as each is made. Repeat until all samosas are formed. At this point the samosas may be frozen, well wrapped, for up to 1 month. Fry directly from the freezer.

5. Preheat oven to 170°F (80°C).

6. Pour canola oil into wok to a depth of 3 inches (7.5 cm) but no higher than half the depth of pan. Attach frying thermometer to side of pan, making sure point is not touching bottom of pan. Heat over medium-high heat until thermometer reads 350°F (180°C). Carefully place 3 or 4 samosas at a time into hot oil and fry, turning once, until golden brown, 4 to 5 minutes per side. Transfer to a plate lined with paper towel and keep warm in oven. Repeat with remaining samosas, adjusting heat as necessary between batches. Serve immediately.

Roasted root vegetable chips

Makes about 2 cups (500 mL)

This simple recipe is a healthy version of everyone's favorite guilty pleasure. The trick to truly crunchy chips is in slicing; the thinner the slices the crisper the chips. Parsnip slices crunch up into adorable little rosettes, and beets are savory and sweet at the same time. Try this with carrots, purple potatoes, winter squash or your favorite root vegetables. Parchment paper or a silicone liner makes cleanup easy but it is not essential to the recipe.

Tip

Slice vegetables using a mandoline for thinnest chips, or slice in a food processor to save time. Slices done in a food processor may be slightly thicker, so adjust roasting times accordingly.

- **2 baking sheets, lined with parchment paper or silicone liner**
- **Preheat oven to 275°F (140°C)**

1/2	garnet yam or sweet potato	1/2
1	parsnip	1
1	beet, trimmed	1
1/2	small celery root, trimmed, peeled and cut into quarters	1/2
7 tsp	olive oil, divided	35 mL
	Salt and freshly ground black pepper	

1. Scrub yam, parsnip and beet well under running water. Slice yam, parsnip, beet and celery root as thin as possible, 1/8 inch (3 mm) or less. Place yam and parsnip slices in a bowl, toss with 3 tsp (15 mL) of the oil and a sprinkle of salt and pepper. Arrange on prepared baking sheet in a single layer. Toss celeriac with 2 tsp (10 mL) of oil and a sprinkle of salt and pepper and arrange at one end of second baking sheet. Repeat process with beet, tossing with 2 tsp (10 mL) of oil and a sprinkle of salt and pepper. Arrange next to celeriac.
2. Bake in preheated oven, until browned and crisp, 1 1/2 to 2 1/2 hours. Check chips a few times, removing any in danger of burning.
3. Let chips cool completely on pans on wire racks (the chips will crisp considerably while cooling). Store chips in a resealable plastic bag at room temperature for up to 3 days.

Variation

Sprinkle with snipped fresh herbs, garlic powder or toasted spices while tossing with oil.

Shanghai shiitake pâté

Makes 1½ cups (375 mL)

Thin, crisp rice crackers, crusty sourdough French bread or fresh crudités are dazzling topped with this heavenly pâté. Serve as a cocktail party appetizer or as a light lunch with a bean and greens salad.

✖ Tip

Reserve water from reconstituting mushrooms to use in broth, stocks, soups or stews. Refrigerate in an airtight container for up to 5 days or freeze for 2 months.

✖ Food processor
✖ 1½- to 2-cup (375 to 500 mL) glass or ceramic dish, lightly oiled

1½ cups	boiling water	375 mL
1½ oz	dried shiitake mushrooms	45 g
Agar		
¼ tsp	agar powder	1 mL
¼ cup	water	60 mL
½ cup	walnut halves	125 mL
2	green onions, white and light green parts only, cut into 2-inch (5 cm) pieces	2
¼ cup	packed fresh basil leaves	60 mL
¼ cup	packed Italian flat-leaf parsley leaves	60 mL
1 tbsp	freshly squeezed lemon juice	15 mL
½ tsp	toasted sesame oil	2 mL
¼ tsp	chile-garlic sauce	1 mL
¼ tsp	salt	1 mL
Pinch	granulated sugar	Pinch
¼ cup	packed arugula leaves	60 mL
2 tbsp	chopped roasted red bell pepper	30 mL

1. In a small heatproof bowl, pour boiling water over mushrooms and let stand until softened, about 30 minutes. Drain mushrooms, reserving liquid if desired (see Tip, left).

2. *Agar:* In a small saucepan, stir agar powder into water and let stand for 10 minutes. Bring to a boil over medium heat. Reduce heat and simmer until mixture begins to thicken, 5 to 6 minutes. Remove from heat and let cool.

3. In food processor, combine mushrooms, walnuts, green onions, basil and parsley and process for 30 seconds. Scrape sides. Add lemon juice, sesame oil, chile-garlic sauce, salt and sugar and process until well blended but not creamy smooth.

4. Add arugula, roasted red pepper and cooled agar to mushroom mixture and pulse until just combined, 10 to 15 times. Transfer pâté to prepared dish, smoothing top. Cover and refrigerate until set, for at least 4 hours or for up to 5 days.

5. To serve, loosen at edges and invert onto a small platter and serve with crackers or crudités.

Spicy, sweet and tart roasted chickpeas

**Makes 1½ cups
(375 mL)**

Splendid for a cocktail party appetizer, an after-school snack, hiking munchies or road trip boredom squelcher.

✴ Tip

Use 2 cans (each 14 to 19 oz/398 to 540 mL) chickpeas in place of freshly cooked, rinsing, draining and drying well.

✴ **Preheat oven to 450°F (230°C)**
✴ **Rimmed baking sheet, lined with parchment paper**

4 cups	cooked chickpeas, well-drained and dried (see Tip, left)	500 mL
½ cup	olive oil	125 mL
½ cup	granulated sugar	125 mL
1 tsp	ground cumin	5 mL
¾ tsp	ground coriander	3 mL
½ tsp	ground ginger	2 mL
½ tsp	ground cloves	2 mL
½ tsp	salt	2 mL
2 tsp	freshly squeezed lime juice	10 mL

1. Spread chickpeas on baking sheet in a single layer. Bake in preheated oven until browned and crunchy and dried in the center, 35 to 40 minutes. Watch carefully during the last 5 minutes as chickpeas quickly go from browned to burnt.

2. While chickpeas are roasting, place oil and sugar in a bowl. In a small bowl, combine cumin, coriander, ginger, cloves and salt. Set aside.

3. When chickpeas are roasted, drizzle with lime juice and immediately add hot nuts to sugar and oil mixture, tossing well to coat. Sprinkle with spice mixture. Let dry completely before serving.

Sticky rice with pineapple dipping sauce

A fun appetizer you eat with your fingers, scooping the tender rice into a ball and dipping into a delicious sauce. This absolute staple in Northern Thailand and Laos is so easy to make without any special equipment. Look for Thai style sticky rice or glutinous rice at Asian markets. Leftover sticky rice can be reheated by gently steaming or reheating in the microwave.

✖ Tips

Rice may be soaked for as little as 6 hours but longer soaking produces tastier rice. Thai cooks use a traditional, conical-shaped steaming basket but a bamboo or stainless-steel steamer basket or insert works well as long as the rice is wrapped in cheesecloth and is not touching the water.

If available, use a garlic press for garlic as pressed garlic is better incorporated into the dipping sauce.

✖ Variation

Garnish rice with chopped fresh pineapple and thinly sliced green onions.

✖ Steamer basket
✖ Cheesecloth

Rice

2 cups	long-grain Thai sticky rice	500 mL

Pineapple Dipping Sauce

6 tbsp	pineapple juice	90 mL
	Grated zest and juice of 2 limes	
2	cloves garlic, minced, grated or puréed (see Tips, left)	2
1	small Thai bird's-eye chile, finely chopped	1
3 tbsp	finely grated carrot	45 mL
3 tbsp	granulated sugar	45 mL
2 tbsp	toasted sesame oil	30 mL
2 tbsp	soy sauce	30 mL
1 tbsp	finely chopped shallot	15 mL
3 tbsp	finely chopped fresh cilantro	45 mL
3 tbsp	coarsely chopped dry roasted peanuts	45 mL

1. *Rice:* In a sieve, rinse rice under running water until water runs clear. Drain and place in large bowl. Add water to cover by 3 inches (7.5 cm), cover bowl and let soak for at least 6 hours or up to 24 hours.

2. Place 2 to 3 inches (5 to 7.5 cm) water in a saucepan with steamer basket, ensuring it is below bottom of steamer. Line steamer basket with cheesecloth. Drain rice and transfer to steamer, spreading evenly. Fold sides of cheesecloth over top of rice. Cover pan and bring water to a boil over medium heat. Reduce heat and steam rice over a low boil until shiny and tender, 25 to 30 minutes.

3. *Pineapple Dipping Sauce:* While rice is cooking, in a small bowl, combine pineapple, lime zest and juice, garlic, chile, carrot, sugar, oil, soy sauce and shallot and whisk until sugar is dissolved. Sprinkle top with cilantro and nuts and set aside.

4. When rice is done, transfer to a covered serving bowl. When ready to eat, remove cover and serve along with dipping sauce. Rice may be served hot, warm or at room temperature.

Tempeh mango lettuce cups with chile-garlic dipping sauce

Spicy and sweet flavors mingle to create an exotic and beautiful dish that is easy to prepare and a fabulous candidate for entertaining. Serve as an appetizer or as a light meal.

✖ Tip

This is great served buffet style: Place a platter of lettuce leaves, a serving bowl of tempeh mixture and a pitcher of ponzu sauce in the center of the table and let guests serve themselves.

3/4 cup	Pantry Ponzu Sauce, omitting cilantro (page 288), or store-bought	175 mL
1 lb	tempeh, crumbled	500 g

Filling

2 tbsp	peanut oil	30 mL
1 tbsp	grated gingerroot	15 mL
3	cloves garlic, minced	3
1/2	red bell pepper, finely chopped	1/2
1	large mango, chopped	1
3/4 cup	unsalted roasted cashews, chopped	175 mL
3/4 cup	chopped drained canned water chestnuts	175 mL
3	green onions, white and light green parts only, minced	3
1/4 cup	chopped fresh cilantro	60 mL
12	iceberg lettuce leaves or butter lettuce leaves	12

1. Pour ponzu sauce into a shallow dish. Add tempeh and let marinate for 30 minutes to 1 hour.

2. *Filling:* Place a large skillet over medium heat and let pan get hot. Add peanut oil and tip pan to coat. Add ginger and garlic and cook, stirring, for about 20 seconds. Add bell pepper and cook, stirring, until it just begins to soften, 3 to 4 minutes. Drain tempeh, discarding marinade, add to skillet and cook, stirring frequently, until browned and crispy around the edges, 4 to 6 minutes. Remove pan from heat and stir in mango, cashews, water chestnuts, green onions and cilantro.

3. To serve, place a lettuce cup on a plate, top with a generous amount of tempeh mixture and drizzle with a spoonful of sauce. Roll and eat.

Toasted tofu with onion miso jam

Serves 4

Delicate toasted tofu is paired with the savory sweetness of the onion jam. Serve as a unique appetizer or for lunch or a light dinner with a butter lettuce salad topped with Champagne Vinaigrette (page 302).

✷ Tip

Tofu may also be toasted on the stove top. Heat a cast-iron skillet over medium-high heat until very hot. Carefully add tofu slices and toast until lightly browned, 2 to 3 minutes per side.

✷ Variation

If vegan sake is unavailable, substitute mirin or white wine.

✷ Rimmed baking sheet, lightly oiled

Tofu

1 lb	extra-firm tofu	500 g
2 tbsp	olive oil	30 mL
	Salt and freshly ground black pepper	
2 tsp	toasted sesame seeds, optional	10 mL

Onion Miso Jam

2 tbsp	olive oil	30 mL
2 tbsp	vegan hard margarine	30 mL
2	large sweet onions, such as Vidalia or Walla Walla, thinly sliced	2
1 tsp	granulated sugar	5 mL
2 tbsp	vegan sake	30 mL
2 tbsp	brown rice syrup	30 mL
2 tbsp	rice wine vinegar	30 mL
1 tbsp	white miso	15 mL

1. *Tofu:* Press tofu according to instructions on page 12. Then cut tofu crosswise into 8 pieces and place on prepared baking sheet. Brush both sides with oil and lightly season with salt and pepper to taste.

2. *Onion Miso Jam:* Meanwhile, place a large nonstick skillet over medium heat and let pan get hot. Add oil and margarine and tip pan to coat. Add onions, stirring to coat. Cook, stirring frequently, about 6 minutes. Add sugar and cook, stirring occasionally, until onions slowly turn golden, 20 to 30 minutes, reducing heat to medium–low, if necessary.

3. In a small bowl, combine sake, brown rice syrup, vinegar and miso, mixing well. Stir mixture into onions. Reduce heat to low and simmer, stirring occasionally, until liquid reduces and mixture thickens, about 30 minutes. Set aside.

4. Preheat oven to 450°F (230°C).

5. Bake tofu in preheated oven for 10 minutes. Carefully flip tofu and bake for 8 minutes more. Remove pan from oven and set oven to broil. Carefully spread a thick layer of jam on each piece of tofu, return to oven and broil until jam begins to bubble, 30 seconds to 2 minutes. Sprinkle with sesame seeds, if using, and serve immediately.

Layered pesto and macadamia nut cream cheese torte

Layers of aromatic pesto and rich, creamy nut cheese may appear complex but come together easily and are well worth the effort. Make the pestos ahead and refrigerate while the cheese is processing.

✖ Tips

Nuts are typically soaked to break down enzymes, which aid digestion, and to soften harder nuts for easier blending. Macadamia nuts are soft and soaking is not advisable for this recipe. If using cashews, soak nuts in water for 2 to 4 hours.

When nuts are to be blended look for halves and pieces as they are less expensive than just halves.

✖ Blender
✖ Food processor
✖ Cheesecloth
✖ 4-cup (1 L) torte mold or bowl, lightly oiled and lined with plastic wrap, ends and sides extending

Nut Cheese

2 cups	raw macadamia nuts or soaked cashews (see Tips, left)	500 mL

Sun-Dried Tomato Pesto

2	cloves garlic	2
1 cup	drained oil-packed sun-dried tomatoes	250 mL
1 cup	walnut halves and pieces (see Tips, left)	250 mL
1/4 cup	olive oil	60 mL
2 tbsp	freshly squeezed lemon juice	30 mL
1 tsp	granulated sugar	5 mL
1/2 tsp	freshly ground black pepper	2 mL
Pinch	salt	Pinch

Basil Pesto

2	cloves garlic	2
2 cups	packed fresh basil leaves	500 mL
1 cup	toasted pine nuts	250 mL
1/4 cup	grated vegan Parmesan cheese alternative, optional	60 mL
2 tbsp	freshly squeezed lemon juice	30 mL
1/2 tsp	salt	5 mL
1/2 cup	olive oil	125 mL
	Sprigs basil, optional	
1/4 cup	finely chopped walnuts, optional	60 mL
	Crackers or baguette	

1. *Nut Cheese:* Place macadamia nuts in a blender, add water to just cover, no more. Starting on a lower speed and increasing gradually as nuts are chopped, blend until thick and completely smooth and creamy. Line a colander with double layers of cheesecloth and set over a plate.

Transfer mixture to colander, folding cheesecloth to wrap thoroughly. Set a plate on top and weigh down with a heavy can. Set aside in a draft-free area until drained, thick and the consistency of cream cheese, for at least 8 hours or overnight. Transfer to an airtight container and refrigerate for at least 4 hours or overnight.

2. *Sun-Dried Tomato Pesto:* In food processor, with motor running, drop garlic through feed tube and process until finely chopped. Scrape sides. Add sun-dried tomatoes, walnuts, oil, lemon juice, sugar, pepper and salt and process into a smooth pesto, stopping to scrape sides as necessary. Taste and adjust seasonings with salt and pepper, if needed, adding additional oil if pesto is dry. Transfer to an airtight container and refrigerate until needed or for up to 5 days.

3. *Basil Pesto:* In clean food processor, with motor running, drop garlic through feed tube and process until finely chopped. Scrape down sides. Add basil, pine nuts, cheese, if using, lemon juice and salt and pulse until roughly chopped, 10 to 15 times. Scrape down sides and, with motor running, drizzle in oil through feed tube and process into a smooth pesto, stopping to scrape sides as necessary. Taste and adjust seasonings with salt and pepper, if needed, adding additional oil if pesto is dry. Transfer to an airtight container and refrigerate until needed or for up to 5 days.

4. Divide nut cheese into thirds and spread one-third of nut cheese in the bottom of prepared torte mold. Spread sun-dried tomato pesto over cheese as the second layer. Top with one-half of remaining nut cheese as the third layer and spread basil pesto as the fourth layer. Spread remaining nut cheese as top layer. Cover and refrigerate to chill completely, 4 to 6 hours.

5. To serve, immerse bottom inch (2.5 cm) of mold in warm water for 30 seconds and pat dry. Invert a serving plate on top of mold, then quickly flip to unmold torte onto plate. Remove cover and garnish torte with basil sprigs and chopped walnuts, if using. Serve with crackers or sliced baguettes.

White bean hummus with spiced baked pita chips

Serves 4

This pleasant change from traditional chickpea hummus benefits from a fresh lemony flavor that balances well with the spicy pita chips. This quick and easy appetizer is also a great picnic take along or a perky addition to school lunch boxes.

Tip

Stack the pita halves and slice into wedges. This will save time and create uniform chips.

- **Preheat oven to 350°F (180°C)**
- **2 baking sheets, lined with parchment paper or silicone liners**
- **Food processor**

Pita Chips

4	6-inch (15 cm) pitas, each split into 2 circles	4
1/4 cup	olive oil	60 mL
1/2 tsp	salt	2 mL
1/2 tsp	smoked paprika	2 mL
1/4 tsp	ground cumin	1 mL

White Bean Hummus

2	cloves garlic, coarsely chopped	2
2 cups	cooked cannellini beans	500 mL
3 tbsp	freshly squeezed lemon juice	45 mL
3 tbsp	tahini	45 mL
2 to 4 tbsp	water	30 to 60 mL
1/2 tsp	salt	2 mL
1/4 cup	olive oil, divided	60 mL
1 tbsp	finely chopped fresh Italian flat-leaf parsley	15 mL
2 tbsp	finely chopped red onion	30 mL

1. *Pita Chips:* Cut each pita half into 6 wedges and place, smooth side up, on prepared baking sheet. Brush tops with oil and sprinkle with salt, paprika and cumin. Bake in preheated oven, for 6 minutes. Remove pan from oven and use tongs to flip chips. Return to oven and bake until chips are crisp, 6 to 8 minutes. Let cool.
2. *White Bean Hummus:* In food processor, with motor running, drop garlic through feed tube and process until finely chopped. Scrape down sides. Add beans, lemon juice, tahini and 2 tbsp (30 mL) water and process until just blended. Scrape down sides. Add salt and 3 tbsp (45 mL) of the oil and process until very smooth, adding additional water if needed.
3. Transfer hummus to a serving bowl, drizzle top with remaining oil and garnish with parsley and red onions. Serve with pita chips.

Breakfast Anytime

Almond bear claw muffins

Makes 12 muffins

Almost as good as those decadent bear claws of yesteryear but quite a bit better for you, these handsome muffins feature a center of streusel as well as layers of almond flavor throughout. For a real treat, add in-season cherries as suggested in the variation, right.

✴ Tip

Muffins are best eaten the day they are made but may be cooled completely, then individually wrapped and frozen for up to 1 month. Reheat directly from the freezer in microwave on High for about 20 seconds.

✴ Preheat oven to 400°F (200°C)
✴ Food processor
✴ 12-cup muffin pan, lightly oiled or lined with paper liners

Streusel

¼ cup	whole wheat flour	60 mL
¼ cup	all-purpose flour	60 mL
3 oz	almond paste	90 g
2 tbsp	packed brown sugar	30 mL
Pinch	salt	Pinch
2½ tbsp	almond or vegetable oil	37 mL
½ cup	sliced almonds, divided	125 mL

Muffins

1 cup	whole wheat flour	250 mL
1 cup	all-purpose flour	250 mL
¾ cup	granulated sugar	175 mL
2 tsp	baking powder	10 mL
½ tsp	salt	2 mL
½ cup	Almond Milk (page 19) or store-bought	125 mL
⅓ cup	almond or vegetable oil	75 mL
½ cup	unsweetened applesauce	125 mL
1 tsp	vanilla extract	5 mL
½ tsp	almond extract	2 mL

1. *Streusel:* In food processor, combine whole wheat flour, all-purpose flour, almond paste, brown sugar, salt and almond oil and pulse until combined. Reserve 2 tbsp (30 mL) of sliced almonds for topping. Remove blade and stir in remaining almonds. Set aside.

2. *Muffins:* In large bowl, stir together whole wheat flour, all-purpose flour, sugar, baking powder and salt. In another bowl, stir together almond milk, oil, applesauce, vanilla and almond extracts. Add wet ingredients to dry ingredients and stir until just combined.

3. Spoon half of batter into prepared muffin cups. Top with half of streusel. Cover with remaining batter. Top with remaining streusel, pressing down lightly. Place reserved sliced almonds sticking up, bear claw-style.

4. Bake in preheated oven until a toothpick inserted in center of muffin comes out clean, 20 to 25 minutes, checking for overbrowning halfway through baking time. If muffins are getting too dark, cover loosely with foil and continue baking. Let cool slightly in pan on a wire rack and serve warm.

❖ Variation

Add cherries to batter in Step 2, after mixing wet and dry ingredients. Add either 1/2 cup (125 mL) chopped dried cherries or 1 cup (250 mL) fresh cherries, pitted and chopped, or 1/2 cup (125 mL) thawed, well-drained and chopped frozen cherries.

Morning millet muffins

Enjoy these hearty little muffins in the morning with a spot of jam and delight in the crunchy bursting of millet in your mouth. Not too sweet, these tasty muffins would be equally at home served with a steaming bowl of chili.

✴ Tip

If you cannot find vanilla-flavored coconut milk, use regular coconut milk with 1 tsp (5 mL) vanilla.

✴ Preheat oven to 400°F (200°C)
✴ 12-cup muffin pan, lined with paper liners

1½ cups	vanilla coconut milk (see Tip, left)	375 mL
¾ cup	millet	175 mL
1 cup	whole wheat flour	250 mL
1 cup	all-purpose flour	250 mL
1 tbsp	ground flax seeds	15 mL
2 tsp	baking powder	10 mL
½ tsp	salt	2 mL
½ cup	brown rice syrup	125 mL
¼ cup	sunflower or vegetable oil	60 mL

1. In a small saucepan, stir together milk and millet. Bring just to a boil over medium heat, stirring occasionally. Remove from heat and let cool completely.

2. In a large bowl, stir together whole wheat flour, all-purpose flour, flax seeds, baking powder and salt.

3. In another bowl, whisk together rice syrup, oil and millet mixture. Add wet mixture to dry and gently fold together until just incorporated (batter will be lumpy). Spoon batter into prepared muffin pan.

4. Bake in preheated oven until a toothpick inserted in center comes out clean, about 15 minutes. Let cool in pan on a wire rack for 5 minutes. Dump muffins upside down onto wire rack and let cool completely.

Raspberry streusel muffins

Seductive muffins bursting with blushing raspberries and topped with sweet crumbly streusel use an overripe banana to replace the egg. Delicious and decadent as those from the best B&B, they are equally good at room temperature or hot with a smear of vegan margarine. These won't last long so eat 'em while you got 'em.

✛ Tip

Muffins are best freshly baked but may be cooled completely, individually wrapped and frozen for up to 1 month. Reheat directly from the freezer in microwave on High for about 20 seconds.

✛ Preheat oven to 400°F (200°C)
✛ 12-cup muffin pan, lightly oiled or lined with paper liners

Streusel

1/4 cup	whole wheat flour	60 mL
1/4 cup	all-purpose flour	60 mL
2 tbsp	packed brown sugar	30 mL
1/4 tsp	ground cinnamon	1 mL
Pinch	salt	Pinch
2 1/2 tbsp	vegetable oil	37 mL

Muffins

1 cup	whole wheat flour	250 mL
1 cup	all-purpose flour	250 mL
3/4 cup	granulated sugar	175 mL
2 tsp	baking powder	10 mL
1/2 tsp	salt	2 mL
1/2 cup	Almond Milk (page 19) or Soy Milk (page 18) or store-bought	125 mL
1/3 cup	coconut oil, melted	75 mL
1	very ripe small banana, mashed (1/3 to 1/2 cup/75 to 125 mL)	1
1 tsp	vanilla extract	5 mL
2 cups	fresh or frozen (not thawed) raspberries	500 mL

1. *Streusel:* In a bowl, stir together whole wheat flour, all-purpose flour, brown sugar, cinnamon, salt and oil. Using fingers, work into large clumps then crumble. Set aside.

2. *Muffins:* In large bowl, stir together whole wheat flour, all-purpose flour, sugar, baking powder and salt and set aside.

3. In another bowl, stir together almond milk, oil, banana and vanilla. Add wet ingredients to dry ingredients and stir just until combined. Gently fold in raspberries.

4. Spoon batter into prepared muffin cups and top with streusel, pressing it lightly into batter. Bake in preheated oven until toothpick inserted into center comes out clean, about 20 minutes. Let cool slightly in pan on a wire rack and serve warm.

Blue cornmeal green chile scones

The easy and the exotic meld in these savory batter-type drop scones. The classic flavor combination of corn and green chile is a natural to accompany Taos Chorizo Scramble (page 97) or Smoky Chipotle Black Bean Chile (page 280).

✖ Tips

Yellow cornmeal is a fine substitute for blue cornmeal.

Scones can wrapped well and stored at room temperature for 1 to 2 days.

✖ Preheat oven to 400°F (200°C)
✖ Baking sheet, lined with parchment paper

2¼ cups	all-purpose flour	550 mL
1 cup	blue cornmeal	250 mL
1 tbsp	granulated sugar	15 mL
1 tbsp	baking powder	15 mL
1 tsp	salt	5 mL
½ tsp	baking soda	2 mL
¾ cup	cold vegan hard margarine, cut into small pieces	175 mL
¼ cup	drained canned diced roasted green chiles	60 mL
2 tbsp	chopped chives	30 mL
¾ cup	Soy Milk (page 18) or store-bought	175 mL

1. In a large bowl, whisk together flour, cornmeal, sugar, baking powder, salt and baking soda. Add margarine and cut into flour mixture using 2 knives or pastry blender until small chunks and smaller crumbs are formed. Stir in green chiles and chives. Add soy milk and quickly mix with a fork until stiff batter is formed.

2. Drop batter by scant ¼ cup (60 mL) measures on prepared baking sheet, about 2 inches (5 cm) apart. Bake in preheated oven until tops and edges are golden brown, 15 to 18 minutes. Let cool on baking sheet on a wire rack for 10 minutes. Serve warm.

> ## ✖ Variation
> Delete chives and add 2 tbsp (30 mL) finely chopped green onions and 3 tbsp (45 mL) toasted pumpkin seeds with the green chiles.

Lemon-glazed ginger scones

Makes 12 scones

Fresh ginger and lemon scent these delicate scones, perfect for an afternoon tea or a Sunday breakfast.

✿ Tip

Scones can be stored at room temperature, well wrapped, for 1 to 2 days.

✿ **Preheat oven to 400°F (200°C)**

Dough

3 cups	all-purpose flour	750 mL
1/3 cup	granulated sugar	75 mL
2 tsp	baking powder	10 mL
1/2 tsp	baking soda	2 mL
1/2 tsp	salt	2 mL
3/4 cup	vegan hard margarine, chilled, cut into small pieces	175 mL
1	piece (1 to 2 inches/2.5 to 5 cm) gingerroot, peeled and grated (2 to 3 oz/60 to 90 g)	1
3/4 to 7/8 cup	Soy Milk (page 18) or store-bought	175 to 220 mL

Glaze

1 cup	confectioner's (icing) sugar	250 mL
1 1/2 tbsp	freshly squeezed lemon juice	22 mL

1. *Dough:* In large bowl, whisk together flour, sugar, baking powder, baking soda and salt. Add chilled margarine and blend using 2 knives or pastry blender until small chunks and smaller crumbs are formed. Place grated ginger in a 2-cup (500 mL) glass measuring cup and add enough soy milk to make 1 cup (250 mL). Add soy milk mixture to crumbs and mix with a fork until a loose dough is formed.

2. Turn dough onto a lightly floured work surface and knead gently for 30 seconds. Divide dough in half. Pat or roll each half into a 5-inch (12.5 cm) circle and cut each circle into 6 wedges. Place wedges on an ungreased baking sheet at least 1 inch (2.5 cm) apart.

3. Bake in preheated oven until tops and edges are golden brown, 18 to 22 minutes. Let cool on baking sheet on a wire rack for 10 minutes. Transfer scones to rack and let cool completely.

4. *Glaze:* In a small bowl, stir together confectioner's sugar and lemon juice. Drizzle glaze over scones and allow glaze to harden. Serve scones at room temperature.

Giant cinnamon rolls

The first taste of these cinnamon rolls will transport you to a decadent cinnamon and brown sugar heaven. Mashed potatoes keep dough moist and light; don't worry about black pepper in leftover spuds, because the ground cinnamon in the dough covers any peppery taste.

✖ Tip

Store in an airtight container at room temperature for up to 3 days.

✖ Stand mixer with dough hook
✖ 13- by 9-inch (33 by 23 cm) glass baking dish, lightly oiled

Dough

1 cup	Soy Milk (page 18) or store-bought	250 mL
3 tbsp	vegan hard margarine	45 mL
¾ cup	mashed potatoes	175 mL
6 tbsp	granulated sugar	90 mL
1 tsp	salt	5 mL
½ tsp	ground cinnamon	2 mL
¼ cup	warm water	60 mL
2 tsp	active dry yeast	10 mL
3½ to 4¼ cups	all-purpose flour	875 mL to 1.06 L

Filling

2 tbsp	vegan hard margarine, melted	30 mL
2 tbsp	pure maple syrup	30 mL
1 cup	packed brown sugar	250 mL
2 tsp	ground cinnamon	10 mL
½ cup	raisins	125 mL
½ cup	chopped pecans	125 mL

Frosting

1½ cups	confectioner's (icing) sugar, sifted	375 mL
¼ cup	vegan hard margarine, melted	60 mL
1 to 2 tbsp	plain soy milk	15 to 30 mL
½ tsp	vanilla extract	2 mL

1. *Dough:* In a small saucepan, heat soy milk over medium heat until steaming and bubbles form around edge to scald. Remove from heat and stir in margarine, mashed potatoes, sugar, salt and cinnamon. Let cool to lukewarm.

2. In bowl of stand mixer, combine warm water and yeast and let stand until foamy, about 5 minutes. Whisk potato mixture into yeast.

3. Attach bowl to mixer and fit with dough hook. On low speed, gradually add 3½ cups (875 mL) of flour to potato mixture. Mix for 2 minutes. Add remaining flour, 1 tbsp (15 mL) at a time, until a sticky dough forms. Beat for 2 minutes. Transfer to a large warm oiled bowl. Turn dough so top is oiled. Cover with a clean kitchen towel and let rise in a warm, draft-free place until doubled in size, about 45 minutes.

4. *Filling:* In a small bowl, combine margarine and maple syrup. (It's okay if they don't blend completely.) Set aside. Turn dough onto a floured work surface. Roll or pat into a rectangle about 18- by 12-inches (45 by 30 cm). Brush margarine mixture over dough, leaving about a ½-inch (1 cm) border all around. Sprinkle brown sugar then cinnamon evenly over margarine. Scatter raisins and pecans over brown sugar. Starting at one long end, roll up jelly-roll fashion, pinching seam to seal. Cut into 12 thick slices. Arrange cut side down in prepared dish, patting back into a roll shape, if necessary. Cover lightly with plastic wrap and let rise until doubled in bulk, 45 minutes to 1 hour.

5. About 10 minutes before rolls have completely risen, preheat oven to 350°F (180°C). Uncover dish and bake in preheated oven until rolls are puffed and tops are golden, 20 to 25 minutes. Let cool in pan for 10 minutes.

6. *Frosting:* In small bowl, stir together confectioner's sugar and melted margarine, adding soy milk a little at a time to help blend. Stir in vanilla. Drizzle frosting over cinnamon rolls. Serve warm.

Blackberry crumble coffee cake

Almost more crumble than cake, this homey dessert will please berry and coffee cake lovers alike.

✖ Tip

This cake is best eaten the day it is made but will keep, covered with plastic wrap at room temperature for up to 2 days.

✖ Preheat oven to 325°F (160°C)
✖ 8-inch (20 cm) square glass baking dish, lightly oiled

Crumble

½ cup	large-flake (old-fashioned) rolled oats	125 mL
¼ cup	whole wheat flour	60 mL
¼ cup	all-purpose flour	60 mL
¼ cup	packed brown sugar	60 mL
¾ tsp	ground cinnamon	3 mL
¼ tsp	salt	1 mL
¼ cup	vegan margarine, melted	60 mL

Cake

¾ cup	all-purpose flour	175 mL
6 tbsp	whole wheat flour	90 mL
½ cup + 2 tbsp	granulated sugar	155 mL
1 tsp	baking powder	5 mL
½ tsp	baking soda	2 mL
½ tsp	salt	2 mL
6 tbsp	almond or soy milk	90 mL
¼ cup	vegetable oil	60 mL
	Grated zest of 1 lemon	
2 tbsp	freshly squeezed lemon juice	30 mL
1 tsp	vanilla extract	5 mL
2 cups	fresh or frozen (not thawed) blackberries	500 mL

1. *Crumble:* In a bowl, combine oats, whole wheat flour, all-purpose flour, brown sugar, cinnamon, salt and margarine. Using your fingers, work into large clumps then crumble. Set aside.

2. *Cake:* In large bowl, stir together all-purpose flour, whole wheat flour, sugar, baking powder, baking soda and salt. In a small bowl or 2-cup (500 mL) glass measuring cup, stir together almond milk, oil, lemon zest, lemon juice and vanilla. Add wet ingredients to dry ingredients and stir until just combined. Fold in berries. Spread in prepared pan and scatter crumble over batter.

3. Bake in preheated oven until a toothpick inserted into the center comes out clean, 45 to 50 minutes, or 10 minutes longer if using frozen berries. Let cool slightly in pan on a wire rack. Serve warm.

Banana-cardamom cornmeal cakes

Sweet spiced cornmeal cakes whip together in a snap. A delicious way to use bananas that are too fast approaching old age. Serve cakes hot, topped with warm maple syrup.

✖ **Preheat oven to 200°F (100°C)**
✖ **Large griddle or nonstick skillet**

1 cup	all-purpose flour	250 mL
1/2 cup	cornmeal	125 mL
1 tbsp	baking powder	15 mL
1 tsp	ground cardamom	5 mL
1/2 tsp	ground cinnamon	2 mL
1/4 tsp	salt	1 mL
1 1/2 cups	non-dairy milk	300 mL
3 tbsp	brown rice syrup	45 mL
	Canola oil	
1 cup	chopped banana	250 mL

1. In a large bowl, combine flour, cornmeal, baking powder, cardamom, cinnamon and salt. In a separate bowl, combine milk, rice syrup and 2 tbsp (30 mL) oil. Add wet ingredients to dry ingredients and stir until just combined. Do not over mix. Gently stir in banana.

2. Place griddle over medium heat and let pan get hot. Add 1 tsp (5 mL) oil, tip pan to coat and let oil heat. Using a 1/4 cup (60 mL) measure for each cake, pour batter into a circle. Cook until bubbles form, tops lose their gloss and edges begin to brown, 2 1/2 to 3 minutes. Flip pancakes and cook until puffed, center springs back when lightly pressed and bottoms are browned, about 2 minutes. Transfer cooked cakes to a platter and hold in warm oven. Repeat with remaining batter, adding oil and adjusting heat as needed between batches.

> ✖ **Variation**
> Substitute chopped very ripe pears for bananas.

Nine-grain griddle cakes

Hearty and delicious from the lovely variety of grains, these petite griddle cakes pack a big nutritional punch and are a great start to a winter's day.

✖ Tip

Find a hot cereal mix from a health food store or local mill, if you're lucky enough to have one. Use either a 7-grain or 9-grain cereal with an assortment of grains such as hard and/or soft wheat, rye, oat bran, oats, corn, barley, millet, flax seeds and spelt. Or create your own mix of favorite grains.

✖ Preheat oven to 200°F (100°C)
✖ Spice or coffee grinder

½ cup	9-grain hot cereal mix (see Tip, left)	125 mL
½ cup	whole wheat flour	125 mL
1 tbsp	baking powder	15 mL
¼ tsp	salt	1 mL
½ cup	cooked brown rice, cooled	125 mL
½ cup	Soy Milk (page 18) or	125 mL
	Almond Milk (page 19) or store-bought	
¼ cup	pure maple syrup	60 mL
4 tbsp	canola oil, divided	60 mL
	Pure maple syrup, optional	

1. In spice grinder, grind 9-grain cereal to a powder. Transfer to a large bowl, add flour, baking powder and salt and whisk to combine. Set aside.

2. In a small bowl, stir together cooked rice, soy milk, maple syrup and 2 tbsp (30 mL) of the oil. Pour milk mixture into dry ingredients and stir just until combined (do not overmix).

3. Place skillet over medium–high heat and let pan get hot. Add 1 tbsp (15 mL) of oil and tip pan to coat. Using 2 tbsp (30 mL) batter for each, form small griddle cakes, spreading batter evenly. Cook until tops lose their gloss and edges begin to brown, 2 to 3 minutes. Flip cakes and cook for an additional 2 to 3 minutes. Transfer to a platter and hold in warm oven. Repeat process with remaining batter, using more oil and adjusting heat between batches as needed. Serve warm topped with maple syrup, if using.

Orange-cranberry breakfast loaf

Serves 8 to 10

A vegan version of a traditional quick bread, this sunny loaf makes a welcome gift during the holidays or a great breakfast treat anytime. A dab of marmalade gives it an extra orange kick.

Tips

Substitute ½ cup (125 mL) chopped dried cranberries if fresh are not available. Add dried cranberries after wet ingredients are mixed with dry ingredients, stirring just to combine.

Store well wrapped at room temperature for up to 4 days.

- **Preheat oven to 350°F (180°C)**
- **9- by 5-inch (23 by 12.5 cm) metal loaf pan, lightly oiled**

2	oranges	2
1 cup	whole wheat flour	250 mL
1 cup	all-purpose flour	250 mL
2 tsp	baking powder	10 mL
½ tsp	baking soda	2 mL
½ tsp	salt	2 mL
1 cup	chopped cranberries (see Tips, left)	250 mL
¾ cup	granulated sugar	175 mL
2 tbsp	canola oil	30 mL
2 tbsp	marmalade	30 mL

1. Grate zest from 1 of the oranges. Squeeze juice from both oranges. Measure ¾ cup (175 mL) juice, adding water if necessary. Set aside.
2. In large bowl, stir together whole wheat flour, all-purpose flour, baking powder, baking soda and salt. Sprinkle orange zest over dry ingredients. Stir in cranberries and set aside.
3. In small saucepan over low heat, heat orange juice just until steaming. Remove from heat and stir in sugar, oil and marmalade. Add orange juice mixture to dry ingredients and stir just until combined.
4. Pour into prepared loaf pan, smoothing top. Bake in preheated oven until toothpick inserted in center comes out clean, 45 to 50 minutes. Let cool in pan on a wire rack for 10 minutes, then remove from pan and let cool completely on rack.

Cinnamon-raisin french toast

Serves 6 to 8

This simply scrumptious and comforting French toast is suitable for any time of the day or night.

✕ Tips

Eggless French toast presents unique challenges for the intrepid breakfast cook. These few simple steps can help greatly improve the result: Dry coated slices for 10 minutes before frying; use a very well-seasoned pan or griddle; and once cooking, don't disturb each slice for a full 4 to 5 minutes before flipping.

After flipping, cook French toast for 4 minutes, which should produce a nicely browned underside. To check, lift a corner but be cautioned that lifting toast off the griddle will stop cooking process.

✕ Preheat oven to 200°F (100°C)
✕ Wire rack
✕ Rimmed baking sheet

1 cup	Soy Milk (page 18) or Almond Milk (page 19) or store-bought	250 mL
2 tbsp	all-purpose flour	30 mL
$\frac{1}{2}$ tsp	ground cinnamon	2 mL
1 tsp	vanilla extract	5 mL
1 lb	sliced vegan cinnamon-raisin bread, day-old	500 g
1 to 2 tbsp	canola oil	15 to 30 mL

1. In a bowl, gradually whisk soy milk into flour, making sure all flour is dissolved. Stir in cinnamon and vanilla. Pour mixture into a shallow dish.

2. Set wire rack on top of baking sheet. Dip each bread slice very briefly in milk mixture and place on rack to catch drips. Let dry for 10 minutes.

3. Place a skillet or griddle over medium-high heat and let pan get hot. Coat pan with a 1 tbsp (15 mL) of the oil. Working in batches to avoid crowding pan, place coated bread in hot pan. Cook until edges begin to brown and coating starts to look dry, 4 to 5 minutes. Flip and cook, for another 4 to 5 minutes (see Tips, left). Transfer to platter and hold in a warm oven. Repeat process with remaining bread, adding more oil to pan and adjusting heat between batches as needed. Serve warm.

Stuffed sourdough french toast

The very picture of a luscious and luxurious Sunday brunch. Serve with Maple Bourbon Tempehacon (page 27) and fresh orange juice Mimosas.

✖ Tip

A well-seasoned cast-iron pan or griddle is worth its weight in gold. The cast iron retains and distributes heat evenly and the "seasoned" coating prevents sticking. For tips on seasoning a cast-iron pan see page 101.

✖ Variation

Change the fruit filling according to the season. For fall, sauté 1 apple, peeled and thinly sliced, in 1 tbsp (15 mL) vegan margarine until soft, 10 to 12 minutes. Mix apple with ½ cup (125 mL) apple butter and stuff as directed.

✖ Preheat oven to 200°F (100°C)
✖ Wire rack
✖ Rimmed baking sheet

1 cup	strawberry jam	250 mL
1 cup	sliced strawberries	250 mL
1	loaf (1 lb/500 g) day-old vegan sourdough bread, cut into 1-inch (2.5 cm) thick slices	1
1 cup	plain soy or almond milk	250 mL
2 tbsp	all-purpose flour	30 mL
½ tsp	ground cinnamon	2 mL
1 tsp	vanilla extract	5 mL
1 to 2 tbsp	canola oil	15 to 30 mL
	Heavy Cream (page 26), optional	

1. In a small saucepan over medium heat, stir strawberry jam until heated through, 2 to 3 minutes. Remove from heat, stir in sliced strawberries and set aside.

2. On cutting board, lay each bread slice, cut side down. Working with one slice at a time, place hand flat on top to steady while making pocket. Using a small sharp knife, cut a deep horizontal slit into bottom crust side of bread slice without slicing through the other side. Stuff 1 to 2 tbsp (15 to 30 mL) strawberry mixture inside, being careful not to overstuff (reserve any extra for topping). Set aside.

3. In a bowl, gradually whisk soy milk into flour, making sure all flour is dissolved. Stir in cinnamon and vanilla. Pour milk mixture into a shallow dish.

4. Set wire rack on top of baking sheet. Dip each slice very briefly in soy mixture and set on rack to catch drips. Repeat with remaining slices and let air dry for 10 minutes.

5. Place a well-seasoned skillet or griddle over medium–high heat and let pan get hot. Add 1 tbsp (15 mL) of the oil and tip pan to coat. In batches to avoid crowding pan, place coated slices on hot pan. Cook until edges begin to brown and coating starts to look dry, 4 to 5 minutes. Flip and cook, for another 4 to 5 minutes (see Tips, page 78). Transfer cooked French toast to a platter and hold in warm oven. Repeat process with remaining slices, adding more oil to pan and adjusting heat as needed.

6. Serve warm, topped with heavy cream, if using, and garnish with any remaining strawberry mixture, if desired.

Gingerbread pancakes with mandarin orange syrup

Makes 6 to 8 griddle cakes

Serve vegan sausage patties with these warm and spicy pancakes for a sunny and elegant brunch. Mandarin syrup will keep for up to a week and is wonderful over ice cream or fruit, especially topped with Easy Homemade Granola (page 87).

✂ **Preheat oven to 200°F (100°C)**

Mandarin Syrup

1/2 cup	packed brown sugar	125 mL
1	can (11 oz or 284 mL) mandarin orange segments in juice or syrup	1
2 tbsp	cornstarch	30 mL
	Grated zest of 1 orange	
1 tbsp	orange-flavored liqueur	15 mL

Pancakes

1/2 cup	all-purpose flour	125 mL
1/2 cup	whole wheat flour	125 mL
1 tbsp	baking powder	15 mL
1 tsp	Autumn Spice Blend (page 309) or store-bought pumpkin pie spice	5 mL
1 tsp	ground ginger	5 mL
1/4 tsp	salt	1 mL
1 cup	Soy Milk (page 18) or Almond Milk (page 19) or store-bought	250 mL
3 tbsp	light (fancy) molasses	45 mL
1	piece (1 inch/2.5 cm) gingerroot, peeled and grated	1
4 tbsp	canola oil, divided	60 mL

1. *Mandarin Syrup:* In a saucepan over medium heat, melt brown sugar, stirring frequently.

2. Pour mandarin juice into small bowl. Stir in cornstarch and add to melted brown sugar in pan, stirring constantly. Bring to boil and boil, stirring, for 1 minute. Stir in orange zest and liqueur and keep warm over low heat.

3. *Pancakes:* In a bowl, whisk together all–purpose flour, whole wheat flour, baking powder, spice blend, ground ginger and salt. Set aside.

✕ Tip

Refrigerate uncooked pancake batter in an airtight container for up to 3 days, adding soy milk to thin batter if necessary.

4. In small bowl, stir together soy milk, molasses, ginger and 2 tbsp (30 mL) of the oil. Pour milk mixture into dry ingredients and stir just until combined (do not overmix).

5. Place skillet over medium-high heat and let pan get hot. Add 2 tsp (10 mL) of oil and tip pan to coat. Using ¼ cup (60 mL) batter for each, form pancakes, spreading batter in an even circle. Cook until tops lose their gloss and edges begin to brown, 3 to 5 minutes. Flip pancakes and cook, for another 3 to 4 minutes (see Tips, page 78). Transfer cooked cakes to a platter and hold in warm oven. Repeat with remaining batter, adding oil and adjusting heat as needed.

6. Serve with warm mandarin syrup.

Go go breakfast bars

These colorful and healthful bars travel far beyond breakfast and make a handy snack for people on the go. The sky is the limit on variations and many suggestions are listed below. Try this with some favorites to create your own signature bar — you could even name it after yourself.

✖ Tips

Flax seeds are available in grocery or natural food stores either raw or toasted, sometimes referred to as roasted. Raw flax seeds may be toasted in a heavy-bottomed skillet over medium-high heat while stirring or shaking the pan constantly to prevent burning until seeds turn a golden brown. Store in an airtight container in the refrigerator for up to 3 weeks.

Refrigerate wrapped bars for up to 1 week or freeze for up to 2 months. Bars wrapped individually in waxed paper squares are perfect to tuck into a backpack, purse or lunch box.

✖ Preheat oven to 325°F (160°C)

✖ 13- by 9-inch (33 by 23 cm) glass baking dish, lined with lightly oiled parchment paper extending up beyond sides

2½ cups	rolled spelt	625 mL
1 cup	chopped raw cashews	250 mL
1 cup	chopped dried apricots	250 mL
½ cup	chopped dried cherries	125 mL
¼ cup	ground almonds (almond meal)	60 mL
¼ cup	oat bran	60 mL
¼ cup	sesame seeds	60 mL
¼ cup	green pumpkin seeds (pepitas)	60 mL
2 tbsp	toasted flax seeds (see Tips, left)	30 mL
1 tbsp	coconut oil	15 mL
¾ cup	packed brown sugar	175 mL
½ cup	agave nectar	125 mL
½ tsp	salt	2 mL

1. In a dry large skillet over medium-high heat, cook spelt, stirring frequently, until lightly toasted, 4 to 5 minutes. Let cool and place in a large bowl along with cashews, apricots, cherries, almond meal, oat bran, sesame seeds, pumpkin seeds and flax seeds.

2. In a saucepan, heat coconut oil over medium-high heat. Add brown sugar, agave and salt and whisk to combine. Bring to a boil and cook, stirring, until sugar is dissolved, 2 to 3 minutes. Remove from heat and add to ingredients in large bowl, stirring well to combine.

3. Transfer mixture to prepared baking dish and use the back of a spoon to spread and compress mixture evenly. Bake in preheated oven until edges brown slightly, about 15 minutes. Let cool completely in dish on a wire rack.

4. Use extended parchment to gently remove from dish and transfer bars to cutting board. Cut into desired size bars.

✖ Variations

Substitute dates, dried papaya, mango, figs, blueberries, cranberries, pecans, walnuts, pine nuts, hemp seeds, sunflower seeds or poppy seeds.

Pioneer buckwheat pancakes

This instant pancake mix is delicious and without all the additives of a commercially prepared mix. Mix dry ingredients and store in the pantry for use when time is short. Add liquid ingredients and breakfast is ready in no time. Because only oil and water are added to the mixed dry ingredients, these are a perfect take-along choice when exploring the great outdoors.

Tips

For 18 pancakes, mix 2 cups + 2 tbsp (530 mL) (half of dry mixture) with 1 tbsp (15 mL) oil and 1 cup (250 mL) water. For 9 pancakes, mix 1 cup + 1 tbsp (265 mL) (one-quarter of dry mixture) with 2 tsp (10 mL) oil and 1/2 cup (125 mL) water.

The griddle will get hotter the longer it has been on the heat. If necessary, remove from heat to let pan cool slightly and reduce stove temperature to prevent pancakes from browning too quickly and being undercooked through the center.

Preheat oven to 200°F (100°C)

1 cup	all-purpose flour	250 mL
1 cup	buckwheat flour	250 mL
2 cups	non-dairy milk powder, such as soy, hemp or nut	500 mL
1/4 cup	packed brown sugar	60 mL
1 tbsp	baking powder	15 mL
1/4 tsp	salt	1 mL
	Canola oil	
2 cups	water	500 mL

1. In a large bowl, combine all-purpose flour, buckwheat flour, milk powder, brown sugar, baking powder and salt, whisking to completely incorporate. At this point, dry mixture may be stored in an airtight container in a cool dark place for up to 3 months.

2. When ready to make pancakes, place dry ingredients in a bowl. In a small bowl, combine 2 tbsp (30 mL) oil and water and add to dry ingredients, stirring just to incorporate (do not overmix).

3. Place griddle or skillet over medium heat and let pan get hot. Add 1 tsp (5 mL) oil, if necessary, and let it get hot. Using 2 tbsp (30 mL) of batter for each, form small pancakes (do not crowd griddle). Cook until bubbles form and burst and outer edge lose their gloss, 2 to 2 1/2 minutes. Flip pancakes and cook until underside is browned and pancake is slightly puffed, 1 to 1 1/2 minutes.

4. Transfer cooked pancakes to platter in warm oven and repeat with remaining batter, adding oil and adjusting heat between batches, as needed.

Variation

If you want less-sweet pancakes, decrease brown sugar to 3 tbsp (45 mL).

Popeye spinach and feta breakfast stack

Serves 4	

Sautéed mushrooms, onions, peppers and spinach are piled high on crispy hash browned potatoes and topped with salty and creamy soy feta. A breakfast that is as good for you as it is good to eat!

⚏ Preheat oven to 200°F (100°C)

1	recipe Pan-Fried Onion and Potato Hash Browns (page 104)	1
2 tbsp	olive oil	30 mL
½	red onion, chopped	½
12 oz	cremini mushrooms, sliced	375 g
3	cloves garlic, chopped	3
½ cup	chopped drained roasted red bell pepper	125 mL
1 lb	fresh spinach, trimmed	500 g
1 cup	drained Greek Herbed Soy Feta in Olive Oil (page 24) or cubed store-bought soy feta	250 mL

1. Cook hash browns according to recipe. Transfer to a baking dish and place in preheated oven.

2. Place a large skillet over medium heat and let pan get hot. Add oil and tip pan to coat. Add red onion and mushrooms, stirring to coat with oil. Cook, stirring occasionally, until mushrooms begin to wilt, about 6 minutes. Add garlic and roasted pepper and cook, stirring, until mushrooms are golden and slightly browned at edges, 4 to 5 minutes. Stir in spinach and cook until just wilted, about 2 minutes.

3. Divide hash browns between 4 plates and top each with one-quarter of sautéed vegetable mixture. Crumble feta over top and serve hot.

Breakfast tacos

The deliciousness of crusty potatoes, tofu and crunchy tempehacon bits in soft hot flour tortillas and topped with rich and zesty tomato salsa can turn any morning into a gourmet delight. This recipe is easily doubled or tripled for a brunch gathering. Serve with Blazing Mary (page 323).

✖ Tip

Parboiling potatoes gives them a head start especially when making fried potatoes. *To parboil potatoes:* Place potatoes in a saucepan, cover with water and bring to a gentle boil over medium-high heat. Gently boil potatoes until a fork inserted pierces the outer potato but meets considerable resistance near the middle, 8 to 10 minutes for small to medium potatoes and 10 to 15 minutes for large potatoes.

2 tbsp	olive oil, divided	30 mL
1/2	small onion, sliced	1/2
2	cloves garlic, minced	2
1 tsp	ground cumin	5 mL
1/2 tsp	dried oregano	2 mL
1/2 tsp	chile powder	2 mL
2	red potatoes, parboiled and cubed (see Tip, left)	2
8 oz	firm tofu, drained and crumbled	250 g
1 tsp	salt	5 mL
1/2 tsp	freshly ground black pepper	2 mL
4	6-inch (15 cm) vegan flour tortillas	4
1/2 cup	Crunchy Tempehacon Bits (page 22) or store-bought vegan bacon bits	125 mL
2	green onions, white and light green parts only, finely chopped	2
1/2 cup	Year-Round Blender Tomato Salsa (page 300) or store-bought	125 mL

1. Place a large skillet over medium heat and let pan get hot. Add 1 tbsp (15 mL) of the oil and tip pan to coat. Add onion and cook, stirring frequently, until softened and slightly browned, 6 to 8 minutes. Stir in garlic, cumin, oregano and chile powder and cook until garlic is softened, about 1 minute.

2. Move garlic and onion to edges of pan. Add 1 tbsp (15 mL) of oil to center of pan and heat for 30 seconds. Add potatoes and tofu, stir in the onion and garlic and cook, turning frequently, until browned with a light crust, 8 to 10 minutes. Stir in salt and pepper.

3. In another large skillet, heat tortillas, one at a time, over medium heat until softened, puffed and browned in a few areas, 1 to 2 minutes per side. Wrap heated tortillas in a clean kitchen towel placed in a basket to keep warm.

4. Divide tofu and potato mixture among tortillas, top with tempehacon bits, green onions and a spoonful of salsa. Fold each tortilla in half and serve immediately.

Pantry muesli

**Makes about
8 cups (2 L)**

This is a very simple muesli made from ingredients you are likely to have in your pantry. It's fun to get creative, adding nuts, flakes, dried fruit or seeds to your liking.

✖ Tip

Make small batches of muesli, experimenting with various flakes such as spelt, barley and rye to discover your favorites.

2 cups	large-flake (old-fashioned) rolled oats	500 mL
1 cup	oat bran	250 mL
1 cup	whole-grain spelt, barley and/or rye flakes	250 mL
1 cup	chopped almonds	250 mL
1 cup	dried apple slices	250 mL
1/2 cup	unsweetened flaked coconut	125 mL
1/2 cup	dried cranberries	125 mL
1/2 cup	dried apricots	125 mL
1/4 cup	toasted flax seeds (see Tips, page 82)	60 mL
1/4 cup	green pumpkin seeds (pepitas)	60 mL

Nut, rice, hemp or soy milk, cold or warmed

1. In a large airtight container, combine oats, oat bran, cereal flakes, almonds, apple slices, coconut, cranberries, apricots, flax seeds and pepitas. Store at room temperature for up to 2 months.

2. To serve hot, bring equal amounts of muesli and nut, rice, hemp or soy milk to a gentle boil and simmer for 3 to 5 minutes. Alternately soak 1/2 cup (125 mL) muesli with warmed or cold nut, rice, hemp or soy milk for 5 minutes to overnight, depending on desired consistency.

Easy homemade granola

With few ingredients, this granola is economical and easy to prepare. Beyond breakfast, a small resealable bag of granola is a great take-along snack or topping for your favorite vegan ice cream.

- Preheat oven to 250°F (120°C)
- Rimmed baking sheet, lined with parchment paper

2 cups	large-flake (old-fashioned) rolled oats	500 mL
¾ cup	slivered almonds	175 mL
½ cup	sunflower seeds	125 mL
¼ cup	green pumpkin seeds (pepitas)	60 mL
2 tbsp	toasted flax seeds (see Tips, page 82)	30 mL
1¼ cups	unsweetened orange juice	300 mL
1 tsp	vanilla extract	5 mL
½ tsp	ground cardamom	2 mL
2 tbsp	sunflower oil	30 mL
¾ cup	dried blueberries	175 mL

1. In a large bowl, combine oats, almonds and sunflower, pumpkin and flax seeds, mixing well to combine.

2. In another bowl, combine orange juice, vanilla and cardamom. Stir into oats, mixing well to blend. Stir in oil and mix well to coat.

3. Spread mixture evenly on prepared baking sheet. Bake in preheated oven, stirring occasionally to ensure even crisping, until granola is crisp, about 1½ hours. Remove from oven, stir in blueberries and let mixture cool. Store in an airtight container for up to 2 weeks or frozen for up to 2 months.

Variation

Use any nuts, seeds or dried fruit you happen to have on hand. Cranberries, raisins, dried apricots, papaya, mango or figs are excellent choices.

Toasted steel-cut oats with apples and walnuts

Steel-cut oats are just that, whole groats that have been steel-cut into a few pieces. Although they do take much longer to cook than oats that have been rolled and flattened, the texture, flavor and nutritional value are worth the effort. Toasting oats before cooking them in liquid brings out their nutty aroma and enhances the flavor.

3 cups	water	750 mL
1 cup	unsweetened apple juice, preferably unfiltered	250 mL
1 cup	steel-cut oats	250 mL
2	apples, peeled and diced	2
1/4 tsp	freshly grated nutmeg	1 mL
Pinch	salt	Pinch
1/2 cup	chopped toasted walnuts	125 mL
4 tbsp	agave nectar	60 mL
2 cups	unsweetened vanilla almond milk	500 mL

1. In a saucepan over medium–high heat, combine water and apple juice and bring just to a boil.

2. Meanwhile, place a saucepan over medium heat and let pan get hot. Add oats and toast lightly, stirring frequently to prevent burning. When liquid comes to a boil, gradually add to oats, about 1 cup (250 mL) at a time, and bring to a boil. Reduce heat and simmer, stirring often, for 10 minutes. Stir in apples, nutmeg and salt and simmer, stirring often, until oats are cooked to desired consistency, about 10 minutes. Serve bowls of cooked oats topped with walnuts, agave and almond milk.

> ### ⊞ Variations
>
> Substitute ripe pears and pear juice for the apples and apples juice, stirring pears into oats during last 3 to 4 minutes of cooking.
>
> Dried fruit such as cranberries or figs are delicious and should be stirred in during first few minutes of cooking.

Moroccan-spiced oatmeal

An absolute must to
fortify the forces before
a day of shopping in
the Kasbah. Toasting
the oats brings out the
best of them, and this
delectable delight will
bring out the best in
you.

✖ Tip

To toast almonds: Spread
nuts on a baking sheet and
bake in a 350°F (180°C)
oven until fragrant and
slightly browned, 6 to
10 minutes, checking often
as they easily burn.

3 cups	plain hemp milk	750 mL
3 tbsp	brown rice syrup	45 mL
1½ cups	large-flake (old-fashioned) rolled oats	375 mL
1 tsp	ground cinnamon	5 mL
1 tsp	ground cardamom	5 mL
½ tsp	ground ginger	2 mL
¼ tsp	ground cloves	1 mL
¼ cup	chopped dates	60 mL
¼ cup	golden raisins	60 mL
¼ cup	chopped dried apricots	60 mL
½ tsp	almond extract	2 mL
Pinch	salt	Pinch
½ cup	chopped toasted almonds (see Tip, left)	125 mL
2 cups	vanilla hemp or other non-dairy milk, optional	500 mL

1. In a small saucepan over low heat, combine milk and
   brown rice syrup and heat until just warmed.

2. Place another saucepan over medium-high heat and let
   pan get hot. Add oats, cinnamon, cardamom, ginger and
   cloves and cook, stirring frequently, until oats are toasted
   and spices are fragrant, 2 to 3 minutes.

3. Gradually stir warmed milk mixture into oatmeal
   mixture, about 1 cup (250 mL) at a time, and bring to a
   boil, stirring occasionally. Stir in dates, raisins, apricots,
   almond extract and salt. Reduce heat and boil gently,
   stirring often, until oats are thickened, 8 to 12 minutes.
   Remove from heat and let stand to thicken to desired
   consistency. Serve oatmeal in bowls topped with toasted
   almonds and hemp milk, if using.

> ## ✖ Variation
> Top with seasonal fresh fruit and Heavy Cream
> (page 26).

Chorizo chile breakfast bake

This is a spicy morning breakfast requiring very little preparation and is easily done the night before. Benefiting from overnight soaking, the bread absorbs the delicious custard and bakes into a beautifully puffed and golden breakfast.

✖ Blender
✖ 10-cup (2.5 L) baking dish, lightly oiled

1	package (12 oz/375 g) vegan soy chorizo, casings removed	1
3/4 cup	chopped roasted red bell pepper	175 mL
1/2 cup	chopped roasted green chile pepper	125 mL
1/2	loaf (about 1 lb/500 g) day-old vegan rustic Italian bread, cut into 2-inch (5 cm) pieces	1/2
1	package (12.3 oz/350 g) firm silken tofu	1
4 oz	medium regular tofu, drained	125 g
1 1/4 cups	plain hemp or other non-dairy milk	300 mL
2 tbsp	cornstarch	30 mL
1 tsp	onion powder	5 mL
1 tsp	ground cumin	5 mL
1/4 tsp	ground turmeric	1 mL
	Salt and freshly ground black pepper	

1. In prepared baking dish, combine chorizo, roasted red pepper, green chile and bread.

2. In blender, combine silken tofu, medium tofu, milk, cornstarch, onion powder, cumin, turmeric and salt and pepper to taste and blend until smooth. Pour mixture over bread mixture and cover dish. Refrigerate for at least 2 hours or up to overnight, allowing bread to absorb custard.

3. Preheat oven to 350°F (180°C).

4. Remove breakfast bake from refrigerator and let warm to room temperature. Uncover and bake until puffed, firm and golden, 45 minutes to 1 hour. Let stand for 5 to 10 minutes before cutting to serve.

Crispy buckwheat tempehacon waffles

Makes about 16 waffles

These rich yet crispy waffles are loaded with crunchy bits of savory tempeh bacon bits. On the slim chance any are leftover, waffles freeze beautifully for up to 1 month. To make a quick-flavored syrup, thin a favorite fruit jam with a little orange juice.

✖ Tip

Cook waffle batter promptly because commercial egg replacer loses its ability to make batters rise shortly after it is mixed with liquids.

✖ Preheat oven to 200°F (100°C)
✖ Waffle iron, preheated

2 cups	buckwheat flour	500 mL
1 cup	all-purpose flour	250 mL
2 tbsp	granulated sugar	30 mL
2 tsp	baking powder	10 mL
1/2 tsp	baking soda	2 mL
1/4 tsp	salt	1 mL
2 3/4 cups	Soy Milk (page 18) or store-bought	675 mL
3/4 cup	coconut oil, melted	175 mL
1 tbsp	powdered egg replacer (see Tip, left)	15 mL
1/4 cup	warm water	60 mL
1/2 cup	Crunchy Tempehacon Bits (page 22) or store-bought vegan bacon bits	125 mL

1. In a large bowl, combine buckwheat flour, all-purpose flour, sugar, baking powder, baking soda and salt. Set aside.

2. In another bowl, whisk together soy milk and coconut oil (it is OK if coconut oil hardens into small chunks). In a small bowl, thoroughly mix egg replacer with warm water and whisk into soy milk mixture. Add soy milk mixture to dry ingredients and stir just until blended. Stir in tempehacon bits.

3. Fill preheated waffle iron with batter, spreading evenly using a heatproof spatula and cook until waffles are browned and crisp, according to manufacturer's instructions. Transfer cooked waffles to baking sheet and hold in warm oven. Repeat process with the remaining batter. Serve hot with your favorite syrup.

Crêpes with sweet ricotta and strawberries

A festive classic is a great make-ahead choice for a busy weekend brunch. Sweetened ricotta and fresh strawberries are rolled in cinnamon almond crêpes for a memorable meal everyone will love.

✖ Tips

It is important to quickly pour measured batter into hot pan all at once. Use a 1/4 cup (60 mL) measure and fill halfway with batter to measure 2 tbsp (30 mL).

Crêpes should not stick in a nonstick pan, but if they do, add 1 tsp (5 mL) canola oil to pan.

Make almond crème fraîche by using Almond Crème Fraîche (page 16) instead of the silken one.

✖ Blender
✖ Baking sheet, lined with parchment paper

Crêpes

1 cup	all-purpose flour	250 mL
3 tbsp	packed brown sugar	45 mL
1/4 tsp	salt	1 mL
1 1/4 cups	plain non-dairy milk	300 mL
1/4 cup	canola oil	60 mL
1 1/2 tsp	vanilla extract	7 mL
1 tsp	almond extract	5 mL

Filling

1 1/2 cups	Basic Ricotta (page 21)	375 mL
3 cups	strawberries, chopped, divided	750 mL
1/4 cup	confectioner's (icing) sugar, or more to taste	60 mL
1 tsp	ground cinnamon	5 mL
1 1/2 cups	Silken Crème Fraîche (page 16) or store-bought vegan crème fraîche (see Tips, left)	375 mL

1. *Crêpes:* In blender, combine flour, brown sugar, salt, milk, oil and vanilla and almond extracts and pulse until just combined, about 10 seconds. Transfer batter to an airtight container and refrigerate for at least 1 hour or up to 24 hours.

2. *Filling:* In a bowl, combine ricotta, 3/4 cup (175 mL) of the strawberries, sugar and cinnamon and set aside.

3. Place nonstick skillet over medium heat and let pan get hot. Pour 2 tbsp (30 mL) batter into center of pan, tipping pan to spread batter out to a 5-inch (12.5 cm) crêpe. (If batter is a little thick, adjust before pouring next crêpe by thinning with milk or water.) Cook until golden, about 30 seconds. Flip and cook for another 15 seconds. Transfer crêpes to prepared baking sheet and let cool. Repeat process with remaining batter adjusting heat as necessary between crêpes.

4. To serve, spoon 2 to 3 tbsp (30 to 45 mL) of ricotta filling down one side of crêpe and roll, starting at filled side. Spoon 2 tbsp (30 mL) of the crème fraîche over each crêpe, top with chopped strawberries and serve immediately.

> ## ⁘ Variation
>
> Substitute figs for strawberries and garnish with Divine Chocolate Sauce (page 22) or Caramel Sauce (page 23).

Tropical paradise parfait

Serves 2

If you can't take the red eye to the islands at least you can enjoy waking up to this tropical refresher.

⁘ 2 parfait glasses

1	kiwi, cut into bite-size pieces	1
1	mango, cut into bite-size pieces	1
1	banana, sliced	1
1	lime	1
2 1/2 cups	vanilla-flavored coconut milk yogurt	625 mL
1/8 tsp	ground ginger	0.5 mL
1/4 cup	unsweetened shredded coconut	60 mL
1/4 cup	chopped macadamia nuts	60 mL

1. In a large bowl, combine kiwi, mango and banana. Squeeze lime over all and gently toss to coat.

2. In a small bowl, blend yogurt with ginger.

3. Into each parfait glass, spoon one-quarter of fruit mixture. Spoon in 1/2 cup (125 mL) of yogurt and top with 1 tbsp (15 mL) each coconut and macadamia nuts. Layer with 1/4 cup (60 mL) of yogurt, half of remaining fruit mixture, 1/2 cup (125 mL) yogurt and end with 1 tbsp (15 mL) each coconut and macadamia nuts. Serve immediately.

French herbed strata

Delicate herbs of the French countryside come together to create a sophisticated and light-as-a-feather strata well suited for a springtime brunch.

❊ Tip

To clean leeks: Leeks are grown in sand and are sometimes difficult to clean. A good method of cleaning is to vertically slice through the white and light green leaves, leaving most of the dark green leaves intact. Grasp the leek by the dark green leaves, fan out the bottom white and light green portions, exposing much of the inside of the leek, and run under cold water.

❊ 10-cup (2.5 L) baking dish, lightly oiled
❊ Food processor

1 tbsp	olive oil	15 mL
2	large leeks, thoroughly washed and sliced (see Tip, left)	2
8 oz	thin asparagus, ends trimmed, cut into 3-inch (7.5 cm) pieces	250 g
3	cloves garlic, chopped	3
1 tbsp	freshly squeezed lemon juice	15 mL
1 tsp	salt, divided	5 mL
$\frac{1}{2}$ tsp	ground black pepper	2 mL
$\frac{1}{2}$	loaf (1 lb/500 g) day-old vegan French bread, cut into 2-inch (5 cm) pieces	$\frac{1}{2}$
1	package (12.3 oz/350 g) firm silken tofu	1
4 oz	medium regular tofu	125 g
1 cup	plain non-dairy milk	250 mL
$\frac{1}{4}$ cup	dry white wine	60 mL
2 tbsp	cornstarch	30 mL
2 tsp	Dijon mustard	10 mL
1 tsp	onion powder	5 mL
$\frac{1}{4}$ tsp	ground turmeric	1 mL
1 tbsp	fresh tarragon leaves	15 mL
1 tsp	herbes de Provence	5 mL

1. Place a large skillet over medium heat and let pan get hot. Add oil and tip pan to coat. Add leeks and cook, stirring occasionally, for 3 to 4 minutes. Add asparagus, garlic, lemon juice, $\frac{1}{2}$ tsp (2 mL) of the salt and pepper and cook until asparagus turns bright green, 2 to 3 minutes. Remove from heat, stir in bread and transfer to prepared baking dish.

2. In food processor, combine silken and medium tofu, milk, wine, cornstarch, mustard, onion powder, $\frac{1}{2}$ tsp (2 mL) of salt and turmeric and process until very smooth. Add tarragon and herbes de Provence and process until blended. Pour mixture over vegetables and bread. Cover strata and refrigerate for at least 2 hours or up to overnight for bread to absorb custard.

3. Preheat oven to 350°F (180°C).

4. Remove strata from refrigerator and allow it to warm to room temperature. Uncover and bake in preheated oven until slightly puffed and firm, 45 minutes to 1 hour. Let stand for 6 to 8 minutes before cutting to serve.

Greek tofu scramble

Serves 4

This vivid scramble features vegetables likely found in many Greek dishes. The addition of the Greek Soy Feta elevates it to divine!

3 tbsp	olive oil, divided	45 mL
1/2	red onion, finely chopped	1/2
1	green bell pepper, finely chopped	1
2	cloves garlic, minced	2
1 lb	firm tofu, drained and crumbled	500 g
1 tbsp	ground turmeric	15 mL
1 tbsp	fresh oregano	15 mL
2 cups	packed baby spinach	500 mL
1	tomato, seeded and chopped	1
1/2 cup	chopped kalamata olives	125 mL
3/4 tsp	freshly ground black pepper	3 mL
3/4 cup	drained and crumbled Greek Herbed Soy Feta in Olive Oil (page 24) or store-bought soy feta	175 mL

1. Place large skillet over medium heat and let pan get hot. Add 1 tbsp (15 mL) of the oil and tip pan to coat. Add red onion, bell pepper and garlic and cook, stirring occasionally, until just beginning to soften, 5 to 6 minutes.

2. Push vegetables to sides of pan, add remaining 2 tbsp (30 mL) of oil to center and heat for 30 seconds. Add tofu, turmeric and oregano, stir in vegetables and cook, stirring frequently, until tofu starts to slightly brown, 6 to 8 minutes. Add spinach, tomato, olives and black pepper and cook, stirring frequently, until spinach is wilted and tomatoes and olives are heated through, 3 to 5 minutes.

3. Top with soy feta and serve immediately.

Sage and savory mushroom frittata

Serves 6 to 8

These full-flavored mushrooms with the rustic scent of sage create a hearty frittata that is well suited for any meal. Serve with Pan-Fried Onion and Potato Hash Browns (page 104) for breakfast or Athenian Roasted Potatoes (page 148) for dinner.

✖ Tip

Substitute 1 tsp (5 mL) dried sage for 1 tbsp (15 mL) fresh sage.

✖ Preheat oven to 350°F (180°C)
✖ Cast-iron or other ovenproof skillet
✖ Food processor

2 tbsp	olive oil	30 mL
1 lb	mushrooms, sliced	500 g
1/4 cup	sliced shallots (about 2 large)	60 mL
1 tbsp	vegan hard margarine	15 mL
1 tbsp	chopped fresh sage leaves (see Tip, left)	15 mL
1 lb	firm tofu, drained and crumbled	500 g
1	package (12.3 oz/350 g) firm silken tofu	1
1/4 cup	plain soy milk	60 mL
2 tbsp	nutritional yeast	30 mL
1 tbsp	cornstarch	15 mL
3/4 tsp	ground turmeric	3 mL
3/4 tsp	salt	3 mL
1/2 tsp	freshly ground black pepper	2 mL

1. Place cast-iron or ovenproof skillet over medium-high heat and let pan get hot. Add oil and tip pan to coat. Add mushrooms and shallots. Reduce heat to medium and cook, stirring, until softened and lightly browned, 6 to 8 minutes. Add margarine, sage and firm tofu and cook, stirring, for 2 to 3 minutes to let flavors combine. Remove from heat and gently distribute mixture evenly in pan.

2. In food processor, combine silken tofu, milk, nutritional yeast, cornstarch, turmeric, salt and pepper and process until smooth. Pour mixture evenly over vegetable mixture in pan, gently lifting and stirring to combine ingredients.

3. Bake in preheated oven until top is firm and golden, 25 to 30 minutes. Let frittata cool slightly, cut into wedges and serve.

Taos chorizo scramble

Spicy soy chorizo is dynamic scrambled into creamy tofu and crispy potatoes. Cool sour cream and the freshness of cilantro provide just the right balance for a simple and memorable meal that will be a hit any time of day.

2	small red potatoes	2
3 tbsp	olive oil, divided	45 mL
8 oz	vegan soy chorizo, casing removed	250 g
3	green onions, white and light green parts only, finely chopped	3
1 lb	firm tofu, drained and crumbled	500 g
½ cup	Basic Sour Cream (page 21) or store-bought vegan sour cream	125 mL
¼ cup	chopped fresh cilantro	60 mL

1. Place potatoes in a small saucepan and cover with water. Bring to a low boil over medium–high heat. Adjust heat to gently boil potatoes until a fork inserted pierces the outer potato but meets considerable resistance near the middle, 8 to 10 minutes. Set aside. When cool enough to handle, cut into large cubes.

2. Place a large skillet over medium heat and let pan get hot. Add 2 tbsp (30 mL) of the oil and tip pan to coat. Add chorizo and cook, stirring frequently, until heated through and slightly browned, 4 to 5 minutes. Add green onions and cook, stirring, until softened, 2 to 3 minutes. Transfer to a bowl and set aside.

3. Add remaining 1 tbsp (15 mL) of oil and heat for 30 seconds. Add potatoes and tofu and cook, turning frequently, until browned with a light crust, 10 to 12 minutes. Stir in chorizo mixing well to combine. Divide between plates and top each with a dollop of sour cream and a sprinkling of cilantro.

Malibu tofu scramble

A veritable garden of vegetables, from golden sautéed mushrooms, ripe tomatoes and breakfast potatoes to tangy sprouts and creamy avocado, is about all the yummy one scramble can handle.

✖ Tip

To bake a medium-size russet potato: Scrub potato well and slice ⅛ inch (3 mm) off each end. Bake directly on the middle rack of a 375°F (190°C) preheated oven until potato feels soft when gently squeezed, 45 to 60 minutes.

3 tbsp	olive oil, divided	45 mL
2	cloves garlic, minced	2
½	onion, chopped	½
1 lb	cremini mushrooms, sliced	500 g
1	zucchini, diced	1
1	russet (Idaho) potato, baked, peeled and chopped (see Tip, left)	1
1 lb	firm tofu, drained and crumbled	500 g
1 tbsp	ground turmeric	15 mL
1	ripe tomato, seeded and chopped	1
1 cup	fresh basil leaves	250 mL
2 tbsp	champagne vinegar	30 mL
1 tsp	salt	5 mL
½ tsp	freshly ground black pepper	2 mL
1 cup	broccoli sprouts	250 mL
1	avocado, sliced	1
¾ cup	Basic Sour Cream (page 21) or vegan store-bought, optional	175 mL

1. Place skillet over medium heat and let pan get hot. Add 1 tbsp (15 mL) of the oil and tip pan to coat. Add garlic, onion, mushrooms and zucchini and cook, stirring occasionally, until vegetables start to soften, 5 to 6 minutes. Transfer vegetables to a bowl and set aside.

2. Increase heat to medium-high. Add 2 tbsp (30 mL) of oil and heat for 30 seconds. Add potatoes and cook, stirring frequently, until beginning to brown, about 6 minutes. Reduce heat to medium. Add tofu and turmeric and cook, stirring frequently, until potatoes are golden brown and tofu is warmed through, 6 to 8 minutes. Add tomato, basil, vinegar, salt and pepper and cooked mushroom mixture. Cook, stirring frequently, until tomatoes are heated through, 3 to 5 minutes. Stir in sprouts and serve topped with avocado slices. Add a dollop of sour cream, if using.

> ## ✖ Variations
> Substitute apple cider vinegar for champagne vinegar if desired.
>
> Any favorite sprout easily replaces the broccoli sprouts.

Texas tofu migas

Serves 6 to 8

This traditional Tex-Mex breakfast is a superb combination of scrambled tofu, onions, peppers and tortilla chips. The recipe calls for a chipotle pepper, which is simply a smoked dried jalapeño. Find them canned in adobo sauce. The smoking reduces the heat of the jalapeño and heightens the flavor.

✖ Tip

Fresh or stale corn tortillas may be cut into strips and fried in hot oil for use in place of tortilla chips.

1 tbsp	olive oil	15 mL
1/2	onion, peeled and chopped	1/2
1/2	green bell pepper, seeded and chopped	1/2
1/2	red bell pepper, seeded and chopped	1/2
1	clove garlic, chopped	1
2 tbsp	vegan hard margarine	30 mL
1 lb	firm tofu, drained and crumbled	500 g
2	canned chipotle peppers in adobo sauce, drained and chopped	2
1 tsp	ground turmeric	5 mL
1 tsp	salt	5 mL
1/2 tsp	freshly ground black pepper	2 mL
1 cup	corn tortilla chips, slightly crushed (see Tip, left)	250 mL
1	tomato, seeded and chopped	1
2 tbsp	chopped fresh cilantro	30 mL
1	avocado, chopped	1
8 to 12	6-inch (15 cm) vegan flour tortillas, heated	8 to 12
1 cup	Year-Round Blender Tomato Salsa (page 300) or store-bought	250 mL

1. Place a large skillet over medium heat and let pan get hot. Add oil and tip pan to coat. Add onion, green and red bell peppers and garlic and cook, stirring, until vegetables are softened, 8 to 10 minutes. Add margarine and when melted, stir in tofu, chipotles, turmeric, salt and pepper and cook, stirring occasionally, until all liquid is evaporated, 8 to 10 minutes. Stir in tortilla chips, tomato, cilantro and avocado and turn off heat.

2. In another large skillet over medium heat, heat tortillas, flipping once, until softened, puffed and browned in a few areas, 1 to 2 minutes per side. Wrap heated tortillas in a clean kitchen towel placed in a basket to keep warm. Serve migas hot while passing basket of tortillas and bowl of salsa.

✖ Variation

If chipotles are unavailable, use 1 or 2 chopped fresh jalapeños or serrano chile peppers.

Grilled sweet polenta with fruit chutney

Serves 8 to 10

Versatile polenta is equally welcome at breakfast, lunch or dinner. This sweet version makes a sophisticated showing at any meal. Kiwi added to the chutney brings a touch of freshness to the fruit medley.

✖ Tip

To toast walnuts: Spread nuts on a baking sheet and bake in a 350°F (180°C) oven until fragrant and golden brown, 6 to 10 minutes, checking often as they easily burn.

✖ 9-inch (23 cm) square glass baking dish, lightly oiled
✖ Well-seasoned cast-iron grill pan or heavy skillet (see Tips, right)

Polenta

4 cups	cold water	1 L
1 tsp	salt	5 mL
1¼ cups	yellow cornmeal	300 mL
2 tbsp	packed brown sugar	30 mL
2 tbsp	vegan hard margarine	30 mL

Chutney

1	apple, peeled and chopped	1
1	pear, peeled and chopped	1
2 tbsp	currants	30 mL
1 tbsp	grated gingerroot	15 mL
⅓ cup	packed brown sugar	75 mL
½ cup	unsweetened apple cider	125 mL
½ tsp	ground cinnamon	2 mL
¼ tsp	ground allspice	1 mL
2 to 3	kiwi, peeled and chopped	2 to 3
2 to 4 tbsp	canola oil	30 to 60 mL
½ cup	chopped toasted walnuts (see Tip, left)	125 mL

1. *Polenta:* In a large saucepan, combine water and salt. Gradually whisk in cornmeal, smoothing out any lumps. Stir in brown sugar and bring to a boil over medium heat, whisking constantly. Reduce heat to low and simmer, stirring, until mixture thickens and pulls away from sides of pan, 8 to 10 minutes. Remove from heat and stir in margarine. Turn into prepared dish, smoothing top. Cover and refrigerate for at least 2 hours or up to overnight.

✖ Tips

A well-seasoned cast-iron skillet is a treasure in the kitchen. Cast-iron pans are excellent heat conductors, heating evenly without hot spots on the stove top and in the oven. With proper care a well-seasoned cast-iron skillet will provide a lifetime of consistent and stick resistant cooking.

To season a cast-iron skillet: Clean the pan well using steel wool to remove any rust. Coat the pan, inside and out, with a light layer of a cooking oil. Wipe all visible oil from the pan and place, upside down over a piece of foil in a 450 to 500°F (230 to 260°C) oven for 30 minutes. Turn the oven off and let the pan cool slowly. Repeat the process 3 or 4 times to create a glossy coating which seals the pores and creates a nonstick cooking surface.

To clean a cast-iron pan: After cooking, wash pan with hot soapy water, but do not soak. Wipe the pan dry and place on a heated stove-top burner for a few minutes to ensure that your pan is very dry.

2. *Chutney:* In large saucepan, stir together apple, pear, currants, ginger, brown sugar and apple cider. Bring to a boil over medium heat, stirring occasionally. Reduce heat to low and cook, stirring often, until apples have softened but not lost their shape, 10 to 12 minutes. Remove from heat and stir in cinnamon, allspice and kiwi. Keep warm.

3. Slice chilled polenta into 3-inch (7.5 cm) squares and brush each with oil. Place grill pan or skillet over medium heat and let pan get hot. Brush ridges of pan with 1 tbsp (15 mL) of the oil. In batches as necessary, set polenta slices diagonally on grill and cook until edges begin to brown, about 10 minutes (do not move polenta or it may stick). Flip polenta and grill other side for 10 minutes. Repeat with remaining polenta squares, oiling pan and adjusting heat as necessary between batches.

4. Serve polenta topped with chutney and a sprinkle of toasted walnuts.

Sunshine polenta with peach compote

Serves 4

Start your day on the sunny side with a bright and beautiful bowl of creamy polenta topped with heavenly spiced fresh peach compote. It's like a bowl of sunshine.

✴ Tip

Technically, polenta is cooked in about 10 minutes, but continues to plump with longer cooking, which creates a more tender polenta. Cook polenta to your desired plumpness.

Compote

3	peaches, chopped, divided	3
1/3 cup	peach nectar or water	75 mL
3 tbsp	pure maple syrup	45 mL
2 tbsp	orange-flavored liqueur	30 mL

Polenta

1 cup	water	250 mL
2 cups	unsweetened vanilla almond milk	500 mL
1/2 tsp	salt	2 mL
1 cup	corn grits (polenta) or stone-ground cornmeal	250 mL
2 tbsp	vegan hard margarine	30 mL
1 tsp	vanilla extract	5 mL

1. *Compote:* In a small saucepan, combine two–thirds of the peaches, peach nectar, maple syrup and orange liqueur and bring to a boil over medium–high heat, stirring frequently. Reduce heat to medium and simmer, stirring occasionally, until compote is thickened and reduced, about 20 minutes.

2. *Polenta:* In a saucepan over medium heat, combine water, almond milk and salt and bring to a gentle boil. Gradually stir in grits, whisking constantly to eliminate lumps. Reduce heat and simmer, stirring occasionally, until thickened, about 15 minutes. Remove from heat, stir in margarine and vanilla, cover and let stand for 5 minutes.

3. Stir remaining one–third of peaches into compote. Serve polenta hot, topped with a large spoonful of peach compote.

> ## ✴ Variation
> Stir 1/4 cup (60 mL) vegan cream cheese into polenta in place of margarine.

New mexican home-fried potatoes

A well-seasoned cast-iron skillet perfectly browns these home fries and moves to the table with ease as a rustic serving dish.

✖ Tips

For very crispy potatoes continue cooking for an additional 10 to 15 minutes, reducing heat to prevent burning, if necessary.

Cilantro may be added at end of cooking for a fresher flavor or scattered on top as a garnish.

8	medium red potatoes, scrubbed	8
1¾ tsp	salt, divided	8 mL
3 tbsp	canola oil	45 mL
1	onion, diced	1
½	green bell pepper, seeded and diced	½
½	red bell pepper, seeded and diced	½
1	clove garlic, chopped	1
6 oz	well-drained canned diced roasted mild or medium green chile	175 g
1 tsp	smoked paprika	5 mL
1 tbsp	chopped fresh cilantro	15 mL

1. Place potatoes in a large pot, cover with water and add 1 tsp (5 mL) of the salt. Bring to a boil over high heat. Reduce heat and simmer until tender but still firm, 10 to 15 minutes. Drain potatoes and let cool. Remove skins and cut potatoes into 1-inch (2.5 cm) cubes.

2. Place skillet over medium–high heat and let pan get hot. Add oil and tip pan to coat. Add onion, red and green bell peppers and cook, stirring, until just softened, 4 to 5 minutes. Add garlic and cook, stirring, for 1 minute. Add potatoes, green chile, paprika, cilantro and remaining ¾ tsp (3 mL) of salt and cook, tossing occasionally with a spatula, until potatoes are browned, 12 to 15 minutes. Serve hot.

> ## ✖ Variation
> Substitute canned chile with ¾ cup (175 mL) fresh Anaheim, poblano or Hatch green chile.
> *To roast chiles:* Broil or grill chiles, turning frequently, until skin is blistered, 10 to 12 minutes. Transfer to a paper bag and let stand for 15 minutes to allow skins to steam and loosen. Remove from bag, peel and chop. Wearing protective gloves while handling chiles is advised as hot chiles can burn skin.

Pan-fried onion and potato hash browns

Serves 4 to 6

Crispy hash browns are the stuff dreams are made of and easily obtainable. The trick is in dry potatoes, relieved of excess moisture.

✖ Tips

I highly recommend a cast-iron skillet if available as heat is evenly distributed and held after the pan is removed from the heat. A cast-iron pan is versatile and goes from the stove top to the oven, where hash browns can be kept warm until ready to serve (see Tips, page 101).

A very thin spread of potato mixture in pan will produce the crispiest hash brown patty but will require more batches.

✖ Preheat oven to 200°F (100°C)

2	large russet (Idaho) potatoes	2
1	onion	1
¾ tsp	salt	3 mL
½ tsp	ground black pepper	2 mL
2 tbsp	chopped fresh chives	30 mL
¼ cup	grapeseed oil, divided	60 mL

1. Grate potatoes on large hole side of a box grater. Transfer to a mesh sieve and gently press out excess moisture. Grate onion. In a large bowl, combine potatoes, onion, salt, pepper and chives.

2. Place a large skillet over medium–high heat and let pan get hot. Add 2 tbsp (30 mL) of the oil and tip pan to coat. Distribute half of potato mixture over bottom of skillet and flatten with a wide spatula. Reduce heat to medium and cook until underside is a crispy golden brown, 6 to 8 minutes. Remove skillet from heat and slide hash browns onto a plate. Invert a second plate on top and flip, inverting hash browns so cooked side is up. Add remaining oil to skillet and when oil is hot, slide hash browns back into pan. Cook until underside is crisp and golden brown, 6 to 8 minutes.

3. Slide hash browns onto a plate and hold in warm oven while repeating process with remaining potato mixture. Serve hot.

> ### ✖ Variation
> Use a blend of russets and sweet potatoes to produce a beautiful and slightly sweet hash brown patty.

Breads, Rolls and Crackers

❌—❌—❌—❌—❌—❌—❌—❌—❌—❌—❌—❌—❌

Cilantro green chile cornmeal focaccia

Topped with a fresh and delicious cilantro pesto, this decidedly southwestern focaccia is the perfect accompaniment to Roasted Poblano Potato Soup (page 275) or Smoky Chipotle Black Bean Chili (page 280).

✖ Tips

As focaccia is very forgiving, use a larger sheet for thinner focaccia or a smaller baking sheet for thicker focaccia. Adjust baking times accordingly, checking thinner focaccia after 15 minutes and letting thicker focaccia bake from 25 to 30 minutes.

Wrap leftovers in plastic wrap and refrigerate for 1 to 2 days.

✖ **18- by 13-inch (48 by 33 cm) rimmed baking sheet, well oiled (see Tips, left)**
✖ **Food processor**
✖ **Stand mixer**

Dough

1⅓ cups	warm water	325 mL
2 tsp	active dry yeast	10 mL
2¾ to 3 cups	all-purpose flour	675 to 750 mL
1 cup	cornmeal	250 mL
1 tbsp	salt	15 mL
3 tbsp	olive oil	45 mL

Topping

1	clove garlic	1
½ cup	fresh cilantro leaves, stems removed	125 mL
¼ cup	olive oil	60 mL
2 tbsp	drained roasted canned diced mild green chile	30 mL
1 tsp	freshly squeezed lemon juice	5 mL
½ tsp	ground cumin	2 mL
¼ tsp	salt	1 mL
⅛ tsp	freshly ground black pepper	0.5 mL

1. *Dough:* Place warm water in a stand mixer bowl. Stir in yeast and let stand until foamy, about 5 minutes. Stir in 2¾ cups (675 mL) of the flour, cornmeal, salt and olive oil and beat on medium speed for 2 minutes. Beat in remaining flour, 1 tbsp (15 mL) at a time, until a sticky dough forms.

2. Scrape dough onto prepared baking sheet and pat out to edges. Loosely cover with plastic wrap and let rise in a warm, draft-free place until dough looks puffy, about 1 hour.

✖ Tip

By applying the topping at two different times, you get the best of both worlds: the rich flavor of cilantro baked into the dough and the freshness of the uncooked cilantro on top.

3. *Topping:* In food processor, with motor running, drop garlic clove through feed tube. When finely chopped, scrape sides and add cilantro, olive oil, green chile, lemon juice, cumin, salt and pepper. Process into a rough paste, scrape down sides and process until almost smooth. Topping can be made up to 1 day in advance and refrigerated in an airtight container.

4. Preheat oven to 350°F (180°C) about 10 minutes before focaccia has completely risen.

5. Dimple dough all over with fingertips. Spread about half of topping on dough. Bake until edges are golden brown and top looks dry, 18 to 20 minutes. Remove from oven and dollop on remaining topping while hot. Serve warm or at room temperature.

✖ Variations

Change the topping to Classic Pesto Sauce (page 286), puréed sun-dried tomatoes packed in oil, or Cremini and Kalamata Olivada (page 43) for different takes on this scrumptious cornmeal focaccia.

Three-olive focaccia

This olivey focaccia is great on its own but really shines when split for a roasted veggie sandwich.

Tips

As focaccia is very forgiving, use a larger sheet for thinner focaccia or a smaller baking sheet for thicker focaccia. Adjust baking times accordingly, checking thinner focaccia after 15 minutes and letting thicker focaccia bake from 25 to 30 minutes.

Substitute 1½ cups (375 mL) store-bought olive tapenade for the homemade olive mixture; just be sure to look for a vegan-friendly version without anchovy paste.

Well wrap any leftovers in plastic wrap and store at room temperature for up to 2 days.

- Stand mixer with dough hook attachment
- 18- by 13-inch (48 by 33 cm) rimmed baking sheet, well oiled (see Tips, left)

Olive Mixture (see Tips, left)

½ cup	roughly chopped pitted kalamata olives	125 mL
½ cup	roughly chopped stuffed green olives	125 mL
½ cup	roughly chopped pitted oil-cured black olives	125 mL
2	cloves garlic, chopped	2
½ tsp	chopped fresh thyme	2 mL
½ tsp	chopped fresh rosemary	2 mL
1 tsp	lemon juice	5 mL
2 tbsp	olive oil	30 mL

Dough

1⅓ cups	warm water	325 mL
2 tsp	active dry yeast	10 mL
3¼ to 3½ cups	all-purpose flour	800 to 875 mL
1½ tsp	salt	7 mL
3 tbsp	olive oil	45 mL

1. *Olive Mixture:* In a bowl, combine kalamata, green and oil-cured olives. Add garlic, thyme, rosemary, lemon juice and olive oil, stirring well to combine and set aside.

2. *Dough:* In bowl of stand mixer, combine water and yeast and let stand until foamy, about 5 minutes. Add 3¼ cups (800 mL) of the flour, salt and olive oil. Attach bowl to mixer and fit with dough hook attachment. Stir on low until flour is incorporated, then increase speed to medium and beat for 2 minutes. With mixer running on low, add remaining flour, 1 tbsp (15 mL) at a time, stirring until a sticky dough forms. Stir in olive mixture. Dough may be sticky, do not be tempted to add more flour.

3. Scrape dough onto prepared baking sheet and pat out to edges. Loosely cover with plastic wrap and let rise in a warm, draft-free place until dough looks puffy, about 1 hour.

4. Preheat oven to 350°F (180°C) about 10 minutes before focaccia has fully risen.

5. Uncover focaccia and dimple dough all over with fingertips. Bake until edges are golden brown and top looks dry, 20 to 25 minutes. Serve warm or transfer to a wire rack and let cool to serve at room temperature.

Dried apricot and walnut sprouted wheat bread

Makes 1 loaf

Plan to start this dense, wheaty loaf two to three days ahead. You'll need time to soak the wheat berries then additional time to sprout them. If there are kids in the house, they will enjoy seeing the tiny sprouts growing in the glass jars. Finally, the sprouted wheat is pulverized in a food processor with dried apricots and walnuts and baked at a low temperature for a couple of hours. The bread forms a browned crust around a delicious inside with a muffin-like texture.

✖ Tips

Any breathable fabric is suitable to cover jars.

Store in a resealable plastic bag at room temperature for up to 3 days or freeze for up to 1 month.

Sprouting grains and beans allow access to an incredible amount of vitamins, amino acids, enzymes and minerals that are unavailable during their dry state or at any other time of the plants life cycle.

✖ Two wide-mouth 1-quart (1 L) glass canning jars with rings or rubber bands
✖ Two 4-inch (10 cm) squares cheesecloth (see Tips, left)
✖ Food processor
✖ 13- by 9-inch (33 by 23 cm) glass baking dish, oiled

2 cups	wheat berries	500 mL
1/3 cup	dried apricots, roughly chopped	75 mL
1/3 cup	walnut halves or pieces	75 mL

1. Place 1 cup (250 mL) wheat berries in each jar and fill each with warm water. Cover jars with cheesecloth squares and secure each with jar rings or rubber bands. Let stand in a warm place for 8 to 12 hours.

2. Pour out water through cheesecloth, gently shaking jar to drain thoroughly and prevent wheat berries from clumping. Refill jars with warm water, swish gently and drain. Set drained wheat berries in a dark, warm or at least room temperature spot. Rinse, swish and drain well at least twice a day to prevent souring and to inhibit bacteria growth. Repeat this process until sprouts are about the same length as wheat berries, 1/4-inch (0.5 cm), for up to 3 days.

3. Preheat oven to 225°F (110°C).

4. Place sprouted berries in food processor and add apricots and walnuts. Process mixture, scraping down sides often, until a thick paste-like dough is formed, 1 to 2 minutes. Turn dough into prepared baking dish. Oil hands and pat dough into a flat loaf approximately 8- by 4-inches (20 by 10 cm) wide by 1½-inches (4 cm) high.

5. Bake in preheated oven until brown crust has formed and bread gives off a bready aroma, 2¾ to 3 hours. Let cool in pan for 5 minutes then transfer bread to a wire rack and let cool completely.

✖ Variation
Use raisins, dates or figs in place of apricots, and almonds, pecans or pistachios in place of walnuts.

Garlic naan

Shaping the naan into traditional ovals is a bit tricky. No worries, as no one will even notice, let alone complain, while eating this absolutely scrumptious naan hot from the oven and brushed with roasted garlic oil.

✹ **Preheat oven to 350°F (180°C)**
✹ **Stand mixer with dough hook attachment**
✹ **Pizza stone or large baking sheet**

1	whole head garlic	1
1¼ cups	warm water, divided	300 mL
1 tsp	active dry yeast	5 mL
2 to 3 cups	all-purpose flour	500 to 750 mL
1½ tsp	salt	7 mL
2 tbsp	olive oil	30 mL
¼ tsp	coarse salt, preferably pink or black	1 mL

1. Wrap whole head of garlic in foil and place on a baking sheet. Bake in preheated oven until soft, about 45 minutes. Turn oven off. Let garlic cool.

2. Meanwhile, in bowl of stand mixer, stir together ¼ cup (60 mL) warm water with yeast and let stand until foamy, 5 minutes. Add remaining water and 2 cups (500 mL) of flour. Attach bowl to mixer and fit with dough hook attachment. Beat on low speed until flour is incorporated, then increase speed to medium for 2 minutes. Add salt and gradually beat in flour, 1 tbsp (15 mL) at a time, until soft dough is formed.

3. Place in a large warmed oiled bowl, flipping dough to coat with oil. Cover bowl and let rise in a warm, draft-free place until doubled in bulk, about 2 hours. Dough may be refrigerated overnight instead of rising in warm place, but bring to room temperature before continuing.

4. In a small bowl, mash cooled roasted garlic into a paste, gradually mix in oil and set aside.

5. Preheat oven to 500°F (260°C) and place pizza stone (if using) in oven to preheat. If using baking sheet, preheat pan upside down on oven rack (the bottom will be used for baking).

6. Turn dough onto floured surface and divide into 8 pieces. Pat each piece into rough rectangles or ovals, each about 6- by 4-inches (15 by 10 cm). Cover lightly with plastic wrap and let rest for 5 minutes. Place a small bowl of water next to work surface. Using wet fingertips, dimple each piece of dough deeply, using plenty of water. Lift one piece of dough and stretch it between your two hands. (It may be easier to stretch it over the backs of your hands.) It is OK if dough tears in spots. Dough should be approximately 10- by 5-inches (25 by 12.5 cm). Working in batches, carefully place stretched naan, one or two at a time, on hot stone or baking sheet and bake in preheated oven until crisp and dark brown in thin spots, about 5 minutes. Repeat process with remaining dough.

7. Transfer naan to a wire rack and immediately brush with roasted garlic-oil and sprinkle with coarse salt. Wrap in a clean kitchen towel to keep warm while repeating process with remaining dough. Serve naan warm.

Homemade flour tortillas

Simple to make,
homemade tortillas
are far superior to
store-bought. Use them
for tacos, enchiladas,
quesadillas or just
smear toasted tortillas
with margarine and
sprinkle with natural
sugar and cinnamon
for a quick treat. Serve
with soups, chilis,
scrambles or wherever
a hot and delicious
"pusher" or "scooper"
might be needed.

✖ Tip

Cooled tortillas can be
stored in a resealable plastic
bag in the refrigerator for
up to 1 week. *To warm
tortillas:* Wrap tortillas
in a clean damp kitchen
towel and microwave for
30 seconds to 1 minute
or reheat in a skillet over
medium heat, flipping
once.

2½ cups	all-purpose flour, divided	625 mL
¼ tsp	salt	1 mL
⅓ cup	vegan shortening	75 mL
½ to ¾ cup	water	125 to 175 mL

1. In a large bowl, stir together 2 cups (500 mL) of the flour and salt. Using fingers, work shortening into flour mixture until coarse crumbs are formed. Using a wooden spoon, mix in water, starting with ½ cup (125 mL), until a ball of dough forms. Transfer dough to a work surface covered with ¼ cup (60 mL) of flour. Knead dough until no longer sticky, 2 to 3 minutes. Cover dough with a clean damp kitchen towel and let rest for about 1 hour.

2. Divide dough into 8 to 12 pieces and cover with a clean kitchen towel. Scatter remaining ¼ cup (60 mL) of flour on work surface and roll each dough ball into a thin flat circle, about 1/16 inch (2 mm) thick.

3. Place a large heavy skillet over medium–high heat and let pan get hot. Cook tortillas, one at a time and flipping once, until bottom is golden and slightly browned in spots, 2 to 4 minutes per side. Wrap cooked tortillas in a kitchen towel to keep warm. Repeat process with remaining tortillas, adjusting heat as necessary between batches.

Pumpernickel bread

This loaf is a medium-dark rye bread with a touch of spice from the caraway seeds, vinegar and molasses. Perfect for a tempeh and sauerkraut Reuben-style sandwich.

✖ Tip

Store bread in a resealable bag at room temperature for up to 1 week.

✖ Stand mixer with paddle attachment
✖ 9- by 5-inch (23 by 12.5 cm) metal loaf pan, oiled

1 cup	warm water	250 mL
2¼ tsp	active dry yeast	11 mL
¼ cup	cold brewed coffee	60 mL
2 tbsp	canola oil	30 mL
2 tbsp	cider vinegar	30 mL
1 tbsp	unsweetened cocoa powder	15 mL
1 tsp	salt	5 mL
2 to 2½ cups	all-purpose flour	500 to 625 mL
2 cups	rye flour	500 mL
1 tbsp	caraway seeds	15 mL

1. In bowl of stand mixer, combine warm water and yeast and let stand until foamy, about 5 minutes. Attach bowl to mixer and fit with paddle attachment. Add coffee, oil, vinegar, cocoa powder and salt and mix on low to combine. Add 2 cups (500 mL) all-purpose flour and mix on low until flour is incorporated, then increase speed to medium and beat for 2 minutes. Add rye flour and mix on low until flour is incorporated, then increase speed to medium and beat until a sticky dough ball forms around paddle, beating in additional all-purpose flour if necessary, for 2 minutes. Mix in caraway seeds on low speed until incorporated.

2. Turn dough out into a large warm oiled bowl, flipping dough to coat with oil. Cover with a clean kitchen towel and let rise in a warm, draft-free place until doubled in size, about 45 minutes.

3. Punch dough down and transfer to a floured work surface. Roll into a cylinder and fit into prepared loaf pan. Loosely cover with plastic wrap or clean kitchen towel and let rise until dough has risen over the top of the pan, about 30 minutes.

4. Preheat oven to 350°F (180°C) about 10 minutes before loaf is fully risen.

5. Uncover and bake until top is well browned and bottom sounds hollow when tapped, about 30 minutes. Remove loaf from pan and place directly on oven rack and bake to crisp up crust for an additional 5 minutes. Let cool completely on a wire rack before slicing.

Rosemary and olive bread

Makes 1 loaf

Big chunks of kalamata olives star in this crisp chewy bread, but a little cornmeal goes a long way in making the golden crumb just as special. No preheating is necessary; the bread starts in a cold oven.

✴ Tip

Store at room temperature in a resealable plastic bag for up to 3 days.

✴ **Stand mixer with dough hook attachment**
✴ **Baking sheet, oiled and sprinkled with cornmeal**

½ cup	pitted kalamata olives	125 mL
1 cup	warm water	250 mL
2 tsp	active dry yeast	10 mL
1 tsp	granulated sugar	5 mL
1 tsp	salt	5 mL
2 to 2¾ cups	all-purpose flour	500 to 675 mL
½ cup	cornmeal	125 mL
2 tsp	chopped fresh rosemary	10 mL

1. Slice olives into 2 to 3 pieces each or roughly chop. Drain on paper towels. Set aside.

2. In bowl of stand mixer, combine water and yeast and let stand until foamy, about 5 minutes. Attach bowl to mixer and fit with dough hook attachment. Add sugar, salt, 2 cups (500 mL) of the flour, cornmeal and rosemary and mix on low until flour is incorporated, then increase speed to medium and beat for 2 minutes. With mixer running on low speed, add remaining flour, 1 tbsp (15 mL) at a time, until a stiff dough is formed, about 2 minutes.

3. Form dough into a ball and place in a large warm oiled bowl, flipping dough to coat with oil. Cover with a clean kitchen towel and let rise in a warm, draft-free place until doubled in size, about 45 minutes.

4. Punch dough down and transfer to a floured work surface. Pat into a rough rectangle, about 12- by 10-inches (30 by 25 cm). Sprinkle olives over dough and roll up jelly-roll fashion, making sure all olives are tucked inside. Pinch ends to seal. Place on prepared baking sheet and let rest for 5 minutes.

5. Brush loaf with water and place in cold oven. Turn oven to 400°F (200°C) and bake until nicely browned and bottom sounds hollow when tapped, 35 to 45 minutes. Transfer to a wire rack to cool completely before slicing.

Rustic walnut bread

Makes 2 loaves

This easy recipe makes two flattish loaves similar to the ciabatta loaf, which means "slipper" in Italian. With an abundance of toasted walnuts and ultra-crisp crust, these loaves look like you bought them at an artisan bakery!

✖ Tip

The key to working with this very sticky dough is to never touch it with your hands. Use a metal or plastic scraper to move and mold dough.

✖ Stand mixer with dough hook attachment
✖ Metal or plastic dough scraper (see Tip, left)

2¼ cups	warm water, divided	550 mL
2¼ tsp	active dry yeast	11 mL
1 tbsp	granulated sugar	15 mL
4 tsp	salt	20 mL
5½ cups	all-purpose flour	4.375 L
1 cup	whole wheat flour	250 mL
1 cup	toasted walnuts	250 mL
1 tsp	canola oil	5 mL
1 to 2 tbsp	cornmeal	15 to 30 mL
1 tsp	cold water	5 mL
2 cups	boiling water	500 mL

1. In bowl of stand mixer, combine ¼ cup (60 mL) of the warm water and yeast and let stand until foamy, about 5 minutes. Attach bowl to mixer and fit with dough hook attachment. Add sugar, salt and remaining 2 cups (500 mL) warm water. Add all-purpose flour, 1 cup (250 mL) at a time, beating on low speed until dry ingredients are incorporated, then medium speed for 2 minutes after each addition. Add whole wheat flour and walnuts and beat until incorporated into a sticky dough.

2. Using a metal or plastic scraper, transfer dough to a large warm oiled bowl and coat top lightly with oil. Cover with plastic wrap and let rise in a warm, draft-free place until doubled in size, 45 to 55 minutes.

3. Sprinkle a baking sheet with cornmeal. Using scraper, turn dough onto baking sheet and divide into two portions. Form each into a loaf shape with scraper (the dough will be soft) and place evenly spaced on the baking sheet. Let rest for 5 minutes. This dough only rises once.

4. Brush loaves with cold water and place in cold oven. Place a small baking pan of boiling water on bottom rack of oven. Turn oven to 400°F (200°C) and bake until well browned and loaves sound hollow when tapped on bottoms, 45 to 55 minutes. Transfer to a wire rack and let cool before slicing.

Seeded five-grain bread

Makes 2 loaves

This is a good, all-purpose grainy loaf to have with breakfast, lunch or dinner.

✖ Tip

Five-grain cereal is a combinations of oats, wheat, rye, barley, spelt or similar mixture intended for hot cereal.

✖ Stand mixer with paddle attachment
✖ Two 9- by 5-inch (23 by 12.5 cm) loaf pans, lightly oiled

1 cup	five-grain hot cereal (see Tip, left)	250 mL
2 cups	boiling water	500 mL
2¼ tsp	dry active yeast	11 mL
¼ cup	warm water	60 mL
½ cup	light (fancy) molasses or agave nectar	125 mL
1 tbsp	vegetable oil	15 mL
2 tsp	salt	10 mL
5 to 6 cups	all-purpose flour, divided	1.25 to 1.5 L
1 tbsp	poppy seeds	15 mL
1 tbsp	sesame seeds	15 mL
1 tbsp	sunflower seeds	15 mL

1. In bowl of stand mixer, cover five-grain cereal with boiling water. Let stand until mixture is barely warm to the touch, 20 to 25 minutes.

2. In a small bowl, combine yeast in warm water and let stand until foamy, about 5 minutes. Add dissolved yeast to cereal mixture. Stir in molasses, oil and salt. Stir in 3 cups (750 mL) of the flour and mix on medium-low speed for 2 minutes. On low speed, beat in about 2 cups (500 mL) of the remaining flour, ¼ cup (60 mL) at a time, then beat in additional flour, 1 tbsp (15 mL) at a time, as necessary, until a smooth dough forms. Beat on medium-low speed for 2 minutes. Stir in seeds.

3. Turn into a large warm oiled bowl, flipping dough to coat with oil. Cover with a clean kitchen towel and let rise in a warm, draft-free place until doubled in size, about 45 minutes.

4. Punch dough down and transfer to a floured surface. Divide in half, roll each up into a cylinder and fit into prepared pans. Loosely cover with plastic wrap and let rise until dough has risen over top of pans, about 30 minutes.

5. Preheat oven to 350°F (180°C) about 10 minutes before loaves have fully risen.

6. Bake until tops are well browned and bottoms sound hollow when tapped, about 30 minutes. Remove loaves from pans and place directly on oven rack and bake to crisp up crust for an additional 5 minutes. Let loaves cool completely on a wire rack before slicing.

Serrano and roasted pepper cornbread

Serves 8

Colorful, with a kick from a roasted serrano, this golden cornbread looks as good as it tastes. It is almost a must with chili or a morning scramble. Try it with Boy Howdy Texas Chili and Beans (page 279).

✖ Tip

Chile oil can easily coat your fingers and is easily transferred to other areas, such as your eyes. To avoid any discomfort, wear kitchen gloves when peeling charred chiles.

✖ Preheat oven to 425°F (220°C)
✖ 8-inch (20 cm) ovenproof skillet

1 tbsp	ground flax seeds (flax seed meal)	15 mL
3 tbsp	cold water	45 mL
1	red bell pepper	1
1	serrano chile pepper	1
1 cup	all-purpose flour	250 mL
¾ cup	cornmeal	175 mL
1 tbsp	baking powder	15 mL
1 tbsp	granulated sugar	15 mL
½ tsp	salt	2 mL
1 cup	Soy Milk (page 18) or store-bought	250 mL
2 tbsp	canola oil	30 mL
½ cup	fresh or canned corn kernels	125 mL

1. In a large bowl, stir together ground flax seeds and water and set aside.
2. Heat ovenproof skillet over medium–high heat. Add bell pepper and serrano chile and char, turning often, until all sides are charred, about 10 minutes. Transfer bell pepper and chile to a clean damp kitchen towel, wrap and let steam for 10 minutes. Remove and discard skin and seeds, finely chop flesh and set aside. Wipe skillet with oiled paper towel.
3. In a medium bowl, stir together flour, cornmeal, baking powder, sugar and salt. Add soy milk and oil to flax mixture and whisk to combine. Add dry ingredients and stir just until moistened. Fold in chopped bell pepper, chile and corn.
4. Spoon batter into prepared skillet, smoothing top. Bake in preheated oven until toothpick inserted in center comes out clean, 20 to 25 minutes. Let cool for 5 minutes and serve warm. Best eaten the day it is made.

> ## ✖ Variation
> For a quick and less spicy but still colorful cornbread, omit bell pepper and serrano and skip Step 2. Use ⅓ cup (75 mL) chopped drained store-bought roasted red bell peppers and 2 tbsp (30 mL) chopped chives.

Cracked pepper biscotti

An unusual accompaniment to soups or spreads, these peppery biscotti will please even the jaded biscotti connoisseur.

✖ Tip

Store biscotti at room temperature in airtight container for up to 1 week.

✖ **Preheat oven to 350°F (180°C)**
✖ **Stand mixer**

2½ cups	all-purpose flour	625 mL
2 tbsp	cornmeal	30 mL
2 tsp	baking powder	10 mL
1½ tsp	cracked black peppercorns	7 mL
½ tsp	salt	2 mL
1 tbsp	powdered egg replacer	15 mL
¼ cup	water	60 mL
¾ cup	vegan hard margarine, softened	175 mL
2 tbsp	coconut oil	30 mL
1 cup	toasted pine nuts	250 mL

1. In a large bowl, stir together flour, cornmeal, baking powder, pepper and salt and set aside. In a small bowl, stir together egg replacer and water and set aside.

2. In stand mixer bowl, beat margarine and coconut oil until fluffy, about 1 minute. Add flour mixture alternating with egg replacer, ending with flour mixture, beating on low speed until blended. Stir in pine nuts.

3. Divide dough in half and shape each into a log. Transfer logs to a baking sheet and shape each log to about 16- by 2-inches (40 by 5 cm), placing evenly spaced on baking sheet. Bake in preheated oven just until logs begin to brown and are firm to the touch, 20 to 25 minutes. Remove from oven and let cool on pan for 5 minutes. Leave oven on.

4. Using a sharp chef's or serrated knife, slice logs on the diagonal into ½-inch (1 cm) slices. Place each slice cut side down on baking sheet and bake for 7 minutes. Flip slices and bake until crisp and dry, about 5 minutes. Transfer biscotti to a wire rack and let cool completely.

> ## ✖ Variation
> For a touch of green and a slightly smoky taste, omit pine nuts and substitute ½ cup (125 mL) each roasted green pumpkin seeds (pepitas) and toasted sliced almonds.

Giant garlicky croutons

Makes 6 to 7 cups (1.5 to 1.75 L)

Who doesn't want croutons on their salad? And who doesn't prefer fresh, homemade croutons? These giant specimens will perk up the most basic salad and will elevate a good salad to rock star status.

✖ Tips

Store croutons at room temperature for up to 1 week.

✖ Preheat oven to 325°F (160°C)
✖ Baking sheet, fitted with wire rack

1 lb	French or Italian bread	500 g
3	cloves garlic, sliced in half	3
⅓ cup	olive oil	75 mL
¼ tsp	garlic salt	1 mL

1. Slice hard crust off bottom of loaf and discard. Slice horizontally into 1-inch (2.5 cm) slices. Place slices on rack set inside baking sheet. Bake slices in preheated oven for 3 minutes. Turn over and bake for 3 minutes more. Rub bread slices with cut side of garlic. Cut slices into 1-inch (2.5 cm) cubes.

2. Place olive oil in a large bowl. Working in 2 batches, toss bread cubes in oil then place on rack so that they do not touch.

3. Bake until golden at edges, 3 to 5 minutes. Remove from oven and sprinkle with garlic salt. Let cool completely.

> ## ✖ Variation
>
> *Panzanella Salad:* In summer, use these croutons for a quick and easy tomato-basil panzanella salad. In a pretty serving bowl, add 3 to 4 heirloom tomatoes, cut into wedges. Add a handful of basil, torn into pieces, a thinly sliced red onion and about half of the crouton recipe. Toss all together with a red wine vinaigrette.

Sopapillas

In New Mexico these little puffed pillows serve a few purposes. They are great for sopping up enchilada sauce and are also served alongside spicy meals with a dab of sweetness as a way of cooling the heat. Dusted with sugar and cinnamon while hot, they become a sweet crisp dessert.

✖ Tip

The oil must not be too hot or the sopapillas will brown before they fully puff up.

✖ Candy/deep-fry thermometer

2 cups	all-purpose flour	500 mL
2 tsp	baking powder	10 mL
1 tsp	salt	5 mL
1 tsp	granulated sugar	5 mL
3 tbsp	vegan shortening	45 mL
$^7/_8$ cup	plain hemp milk, warmed (approx.)	220 mL
	Canola oil	

1. In a large bowl, sift together flour, baking powder, salt and sugar. Using fingers, work in shortening until incorporated. Add warm milk and mix with a wooden spoon until a slightly sticky dough ball forms (similar to pie crust dough). Add additional heated milk, 1 tsp (5 mL) at a time, if dough is too dry. Cover bowl with a clean damp kitchen towel and let rest for 30 minutes.

2. Divide dough into 4 equal pieces. On a lightly floured surface, roll each piece into a rectangle, $^1/_8$- to $^1/_4$-inch (3 mm to 0.5 cm) thick. Cut dough into 2- to 3-inch (5 to 7.5 cm) triangles and cover with clean damp kitchen towel and let stand for 5 minutes.

3. In a deep saucepan, heat 2 inches (5 cm) of oil over medium–high heat to 325°F (160°C). Carefully place 2 sopapillas at a time into hot oil and fry, turning once, until puffed and golden brown, about 30 seconds per side. Transfer with a slotted spoon to a plate lined with paper towel to drain. Repeat process with remaining sopapillas adjusting heat as necessary between batches. Serve hot, but also good at room temperature.

British four o'clock tea biscuits

Makes 13 to 15

The goodness of toasted oats adds to the appeal of these slightly sweet tea cookies, or biscuits, as they are known in Britain. With a cup of hot tea, they are just the thing to get one through a chilly winter's afternoon.

✖ Tip

Store in an airtight container at room temperature for up to 1 week.

✖ Preheat oven to 350°F (180°C)
✖ Food processor
✖ 3-inch (7.5 cm) biscuit cutter

1 cup	large-flake (old-fashioned) rolled oats	250 mL
1 cup	whole wheat flour	250 mL
1/3 cup	packed brown sugar	75 mL
1/4 cup	all-purpose flour	60 mL
1/2 tsp	salt	2 mL
1/4 tsp	ground cinnamon	1 mL
1/2 cup	vegan hard margarine, cut into pieces	125 mL
2 tbsp	ice water	30 mL

1. Spread oats on a baking sheet. Toast in preheated oven, stirring every 2 minutes, until golden and fragrant, 7 to 9 minutes. Let cool completely.

2. In food processor, combine whole wheat flour, brown sugar, all-purpose flour, salt and cinnamon. Add margarine and pulse until it resembles fine crumbs. Add cooled oats and pulse briefly. Gradually pour ice water through the feed tube, pulsing just until dough comes together. Gather into a ball, press into a disk, wrap in plastic wrap and refrigerate for 30 minutes.

3. On a floured surface, roll out dough to 1/8-inch (3 mm) thickness and cut out biscuits using 3-inch (7.5 cm) cutter. Gather scraps and repeat process. Place on a baking sheet, at least 1/2 inch (1 cm) apart. Bake in preheated oven until edges are browning slightly, 12 to 15 minutes. Let cool completely on pan.

Savory onion biscuits

Makes 8

Here you'll find all the goodness of a biscuit with the added savor of caramelized onion. Wonderful by themselves with a bowl of soup, they also make tasty little sandwiches for teatime or hors d'oeuvres when spread with Maple Rhubarb Jam (page 297) or Mango Habanero Chutney (page 296).

- **Preheat oven to 425°F (220°C)**
- **2-inch (5 cm) cookie cutter, optional**

5 tbsp	canola oil, divided	75 mL
1 cup	chopped onion (about 1 medium)	250 mL
2 cups	all-purpose flour (approx.)	500 mL
4 tsp	baking powder	20 mL
1/2 tsp	salt	2 mL
1/8 tsp	freshly ground black pepper	0.5 mL
1/4 cup	cold vegan hard margarine	60 mL
1/2 cup	Soy Milk (page 18) or store-bought	125 mL
2 tbsp	chopped chives	30 mL

1. Place a skillet over medium heat and let pan get hot. Add 2 tbsp (30 mL) of the oil and tip pan to coat. Add onion and cook, stirring occasionally, until golden, 15 to 20 minutes. Let cool completely.
2. In a large bowl, combine flour, baking powder, salt and pepper. Cut in chilled margarine with two knives or a pastry blender until mixture is the size of peas. With fork, stir in remaining 3 tbsp (45 mL) of canola oil, soy milk, cooled onion mixture and chives, just until blended.
3. Turn dough onto floured work surface and knead 10 to 12 times just until dough holds together. Roll or pat to a thickness of 1/2 inch (1 cm). Using cookie cutter, cut dough into circles or simply cut into 8 squares with a knife. Gather scraps and repeat process. Place on an ungreased baking sheet, at least 1/2 inch (1 cm) apart.
4. Bake in preheated oven until just golden around the edges, 10 to 12 minutes. Let cool slightly on pan. Serve warm.

Potato rolls

These soft rolls are a wonderful way to use up leftover mashed potatoes! Even better with garlic or herbed mashed potatoes.

✖ Tip

Store rolls in resealable plastic bags at room temperature for up to 3 days.

✖ Stand mixer with dough hook attachment
✖ 2 baking sheets, lined with parchment paper

1 cup	Soy Milk (page 18) or store-bought	250 mL
3 tbsp	vegan hard margarine	45 mL
¾ cup	cooked mashed potatoes	175 mL
2 tsp	granulated sugar	10 mL
1 tsp	salt	5 mL
¼ cup	warm water	60 mL
2 tsp	active dry yeast	10 mL
3½ to 4 cups	all-purpose flour	875 mL to 1 L

1. In a small saucepan, heat soy milk over medium heat until steaming and bubbles form around edge to scald. Remove from heat and stir in margarine, mashed potatoes, sugar and salt. Set aside and let cool to lukewarm.

2. In bowl of stand mixer, combine warm water and yeast and let stand until foamy, about 5 minutes. Add potato mixture. Attach bowl to mixer and fit with dough hook attachment. On low speed, gradually beat in 3½ cups (875 mL) of the flour. Beat for 2 minutes. Beat in remaining flour, 1 tbsp (15 mL) at a time, until a sticky dough forms, then beat for 2 minutes more. Transfer to a large warm oiled bowl, flipping dough to coat with oil. Cover with a clean kitchen towel and let rise in a warm, draft-free place until doubled in size, about 45 minutes.

3. Punch dough down and divide into about 18 golf ball–size pieces. Shape each piece into a round bun and arrange on prepared baking sheets, at least 1 inch (2.5 cm) apart. Cover loosely with plastic wrap and let rise until doubled, about 45 minutes.

4. Preheat oven to 350°F (180°C) about 10 minutes before rolls have completely risen.

5. Uncover rolls and bake until puffed and tops are golden, 10 to 15 minutes. Let cool slightly on pan. Serve warm or let cool completely.

Saffron squash rolls

Makes 15 rolls

These rolls get their beautiful golden color from the butternut squash and subtle spice from the saffron.

❖ Tip

Store rolls in an airtight container at room temperature for up to 3 days.

❖ Stand mixer with dough hook attachment
❖ Baking sheet, lined with parchment paper

1 cup	Soy Milk (page 18) or store-bought	250 mL
$\frac{1}{4}$ tsp	saffron threads	1 mL
3 tbsp	vegan hard margarine	45 mL
$\frac{3}{4}$ cup	mashed cooked butternut squash	175 mL
1 tbsp	granulated sugar	15 mL
1 tsp	salt	5 mL
$\frac{1}{4}$ cup	warm water	60 mL
2 tsp	active dry yeast	10 mL
$3\frac{1}{2}$ to 4 cups	all-purpose flour	875 mL to 1 L

1. In a small saucepan, heat soy milk and saffron over medium heat until steaming and bubbles form around edge to scald. Remove from heat and stir in margarine, squash, sugar and salt. Set aside and let cool to lukewarm.

2. In bowl of stand mixer, combine warm water and yeast and let stand until foamy, about 5 minutes. Add squash mixture. Attach bowl to mixer and fit with dough hook. On low speed, gradually add $3\frac{1}{2}$ cups (875 mL) of the flour. Beat for 2 minutes. Add remaining flour, 1 tbsp (15 mL) at a time, until a sticky dough forms, then beat for 2 minutes more. Transfer to a large warm oiled bowl, flipping dough to coat with oil. Cover with a clean kitchen towel and let rise in a warm, draft-free place until doubled in size, about 45 minutes.

3. Punch dough down and transfer to a floured surface. Divide into 15 pieces. Shape each piece into a round bun and arrange on prepared baking sheet in even rows. Rolls may touch while rising but this will not affect outcome. Cover loosely with plastic wrap and let rise until doubled in size, about 45 minutes.

4. Preheat oven to 350°F (180°C) 10 minutes before rolls have completely risen.

5. Bake until rolls are puffed and tops are golden, 15 to 18 minutes. Transfer to a wire rack and let cool slightly. Serve warm or let cool completely.

> ## ❖ Variation
> Add 1 tsp (5 mL) chopped rosemary, sage or whole fresh thyme to squash mixture.

Seeded flatbread

Makes 8

These flat, sturdy cracker-like breads go well with soups and make great dippers. Each can be broken into 12 rustic pieces to serve with White Bean Hummus (page 64) or Herbed Golden Tofu Spread (page 51).

✖ Tip

Store flatbread well wrapped in plastic wrap or an airtight container at room temperature for up to 1 week.

✖ Preheat oven to 400°F (200°C)

2 cups	whole wheat flour	500 mL
1 cup	all-purpose flour (approx.)	250 mL
1 tbsp	sesame seeds	15 mL
1 tbsp	poppy seeds	15 mL
1 tbsp	flax seeds	15 mL
2 tsp	baking powder	10 mL
2 tsp	salt	10 mL
$1/8$ tsp	baking soda	0.5 mL
3 tbsp	canola oil	45 mL
1 cup	ice water	250 mL

1. Place a well-seasoned griddle or skillet in preheated oven to heat (see Tips, page 101).

2. In a large bowl, mix together whole wheat flour, all-purpose flour, sesame seeds, poppy seeds, flax seeds, baking powder, salt and baking soda. Stir in oil until well mixed. Using a wooden spoon, add ice water all at once and beat until mixture forms a ball.

3. Transfer dough to a floured work surface, and using floured hands, knead just until dough is no longer sticky, 2 to 3 times. Divide dough into 8 equal portions. Flatten each into disks and roll out into 7-inch (18 cm) rustic, imperfect circles. Sprinkle liberally with flour and let rest for 5 minutes.

3. Working with one circle at a time, roll rested dough out thinner, to about 9 inches (23 cm) or as big as your griddle can accommodate. Brush off any remaining flour before baking.

4. Carefully place one portion of rolled-out dough into oven, onto heated griddle and bake until flatbread blisters, 3 to 4 minutes. Flip over and bake until bread blisters, 1 to 2 minutes. Do not underbake. Using tongs, transfer to a wire rack. Repeat process with remaining dough. Serve warm or at room temperature.

Caraway rye crackers

You don't need to make crackers, but it is one of those extra special touches you do to accompany a homemade soup on a wintery day or tuck into a loved one's lunchbox. Homemade crackers are not only delicious but they also are a little homespun Valentine.

✪ Tips

Store in an airtight container at room temperature for up to 1 week.

Use cookie cutters to create fun and whimsical shaped crackers.

✪ Preheat oven to 400°F (200°C)
✪ Food processor

1/2 cup	rye flour	125 mL
1/2 cup	all-purpose flour	125 mL
1 tsp	baking powder	5 mL
1/2 tsp	salt	2 mL
1/4 cup	coconut oil	60 mL
2 tbsp	soy milk or other non-dairy milk	30 mL
1 tbsp	light (fancy) molasses	15 mL
1 tbsp	caraway seeds	15 mL

1. In food processor, combine rye flour, all-purpose flour, baking powder and salt and pulse to blend. Add coconut oil and process until mixture resembles fine crumbs. Add soy milk and molasses and pulse to incorporate. Sprinkle caraway seeds over dough and pulse 3 to 4 times until distributed.

2. Gather dough into ball and roll out between sheets of waxed paper or parchment paper to $\frac{1}{16}$-inch (2 mm) thickness. Remove top layer of waxed paper and cut dough using a pastry wheel or knife into $1\frac{1}{2}$-inch (4 cm) squares or other desired shape. Prick all over with fork tines and transfer to a baking sheet. (It's easier to maneuver the pricking of the crackers if the sheet is not lined with parchment but lining is an option, if desired.)

3. Bake in preheated oven until edges begin to brown, 5 to 6 minutes. Transfer to a wire rack and let cool completely.

> ## ✪ Variation
> *Rye Sesame Crackers:* Substitute sesame seeds for the caraway seeds and replace 1 tbsp (15 mL) of the coconut oil with 1 tbsp (15 mL) toasted sesame oil.

Super simple crackers

Makes 30

These crackers are a great use for wonton wrappers leftover from making ravioli or wontons. Just paint on a little soy and sesame "glue" and sprinkle with sesame seeds and salt. It's a fun kitchen activity for little helpers.

Tip

Store crackers in an airtight container at room temperature for up to 1 week.

- **Preheat oven to 300°F (150°C)**
- **Baking sheet, lined with parchment or foil**

2 tbsp	plain soy milk	30 mL
1 tbsp	cornstarch	15 mL
1 tsp	sesame oil	5 mL
1/2 tsp	soy sauce	2 mL
15	vegan 3-inch (7.5 cm) square or round wonton wrappers	15
1 tbsp	black and/or white sesame seeds	15 mL
1/4 tsp	sea salt flakes, optional	1 mL

1. In small bowl, blend soy milk and cornstarch until smooth. Stir in sesame oil and soy sauce and set aside.
2. Cut wonton wrappers in half (on the diagonal, if square). Place in a single layer on prepared baking sheet. Using a basting brush, paint one side of wonton with soy mixture. Sprinkle with sesame seeds and salt flakes, if using.
3. Bake in preheated oven for 5 minutes. Rotate pan front to back and bake until golden brown, about 5 minutes more. Let cool completely on pan on a wire rack.

Scattered-seed crackers

Makes about 80

Packed with whole grain inside, these rustic crackers have seeds inside and out, with a salty-sweet glaze over all.

✖ Tip

Store crackers in an airtight container for up to 1 week.

✖ Preheat oven to 375°F (190°C)
✖ Two 18- by 13-inch (45 by 33 cm) baking sheets

Crackers

$1\frac{3}{4}$ cups	whole wheat flour	425 mL
6 tbsp	ground sunflower seeds	90 mL
3 tbsp	ground flax seeds (flax seed meal)	45 mL
4 tbsp	flax seeds, divided	60 mL
3 tbsp	sesame seeds, divided	45 mL
2 tbsp	poppy seeds, divided	30 mL
1 tsp	coarse salt, divided	5 mL
$\frac{2}{3}$ cup	water	150 mL
2 tbsp	coconut oil	30 mL
$1\frac{1}{2}$ tbsp	agave nectar	22 mL

Glaze

$1\frac{1}{2}$ tbsp	water	22 mL
$1\frac{1}{2}$ tbsp	agave nectar	22 mL

1. *Crackers:* In large bowl, combine flour, ground sunflower seeds, ground flax seeds, 3 tbsp (45 mL) of the flax seeds, 2 tbsp (30 mL) of the sesame seeds, 1 tbsp (15 mL) of the poppy seeds and $\frac{1}{2}$ tsp (2 mL) of the salt. Add water, coconut oil and agave and stir to form a stiff dough. Turn out unto floured work surface and knead until smooth, 3 to 4 minutes. Let dough rest for 20 minutes.

2. Divide dough into 2 equal pieces. Roll out one piece of dough very thinly to a rough rectangle almost as large as baking sheet. Carefully transfer dough to baking sheet and repeat process with second piece. Use a sharp knife to cut dough into diamond or rectangle shapes of approximately 2- by $1\frac{1}{2}$-inches (5 by 4 cm). Bake one sheet at a time in preheated oven until a dark golden brown, 10 to 12 minutes.

3. *Glaze:* In a small bowl, mix together water and agave. In another small bowl, combine remaining flax seeds, sesame seeds and poppy seeds. When crackers come out of the oven, brush lightly with agave mixture then immediately scatter seed mixture over top. Sprinkle with remaining $\frac{1}{2}$ tsp (2 mL) of salt. Let cool completely on a wire rack. Separate crackers.

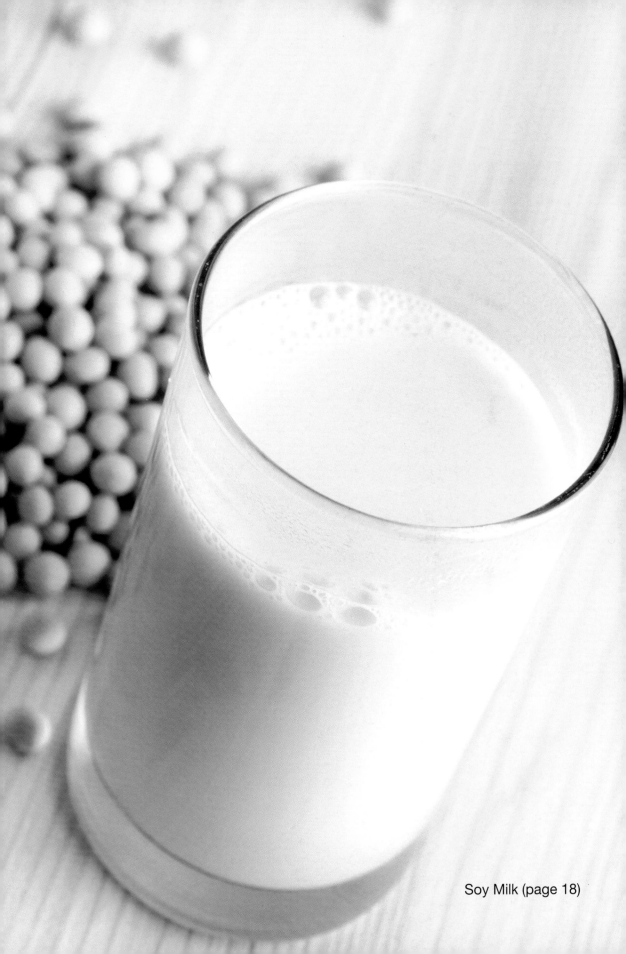

Soy Milk (page 18)

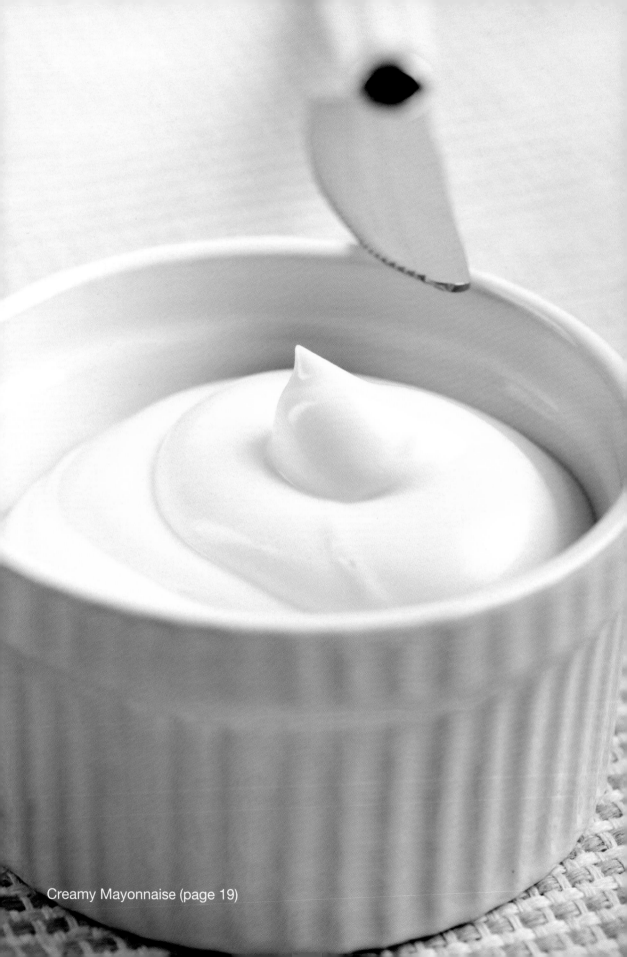

Creamy Mayonnaise (page 19)

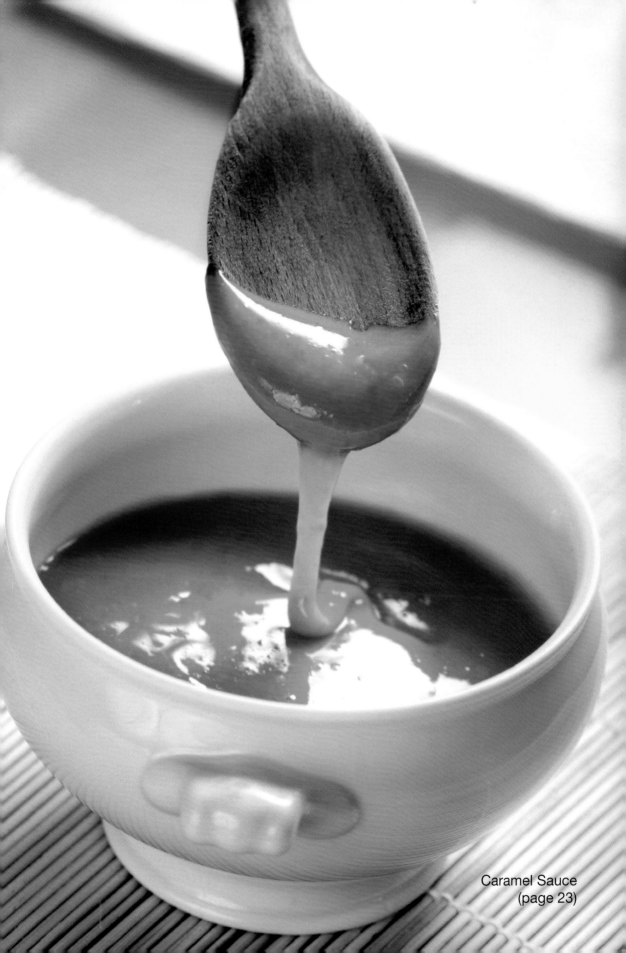

Caramel Sauce
(page 23)

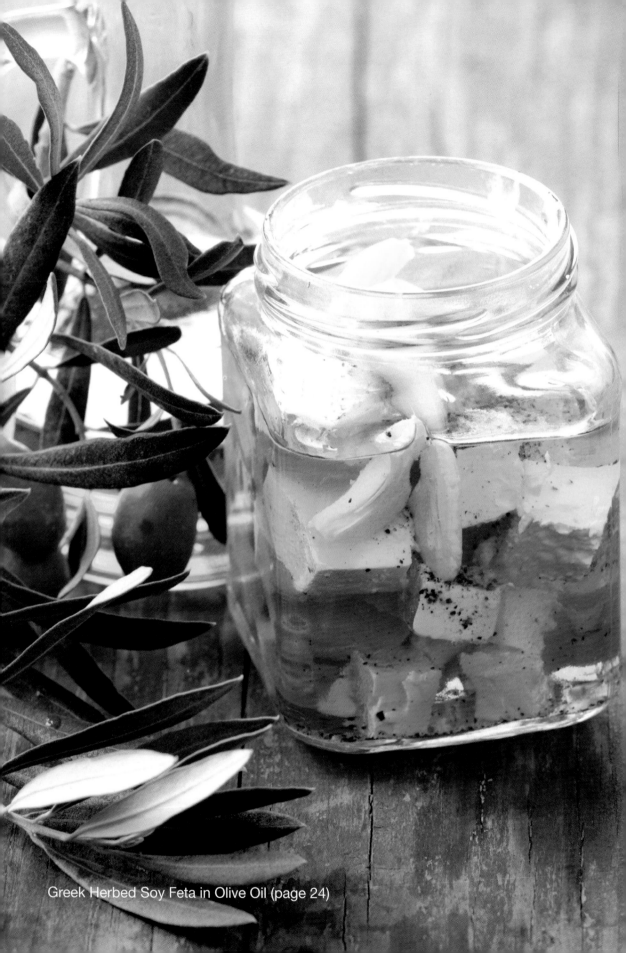
Greek Herbed Soy Feta in Olive Oil (page 24)

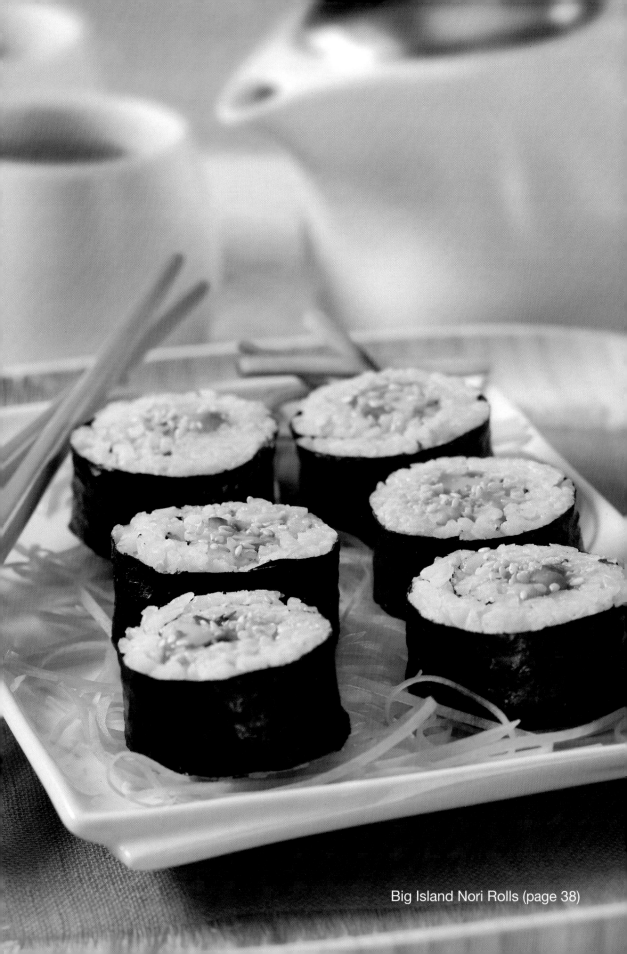

Big Island Nori Rolls (page 38)

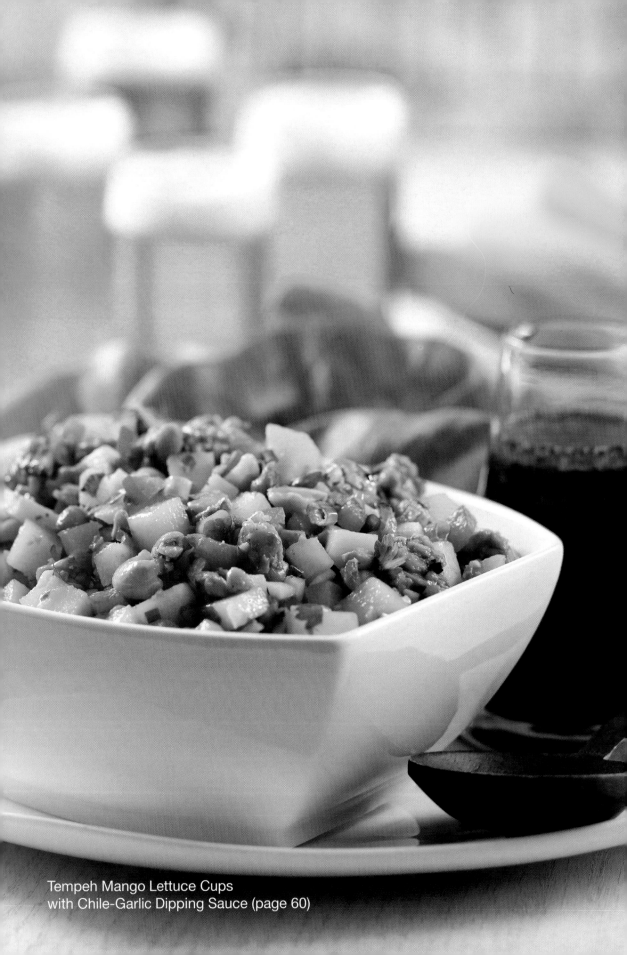

Tempeh Mango Lettuce Cups
with Chile-Garlic Dipping Sauce (page 60)

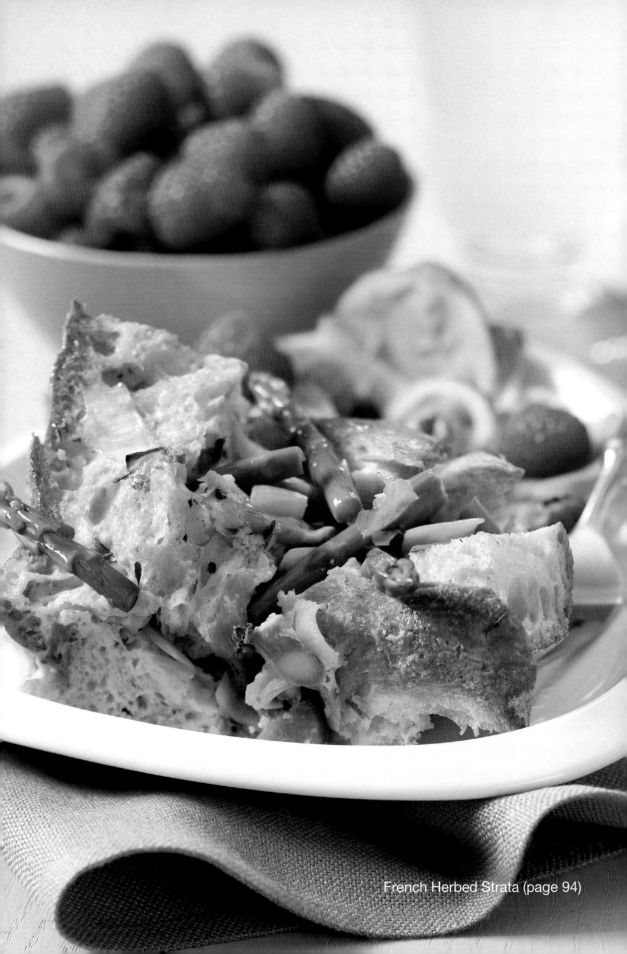

French Herbed Strata (page 94)

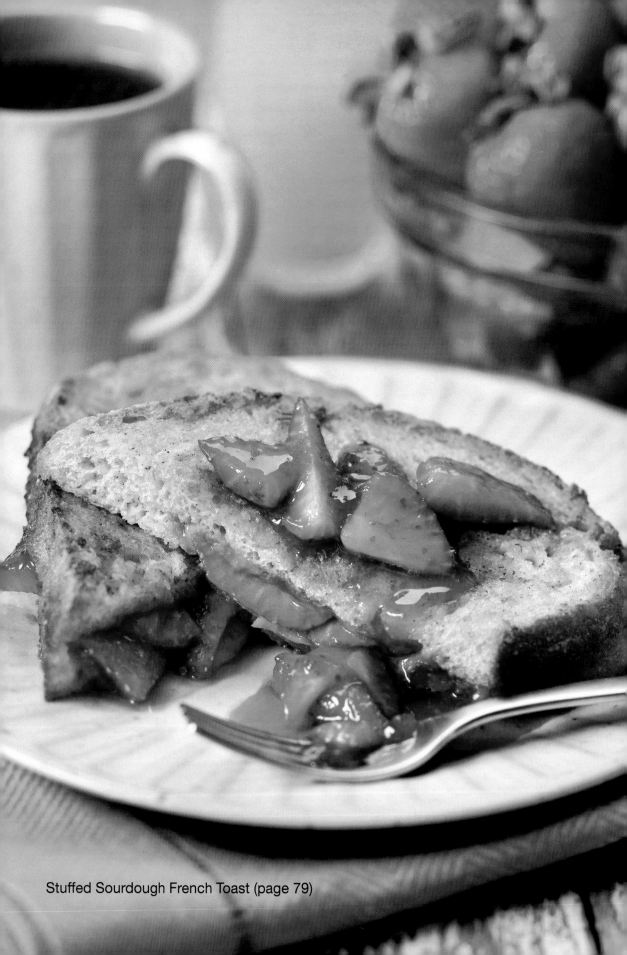

Stuffed Sourdough French Toast (page 79)

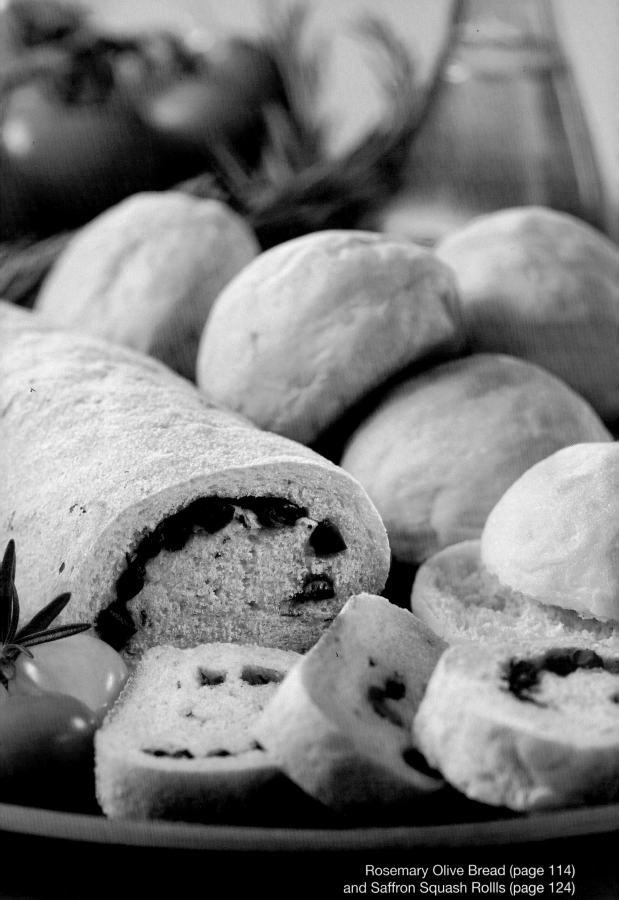

Rosemary Olive Bread (page 114)
and Saffron Squash Rollls (page 124)

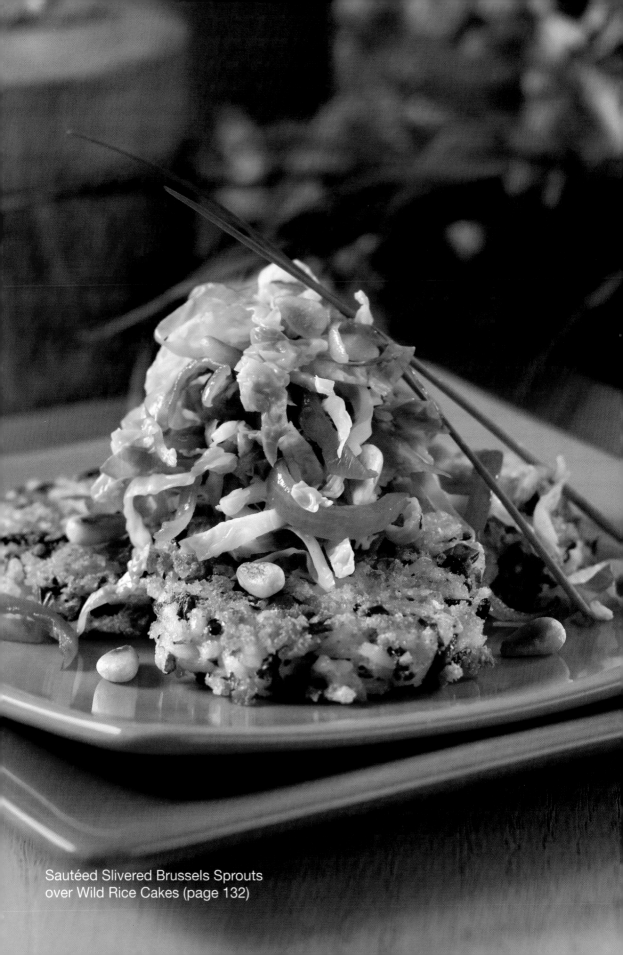

Sautéed Slivered Brussels Sprouts
over Wild Rice Cakes (page 132)

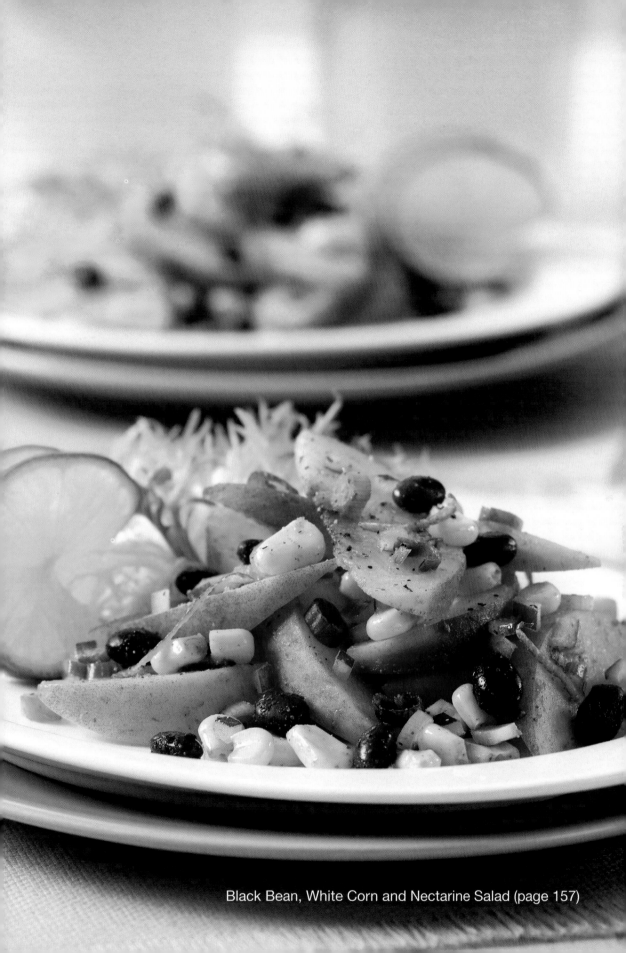

Black Bean, White Corn and Nectarine Salad (page 157)

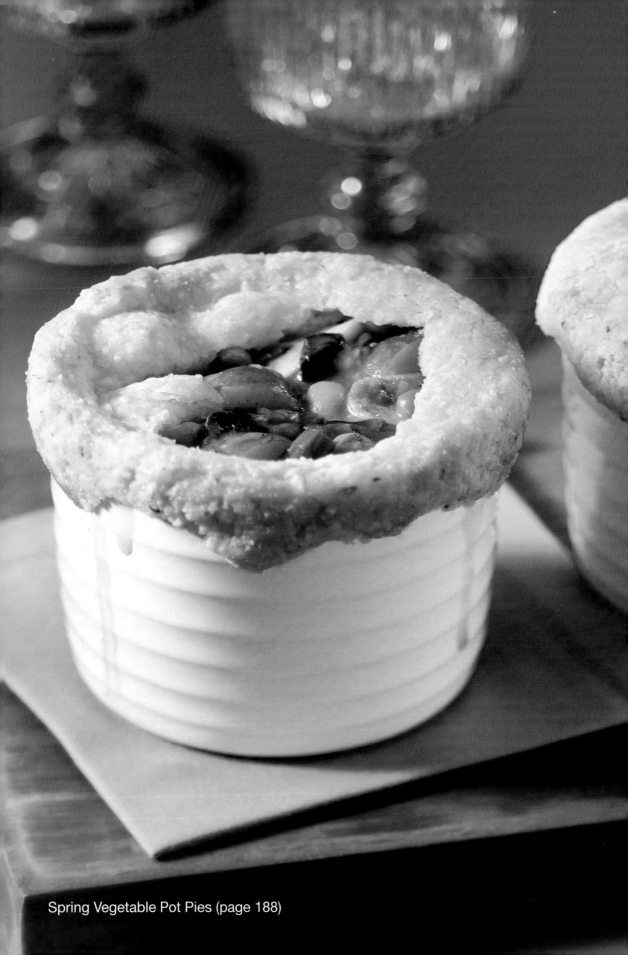

Spring Vegetable Pot Pies (page 188)

Hot Vegetables and Cool Salads

❌—❌—❌—❌—❌—❌—❌—❌—❌—❌—❌—❌—❌

Mediterranean vegetable casserole

This delectable combination of vegetables seasoned with fresh oregano bakes into a mouthwatering lunch or dinner. Serve with a huge Greek salad. Opa!

✖ Tip

Salting and sweating eggplant leaches moisture and some of the bitterness from the eggplant as well as reducing the spongy texture that is likely to absorb grease while cooking. Rinse salt from eggplant and dry with a kitchen towel to eliminate as much moisture as possible before cooking.

✖ Preheat oven to 350°F (180°C)
✖ 13- by 9-inch (33 by 23 cm) baking pan, lightly oiled

1	large eggplant, peeled and cut into 1/2-inch (1 cm) slices (see Tip, left)	1
	Salt	
1	red onion, sliced	1
8 oz	cremini mushrooms, sliced	250 g
1	green bell pepper, sliced	1
2	tomatoes, sliced	2
1/4 cup	olive oil, divided	60 mL
2 tbsp	chopped fresh Greek oregano, divided	30 mL
1 tsp	freshly ground black pepper	5 mL

1. Arrange eggplant slices in colander, sprinkle with 2 tsp (10 mL) salt and set aside to drain for about 20 minutes. Rinse and pat dry.

2. In prepared baking pan, layer half each of eggplant, red onion, mushrooms, bell pepper and tomatoes. Drizzle with 2 tbsp (30 mL) of the oil and sprinkle with 1 tbsp (15 mL) of the oregano and 1/2 tsp (2 mL) each salt and pepper. Repeat with remaining ingredients.

3. Bake casserole in preheated oven until vegetables are tender and top is slightly browned with crisp edges, 40 to 45 minutes. Let stand for 10 minutes before serving.

> ## ✖ Variation
> Fry eggplant slices in olive oil before layering in baking pan.

Oven-baked gnocchi and butternut squash

Serves 4	

Roasting the butternut squash brings out its wonderful sweet flavor as it caramelizes, not to mention filling the house with tantalizing hints of what's to come.

✂ **Preheat oven to 425°F (220°C)**
✂ **2 baking sheets, lined with parchment paper**

1½ lbs	butternut squash, peeled, seeded and cut into ½-inch (1 cm) cubes	750 g
⅓ cup	olive oil, divided	75 mL
6	fresh sage leaves, thinly sliced	6
1½ tsp	fresh thyme leaves	7 mL
½ tsp	salt	2 mL
¼ tsp	freshly ground black pepper	1 mL
1	package (1 lb/500 g) fresh gnocchi	1
½ cup	chopped onion	125 mL
¾ cup	white wine	175 mL

1. In a large bowl, toss together butternut squash, 2 tbsp (30 mL) of the oil, sage, thyme, salt and pepper. Spread evenly onto one baking sheet and place on bottom rack in oven. Bake in preheated oven until squash is softened and beginning to brown, about 30 minutes. Flip cubes after 15 minutes.

2. In same large bowl, toss gnocchi with 1 tbsp (15 mL) of oil. Spread evenly onto other baking sheet and place on middle rack in oven. Bake until heated through and a bit crusty, about 15 minutes.

3. Meanwhile, place a large skillet over medium-low heat and let pan get hot. Add 1 tbsp (15 mL) of oil and tip pan to coat. Add onion and cook, stirring occasionally, until soft, 4 to 6 minutes. Remove from heat. When squash and gnocchi come out of oven, return pan to stove top and increase heat to medium-high. Add squash, gnocchi and wine, stirring to combine. Cook, stirring frequently, until wine reduces slightly, 3 to 5 minutes. Serve immediately.

Sautéed slivered brussels sprouts over wild rice cakes

Serves 4		

Heightened flavors and a vibrant presentation make this dish a real star. It is doubtful there will be any leftover, but if so, chill the shredded Brussels sprouts, dress with balsamic vinaigrette and serve as a memorable side dish.

✖ **Preheat oven to 200°F (100°C)**
✖ **Blender**

1 lb	Brussels sprouts, bottoms and outer leaves trimmed	500 g
2 tbsp	olive oil, divided	30 mL
2	onions, thinly sliced	2
3	cloves garlic, sliced	3
1¼ tsp	salt, divided	6 mL
½ tsp	Dijon mustard	2 mL
½ cup	firm or extra-firm silken tofu	125 mL
2 cups	cooked mixed wild and brown rice	500 mL
2 tbsp	chopped chives	30 mL
1 tbsp	chopped basil	15 mL
1 tbsp	minced Italian flat-leaf parsley	15 mL
⅛ tsp	freshly ground black pepper	0.5 mL
⅓ cup	fresh bread crumbs	75 mL
	Canola oil	
2 tbsp	pine nuts, lightly toasted	30 mL

1. Finely slice sprouts about ¹⁄₁₆-inch (2 mm) thick. Separate slices into shreds and set aside.

2. Place a large nonstick skillet over medium heat and let pan get hot. Add 1 tbsp (15 mL) of the olive oil and tip pan to coat. Add onions and cook, stirring frequently, for 5 minutes. Stir in garlic, ¾ tsp (3 mL) of the salt and mustard and cook, stirring often, until onions are golden and caramelized, about 20 minutes.

3. In a blender, purée tofu until smooth. In a bowl, gently fold together puréed tofu and rice. Mix in chives, basil, parsley, black pepper and remaining ½ tsp (2 mL) of salt. Place bread crumbs in a shallow bowl and, using a tablespoon, drop rice mixture into bread crumbs, patting gently to form a cake. Press additional crumbs on top and use a small spatula to transfer cake to a plate lined with waxed paper. Repeat with remaining rice mixture.

For those who think they don't like Brussels sprouts, think again! Shredded and sautéed, they can be a delicious part of your regular diet so you'll get their fantastic health benefits. Brussels sprouts are nutritious and contain lots of fiber.

4. Place another skillet over medium-high heat and let pan get hot. Add about ¼ inch (0.5 cm) canola oil. When oil is hot, place 3 or 4 rice cakes in pan and cook until edges begin to brown, 4 to 5 minutes. Carefully flip cakes and cook until underside is browned, 2 to 3 minutes. Transfer to a plate lined with paper towels and keep warm in preheated oven. Repeat process with remaining rice mixture.

5. In pan with onions, heat remaining 1 tbsp (15 mL) of olive oil over medium-high heat, pushing onions to one side of pan. Add Brussels sprouts and cook, stirring frequently, until shreds are bright green and just beginning to wilt, about 5 minutes.

6. Arrange 2 to 3 rice cakes on a plate and top each with a little pile of sprouts. Sprinkle with pine nuts and serve.

Summer squash primavera with curried butter sauce

This light and colorful, all-vegetable dish is perfect for dinner on the patio.

:: Tip

A julienne peeler is a hand-held peeler that is used in the same manner as a vegetable peeler but produces results more like a mandolin. It is an inexpensive tool that will create uniform strips of vegetables to be used in cooking, salads or as a garnish.

:: Preheat oven to 200°F (100°C)
:: 16-cup (4 L) baking dish, lightly oiled
:: Julienne peeler (see Tip, left)

2	large zucchini	2
2	large yellow summer squash (yellow zucchini)	2
2 tbsp	olive oil, divided	30 mL
3 tbsp	vegan hard margarine, divided	45 mL
4	green onions, white and green parts, slivered lengthwise and cut into 2-inch (5 cm) pieces	4
1/2 tsp	salt	2 mL
1/2 tsp	freshly ground black pepper	2 mL
1/2	head broccoli, cut into small florets	1/2
1/2	head cauliflower, cut into small florets	1/2
1	medium pattypan squash, cut into large dice	1
1	fresh ear corn, kernels cut from cob	1
1/2	red bell pepper, diced	1/2
1/4 cup	water	60 mL
3 tbsp	dry white wine	45 mL
1 tsp	curry powder	5 mL
1/2 tsp	ground turmeric	2 mL
2 tbsp	golden raisins	30 mL
1/2 cup	toasted walnuts	125 mL

1. Use a julienne peeler to create long strands of zucchini and yellow squash, moving lengthwise, avoiding seeds in center of squash.

2. Place baking dish in preheated oven. Place a large skillet over medium heat and let pan get hot. Add 1 tbsp (15 mL) of the oil and 1 tbsp (15 mL) of the margarine and tip pan to coat. Add green onions and cook, stirring constantly, for 30 seconds. Add zucchini and yellow squash shreds and cook, stirring frequently, just until squash becomes limp, 3 to 4 minutes. Add salt and pepper. Transfer to heated baking dish and return to oven.

As cooking time is short, have vegetables prepped and ready to add at the proper time.

Refrigerate in an airtight container for up to 2 days.

3. Place same pan over medium-high heat and let pan get hot. Add remaining 1 tbsp (15 mL) of oil and tip pan to coat. Add broccoli, cauliflower and pattypan squash. Cover and cook, stirring occasionally, about 5 minutes. Stir in corn, bell pepper and water. Cover pan, reduce heat to medium and cook until vegetables are softened, 2 to 3 minutes.

4. In a bowl, mix together white wine, curry powder and turmeric and stir into vegetables. Add raisins and remaining 2 tbsp (30 mL) of margarine, stirring constantly. Pour mixture over squash in baking dish, sprinkle walnuts over top and serve hot.

Mandarin rice and walnut-stuffed acorn squash

Serves 4 to 8

A delightfully unexpected combination of exotic aromas and fragrant flavors combine in this hearty and warm stuffed squash.

✷ Preheat oven to 375°F (190°C)
✷ 13- by 9-inch (33 by 23 cm) glass baking dish

1	acorn squash, halved lengthwise, seeds and pulp removed	1
2 tsp	olive oil	10 mL
2 tsp	maple syrup	10 mL

Stuffing

1/4 cup	dried figs, diced	60 mL
1	can (11 oz or 284 mL) unsweetened mandarin oranges with juice	1
1 tbsp	olive oil	15 mL
2	shallots, chopped	2
1 tsp	grated gingerroot	5 mL
2 tsp	garam masala	10 mL
1/4 cup	toasted walnuts	60 mL
2 tbsp	golden raisins (sultanas)	30 mL
1 cup	cooked long-grain brown rice	250 mL
2 tbsp	chopped cilantro	30 mL
	Salt and freshly ground black pepper	

1. Place squash in baking dish cut side up and drizzle inside of each half with 1 tsp (5 mL) of the oil and 1 tsp (5 mL) of the maple syrup. Add 1/2 inch (1 cm) water and bake in preheated oven for 45 minutes.

2. *Stuffing:* In a small bowl, combine figs and oranges with juice. Set aside.

3. Place a skillet over medium heat and let pan get hot. Add oil and tip pan to coat. Add shallots, ginger and garam masala and cook, stirring occasionally, until shallots are softened, 2 to 3 minutes. Stir in walnuts, raisins, rice and cilantro. Remove from heat and season with salt and pepper to taste. Mix in fig and orange mixture.

4. Transfer par-cooked squash to a cutting board and when cool enough to handle stuff each half with rice mixture, mounding high without compacting. Return squash to baking dish, cover loosely with foil and bake until squash is tender and stuffing is slightly crunchy on top, 10 to 15 minutes. Let cool slightly before serving.

Lime and saffron caramelized carrots

Serves 4 to 6

Before all oil became the enemy, caramelized carrots were de rigueur. Now that we realize that excess consumption and saturated fats are the culprit, it is once again time to enjoy the sweet and savory delights of candied carrots, using only a good oil, and in moderation, of course.

2 tbsp	olive oil	30 mL
2 tbsp	vegan hard margarine	30 mL
6	carrots, peeled and thinly sliced into coins	6
	Zest and juice of 1 lime	
1/2 tsp	freshly ground black pepper	2 mL
1/4 tsp	salt	1 mL
Pinch	saffron	Pinch

1. Place a large skillet over medium-high heat and let pan get hot. Add oil and when hot, add margarine to melt, tipping pan to coat. Add carrots, lime zest, 2 tsp (10 mL) of lime juice, pepper, salt and saffron and toss to coat. Reduce heat to medium and cook, stirring frequently, until carrots are tender and very caramelized, 10 to 12 minutes. Serve hot.

Variation

Omit the saffron, lime zest and juice and simply sprinkle with chopped fresh parsley and a drizzle of lemon juice.

Balsamic asparagus with walnuts

Fresh asparagus sautéed with a splash of tangy balsamic vinegar and the rich flavor of walnuts are all it takes to create a memorable and very simple summertime side.

2 tbsp	olive oil	30 mL
1	shallot, minced	1
2 lbs	asparagus (about 16 to 20 spears), trimmed and cut into 2-inch (5 cm) pieces	1 kg
1/2 cup	toasted walnut halves	125 mL
3 tbsp	balsamic vinegar	45 mL
3/4 tsp	salt	3 mL
1/2 tsp	freshly ground black pepper	2 mL

1. Place a large nonstick skillet over medium–high heat and let pan get hot. Add oil and tip pan to coat. When hot, add shallots and cook, stirring frequently, until slightly softened and slightly browned, 3 to 5 minutes. Add asparagus, tossing to coat, and cook, turning occasionally, for 5 to 6 minutes. Add walnuts and balsamic vinegar and cook until al dente and slightly browned, 3 to 4 minutes. Sprinkle with salt and pepper and serve immediately.

Italian tomato–braised white cannellini and green beans

Serves 4

The delicious thick herbed tomato sauce is the perfect complement to white and green beans. This quick and easy recipe will soon become a favorite.

8 cups	water	2 L
3 tsp	salt, divided	15 mL
1 lb	green beans, trimmed	500 g
1/4 cup	olive oil	60 mL
1/4 tsp	hot pepper flakes	1 mL
2 1/2 cups	chopped drained tomatoes	625 mL
1/4 cup	minced fresh parsley	60 mL
2	cloves garlic, minced	2
1 tbsp	minced fresh basil	15 mL
1 tbsp	minced fresh thyme	15 mL
1 tbsp	minced fresh oregano	15 mL
1	minced fresh sage leaf	1
1/4 tsp	freshly ground black pepper	1 mL
2 cups	cooked white cannellini beans (if canned, rinsed and drained)	500 mL

1. Fill a large stockpot with water. Add 2 tsp (10 mL) of the salt and bring to a boil over high heat. Add green beans and cook until tender, 6 to 8 minutes. Transfer to a colander and rinse under cold running water. Set aside to drain.

2. Place a large skillet over medium heat and let pan get hot. Add oil and tip pan to coat. Add hot pepper flakes and brown for about 10 seconds. Add tomatoes, parsley, garlic, basil, thyme, oregano, sage, remaining 1 tsp (5 mL) of salt and black pepper. Bring mixture to a boil, partially covered. Reduce heat and simmer until sauce is reduced and thickened, about 20 minutes.

3. Gently fold in green beans and white beans, turning carefully to cover with sauce. Cover pan and simmer until flavors are combined, about 10 minutes. Serve immediately.

> ### ✖ Variation
> Add cooked pasta or wild rice for a hearty meal.

Chestnut and cranberry holiday non-stuffed stuffing

Stuffing is always better when it is not stuffed but rather oven-baked with a crisp golden top and soft savory center. Fresh chestnuts are delightful but only available in the fall. By using jarred chestnuts you can make this lovely dish any day of the year.

✖ Tip

In place of day-old bread cubes, spread fresh cubed bread on baking sheets and bake in a 275°F (140°C) oven until dried with golden edges, 20 to 30 minutes.

✖ 13- by 9-inch (33 by 23 cm) baking dish, lightly oiled with margarine
✖ Foil, one side lightly oiled with margarine

2 tbsp	olive oil	30 mL
5 tbsp	vegan hard margarine, divided	75 mL
12 oz	cremini mushrooms, sliced	375 g
2	stalks celery with leaves, chopped	2
1	onion, chopped	1
1 cup	chopped celery root	250 mL
½ cup	dried cranberries	125 mL
½ cup	freshly squeezed orange juice	125 mL
1 cup	chopped jarred roasted chestnuts or fresh (see Tip, right)	250 mL
½ cup	chopped Italian flat-leaf parsley	125 mL
1 tsp	Sage Seasoning Blend (page 314) or store-bought sage-based seasoning blend	5 mL
2 to 2½ cups	Vegetable Broth (page 31) or store-bought, heated, divided	500 to 625 mL
½ tsp	salt	2 mL
½ tsp	freshly ground black pepper	2 mL
1 lb	loaf day-old, sourdough French bread, cut into 1-inch (2.5 cm) pieces (see Tip, left)	500 g

1. Heat a large skillet over medium–high heat. Add oil and 1 tbsp (15 mL) of the margarine and tip pan to coat. Add mushrooms and cook, stirring frequently, until golden with browned edges, 4 to 5 minutes.

2. Move mushrooms to sides of pan and add 2 tbsp (30 mL) of margarine. When melted, add celery, onion and celery root. Cook, stirring frequently, until softened, 6 to 8 minutes. Add 2 tbsp (30 mL) of margarine and when melted, stir in cranberries, orange juice, chestnuts, parsley and Sage Seasoning Blend. Stir in 2 cups (500 mL) of the vegetable broth, salt and pepper, scraping up any browned bits from the bottom of the pan.

✖ Tip

Roasting fresh chestnuts brings great bragging rights and an incredible cozy winter aroma to your kitchen. *To roast chestnuts:* Choose heavy and firm, deep rich glossy brown chestnuts with a shiny sheen. When gently squeezed the shell should give slightly. Wash chestnuts to eliminate any dirt or mold and cut an X in the flat side. Place chestnuts, slit side up, in a preheated 400°F (200°C) and roast until tender. Test by inserting a fork through slit cut in shell. Transfer chestnuts to a kitchen towel, pressing to crush shells and release chestnuts. Wrap in towel and when cool enough to handle, remove shells.

3. Place bread cubes into a large bowl. Pour broth and vegetable mixture over bread cubes, tossing lightly, allowing cubes to absorb broth. Cover bowl with a clean kitchen towel and set aside for 1 hour. Check cubes after 30 minutes. Cubes should be softened but not soggy. Add up to ½ cup (125 mL) of heated broth, if necessary. Taste stuffing and adjust seasoning.

4. Preheat oven to 350°F (180°C). Transfer stuffing to prepared baking dish and cover with prepared foil, greased side down. Bake in preheated oven for 30 minutes. Remove foil and continue baking until top is golden and crisp, about 15 minutes.

Grilled artichokes with jalapeño mignonette sauce

Choose artichokes with tight leaves, indicating young and fresh artichokes because the leaves begin to spread with age. Serve with Northwest Passage Cedar-Planked Tofu (page 214) and a nice bottle of Pinot Noir.

⚃ Tips

Cook artichokes without a steamer basket by reducing water level to 2 inches (5 cm) and placing artichokes, stems trimmed at base, upright and snug in the bottom of the pan. Simmer for 35 to 40 minutes, checking water level frequently.

If citrus Champagne vinegar is unavailable, substitute Champagne vinegar or white wine vinegar (not as mild) flavored with lemon, orange or grapefruit juice. Leftover and slightly flat Champagne is also a great substitute.

⚃ Large stockpot with steamer basket
⚃ Charcoal or gas grill

2	artichokes, trimmed (see Tips, left)	2
	Half of 1 lemon	
2 tbsp	salt	30 mL
1/4 cup	citrus Champagne vinegar (see Tips, left)	60 mL
1/3 cup	rice wine vinegar	75 mL
2 tbsp	minced shallot	30 mL
2 tbsp	freshly squeezed lime juice	30 mL
1 tbsp	minced jalapeño	15 mL
1/2 tsp	granulated sugar	2 mL
1/2 tsp	freshly ground black pepper	2 mL
2 tbsp	olive oil	30 mL

1. Rub trimmed edges of artichokes with lemon. Fill a large pot with 3 inches (7.5 cm) of water, add salt and insert steamer basket. Place artichokes, cut side down, in steamer basket. Cover pan and simmer until stems are tender and outer leaves are easily dislodged, 25 to 40 minutes, depending on size. Place artichokes upside down in a colander and drain. When cool, cut in half, vertically and remove furry choke.

2. In a large shallow bowl, whisk together Champagne vinegar, rice wine vinegar, shallot, lime juice, jalapeño, sugar and pepper. Add artichokes, turning to coat well with dressing. Cover and refrigerate, turning occasionally, for 1 to 2 hours.

3. Preheat grill to medium–high heat (375 to 400°F/ 190 to 200°C). Remove artichokes from marinade, reserving marinade. Brush artichokes with oil and place on grill. Grill with lid closed, turning once or twice, until heated through and grill marks are visible, 10 to 15 minutes. Serve artichokes hot with a drizzle of reserved marinade.

Braised baby artichokes with wine and herbs

When choosing baby artichokes look for firm compact produce that carry weight because this indicates the artichokes are not dried out. This dish is rustic yet elegant and equally delicious hot or cold; the perfect picnic take along.

2 cups	water	500 mL
1/4 cup	freshly squeezed lemon juice	60 mL
20	baby artichokes	20
2 tbsp	olive oil	30 mL
2	shallots, finely chopped	2
2	cloves garlic, minced	2
1 cup	dry white wine	250 mL
1 tsp	finely chopped basil	5 mL
1 tsp	finely chopped oregano	5 mL
1 tsp	finely chopped thyme	5 mL
1/2 tsp	salt	2 mL
1/2 tsp	freshly ground black pepper	2 mL
2 tbsp	finely chopped parsley	30 mL

1. In a large bowl, combine water and lemon juice. Prepare artichokes one at a time by snapping off all dark green leaves. Cut top off where yellow turns pale green, trim bottom stem, quarter artichokes and drop into lemon water.

2. Place a large skillet over medium heat and let pan get hot. Add oil and tip pan to coat. Add shallots and cook, stirring occasionally, until softened, 2 to 3 minutes. Drain artichokes and pat dry. Add garlic and artichokes to pan and cook, stirring occasionally, until beginning to soften, about 6 minutes.

3. Stir in wine, basil, oregano, thyme, salt and pepper. Cover pan and bring to a boil. Reduce heat to low and simmer, partially covered, until artichokes are tender, 10 to 15 minutes. Taste and adjust seasoning. Serve hot, garnished with fresh parsley or refrigerate and serve chilled.

Purple potato, artichoke and zucchini bake

Serves 4

This easy, one-dish casserole can be served for lunch with a crisp green salad or as a tasty side dish for dinner.

✘ Tip

Frozen artichoke hearts are less expensive and a great substitute. If available, use 1 package (9 to 12 oz/270 to 375 g), thawed and patted dry.

✘ Preheat oven to 350°F (180°C)
✘ 8-cup (2 L) baking dish, lightly oiled

1	can (14 oz/398 mL) artichoke hearts, well drained (see Tip, left)	1
3	purple potatoes, cut into 1-inch (2.5 cm) cubes	3
1	zucchini, cut into 1-inch (2.5 cm) cubes	1
2	cloves garlic, minced	2
1/4 cup	dry white wine	60 mL
3 tbsp	Crunch (page 31) or store-bought bread crumbs	45 mL
2 tbsp	freshly squeezed lemon juice	30 mL
1 tbsp	olive oil	15 mL
1 tsp	dried Mediterranean Seasoning (page 313) or store-bought	5 mL
1/4 cup	Greek Herbed Soy Feta in Olive Oil (page 24), crumbled, optional, or store-bought vegan feta	60 mL

1. In prepared baking dish, combine artichoke hearts, potatoes, zucchini and garlic. Pour wine over all. In a small bowl, combine Crunch, lemon juice, oil and seasoning, mixing well. Scatter over vegetables. Cover with foil and bake in preheated oven for 15 minutes.

2. Remove foil and continue cooking until potatoes are tender and topping is browned, 10 to 15 minutes. Crumble soy feta over top and serve.

> ## ✘ Variation
> This dish is delicious served chilled if you omit the bread crumb topping.

Cuban-spiced corn on the cob

Serves 4

Sweet corn charred
to perfection and
slathered in goodness
comes sans the
cholesterol usually
associated with this
summer barbecue
classic.

✖ Tip

This recipe makes use of
a charcoal or gas grill but
it is possible to oven-roast
corn at 450°F (230°C) for
15 to 20 minutes until
nicely browned.

✖ **Charcoal or gas grill (see Tip, left)**

Sauce

½ cup	vegan hard margarine, melted	125 mL
2 tbsp	All-Purpose Spicy Barbecue Dry Rub (page 308) or store-bought	30 mL
2 tbsp	freshly squeezed lime juice	30 mL
4	ears of corn, shucked	4
2 tsp	nutritional yeast powder	10 mL

1. *Sauce:* In a small bowl, combine margarine, dry rub
   and lime juice, mixing well to incorporate. Cover and
   refrigerate to let flavors combine for at least 1 hour.

2. Heat grill to medium-high heat (375 to 400°F/190 to
   200°C). Place corn on grill rack and cook, with lid
   closed, turning occasionally, until browned and charred,
   about 10 minutes.

3. Spread each grilled ear of corn with about 1 tbsp
   (15 mL) of sauce and a sprinkle of nutritional yeast
   powder. Serve immediately.

Sautéed bitter greens with walnuts

Serves 4

Simple and simply delicious, this is a versatile go-to dish that is a guaranteed winner every time.

¼ cup	olive oil, divided	60 mL
8 cups	kale, trimmed and sliced	2 L
8 cups	baby arugula	2 L
1	shallot, finely chopped	1
3	cloves garlic, finely chopped	3
½ tsp	salt	2 mL
½ tsp	freshly ground black pepper	2 mL
2 tbsp	apple cider vinegar	30 mL
1 cup	cooked white cannellini beans (if canned, rinsed and drained)	250 mL
½ cup	chopped toasted walnuts	125 mL

1. Place large skillet over medium–high heat and let pan get hot. Add oil and tip pan to coat. Add kale, arugula, shallot, garlic, salt and pepper and cook, stirring frequently, until greens slightly diminish in volume, 2 to 3 minutes. Add vinegar, beans and walnuts and gently toss to incorporate. Cook, gently tossing, until beans are warmed through and greens are wilted, 2 to 3 minutes. Remove from heat and serve.

> ## ⚙ Variation
> Substitute Swiss chard, spinach, mustard greens, collard greens, beet greens or turnip greens for kale and arugula.

Smashed russets and garnet yams

A rich and delicious version of everyone's favorite comfort food is made easy by baking the potatoes and garlic. No huge pots to wash, just a baking dish and a bowl. Couldn't get much easier, unless you go out to dinner.

✖ Tips

To roast garlic: Preheat oven to 350°F (180°C). Slice off top ½ inch (1 cm) of garlic head to expose tops of individual cloves. Place garlic head on a piece of foil and drizzle with 1 tsp (5 mL) olive oil. Pull foil sides up and twist ends together to form a loose, sealed puffy pod. Roast in preheated oven until garlic cloves are lightly browned and very tender, 35 to 40 minutes.

Reheat this dish, covered with foil, in a 250°F (120°C) oven until hot, 15 to 20 minutes.

✖ Potato masher

2	large garnet yams or sweet potatoes	2
2	large russet (Idaho) potatoes	2
1	head garlic, wrapped in foil and roasted (see Tips left)	1
2 tbsp	vegan hard margarine	30 mL
2 tbsp	olive oil	30 mL
½ to ¾ cup	plain hemp milk, heated	125 to 175 mL

Salt and freshly ground black pepper

1. Place a 12-inch (30 cm) piece of foil on bottom rack of oven to catch any drips from cooking yam. Place yams and potatoes directly on middle rack. Set oven to 400°F (200°C) and bake until tender, 30 to 45 minutes depending on size. While yams and potatoes are still very warm but cool enough to handle, peel and place in large bowl. Add cooled roasted garlic and mash, until very chunky. Mash in margarine and oil until still chunky but slightly combined. Add ½ cup (125 mL) of the warm hemp milk and mash, adding more milk, 2 tbsp (30 mL) at a time, until desired consistency is achieved. Season with salt and pepper to taste and serve immediately.

Athenian roasted potatoes

A little soak in lemon juice before baking adds a fresh hint of citrus. The olive oil, garlic and oregano form a crisp crust around the creamy and delicious tender potatoes.

- Preheat oven to 400°F (200°C)
- 13- by 9-inch (33 by 23 cm) baking dish

6	russet (Idaho) potatoes, peeled and each sliced into 6 wedges	6
½ cup	freshly squeezed lemon juice, divided	125 mL
3	cloves garlic, finely minced	3
1 tbsp	dried oregano	15 mL
½ cup	olive oil, divided	125 mL
1 tsp	salt	5 mL
¾ tsp	freshly ground black pepper	3 mL
2 tbsp	chopped fresh parsley	30 mL

1. In baking dish, combine potatoes, ¼ cup (60 mL) of the lemon juice, garlic and oregano, tossing to coat. Let stand for 10 minutes. Drizzle potatoes with ¼ cup (60 mL) of the oil and toss. Sprinkle with salt and pepper.

2. Cover pan with foil and bake in preheated oven until potatoes are tender, 20 to 25 minutes. Remove foil and roast, uncovered, until outsides are browned and with slightly crispy edges, about 10 minutes.

3. Whisk together remaining ¼ cup (60 mL) of lemon juice, ¼ cup (60 mL) of oil and parsley and drizzle over crisp potatoes. Season with additional salt and pepper to taste.

Yukon gold potatoes with garlic and rosemary sauce

Steamed tender Yukons are gently tossed in a creamy stove top sauce of roasted garlic, shallot, rosemary and white wine. This rich dish adds huge flavor to any meal.

✖ Preheat oven to 350°F (180°C)
✖ 8-cup (2 L) baking dish
✖ Steamer basket

2	heads garlic	2
2	shallots, roughly chopped	2
2 tbsp	olive oil	30 mL
1 tbsp	finely chopped fresh thyme	15 mL
1 tbsp	finely chopped fresh rosemary	15 mL
	Salt and freshly ground black pepper	
4 lbs	Yukon gold potatoes, quartered	2 kg
1/2 cup	dry white wine	125 mL
3 tbsp	vegan hard margarine	45 mL

1. Slice off top 1/2 inch (1 cm) of garlic heads and place garlic in baking dish. Pile shallot pieces close together and drizzle oil over all. Sprinkle thyme, rosemary, 1/2 tsp each (2 mL) salt and pepper over shallots and cover with foil, crimping to form a dome. Bake in preheated oven until garlic and shallots are softened and lightly browned and very tender, 40 to 50 minutes.

2. About 25 minutes before garlic is done, place steamer basket into a large stockpot and add water to 1 inch (2.5 cm) below basket. Add potatoes and cook until tender, 15 to 18 minutes.

3. Squeeze garlic pulp from skins and place back into baking dish. Add shallots and use a fork to roughly mash. Transfer to a skillet over medium heat. Add wine and margarine and whisk until blended. Bring just to a simmer and cook, stirring frequently, until slightly thickened. Taste and adjust seasonings. Add hot potato quarters and toss to coat. Season with salt and pepper to taste. Serve hot.

Root vegetable latkes with crème fraîche and chives

Crispy potato and root vegetable latkes served with tart and creamy crème fraîche make a delicious appetizer or side dish. Besides the beautiful presentation, the crunchy outside is only upstaged by a creamy satisfying center. Prepare this dish last because it will hold in a warm oven but is best served hot from the pan.

✖ Tip
Removing excess liquid from vegetables helps prevent sticking.

✖ Variation
Use any combination of root vegetables, making sure russet potatoes make up at least half for the best flavor.

✖ Food processor with shredding disk or box grater

2	russet (Idaho) potatoes, peeled	2
1	garnet yam or sweet potato, peeled	1
1	small celery root, peeled	1
2	shallots, finely chopped	2
3 tbsp	chickpea flour	45 mL
¼ cup	all-purpose flour	60 mL
¼ cup	cornstarch	60 mL
1 tsp	salt	5 mL
½ tsp	freshly ground black pepper	2 mL
¾ tsp	smoked paprika	3 mL
⅓ cup	water	75 mL
¼ cup	grapeseed oil, divided	60 mL
1 cup	Silken Crème Fraîche (page 16) or store-bought vegan alternative sour cream	250 mL
¼ cup	minced chives	60 mL
¼ cup	Sprinkle (page 30), optional	60 mL

1. In a food processor with shredding disk, shred potatoes, yam and celery root. Place shredded vegetables in a clean kitchen towel and squeeze to remove any excess liquid. Transfer to a large bowl. Add shallots and stir to combine. In a small bowl, combine chickpea flour, all-purpose flour, cornstarch, salt, pepper and paprika. Using clean hands toss with vegetables, coating well. Drizzle in water and mix with clean hands until mixture is slightly moistened.

2. Place a large skillet over medium heat and let pan get hot. Add 2 tsp (10 mL) of the oil and tip pan to coat. When oil is hot, place large rounded spoonfuls of the vegetable mixture into skillet and flatten each with a spatula. Cook until golden brown, 2 to 3 minutes. Carefully flip and cook until bottom is crisp and golden brown, 1 to 2 minutes. Transfer to plate lined with a double layer of paper towels. Repeat process, adding more oil as needed.

3. Serve latkes topped with a spoonful of crème fraîche, a scattering of minced chives and a sprinkle of Sprinkle, if using.

Cauliflower and leeks with tomato herb sauce

Sweet tomatoes, fragrant herbs, rich roasted cauliflower and leeks come together to create an unusual dish with a huge flavor.

✖ Tips

To easily remove tomato skins: Place tomatoes in gently boiling water until tomato skin begins to split in places, 3 to 4 minutes. Remove with a slotted spoon and peel when cool enough to handle.

Sauce will keep refrigerated in an airtight container for up to 3 days.

✖ Variation

Baked Cauliflower and Leeks with Bread Crumb Topping: Place cauliflower and leeks in a lightly oiled casserole dish, pour sauce over all and toss to coat. Place in a 400°F (200°C) oven for 20 minutes. Mix pine nuts and ¾ cup (175 mL) dried seasoned bread crumbs with 2 tbsp (30 mL) melted vegan margarine and sprinkle over vegetables. Return to oven, reduce heat to 350°F (180°C) and bake until cauliflower is golden brown and top is crunchy, 10 to 15 minutes. Transfer to a platter and serve.

✖ Preheat oven to 400°F (200°C)
✖ Blender
✖ Baking sheet, lined with parchment paper
✖ Warmed mixing bowl

Sauce

3	tomatoes, skinned and seeded (see Tips, left)	3
2	cloves garlic, chopped	2
3 tbsp	red wine vinegar	45 mL
1 tbsp	chopped Italian flat-leaf parsley	15 mL
1 tbsp	chopped basil	15 mL
1 tbsp	chopped oregano	15 mL
½ tsp	salt	2 mL
½ tsp	freshly ground black pepper	2 mL
⅛ tsp	cayenne pepper	0.5 mL
¾ cup	olive oil	175 mL

Vegetables

1	head cauliflower, trimmed into florets	1
1	leek, white and light green parts only, washed very well and thinly sliced (see Tip, page 94)	1
2 tbsp	olive oil	30 mL
1 tsp	salt	5 mL
1 tsp	freshly ground black pepper	5 mL
½ tsp	sweet paprika	2 mL
½ cup	toasted pine nuts	125 mL

1. *Sauce:* In a blender, blend tomatoes, garlic, vinegar, parsley, basil, oregano, salt, black pepper and cayenne pepper until combined, scraping down sides as necessary. Drizzle in oil and blend until almost smooth. Let stand in blender, do not refrigerate. Just before using, pulse once or twice to recombine.

2. *Vegetables:* In a large bowl, combine cauliflower and leeks. Toss with oil, salt, pepper and paprika. Transfer to prepared baking sheet and roast in preheated oven until cauliflower is golden and browned in places, 30 to 40 minutes. Transfer to warm bowl, pour sauce over all and toss to coat. Transfer to serving platter and top with toasted pine nuts and serve immediately.

Chinese long beans with orange sesame glaze

Serves 2 to 4

Chinese long beans will grow up to a yard long but can become tough. Foot-long beans are young and therefore usually tender. Long beans are delicious stir-fried until crispy. If a more-tender bean is desired, parboil beans for 4 to 5 minutes before stir-frying.

❖ Variations

Add 1 cup (250 mL) stir-fried mushrooms or substitute roasted peanuts for sesame seeds.

1 tbsp	peanut oil	15 mL
3 lbs	Chinese long beans, cut into 4-inch (10 cm) pieces	1.5 kg
1	shallot, thinly sliced	1
2	cloves garlic, minced	2
1 tsp	toasted sesame oil	5 mL
1 tbsp	freshly squeezed orange juice	15 mL
1 tbsp	freshly squeezed lime juice	15 mL
1 tbsp	tamari	15 mL
2 tbsp	toasted sesame seeds	30 mL

1. Place a large skillet over high heat and let pan get hot. Add peanut oil and tip pan to coat. Add long beans and stir-fry until beans start to brown, about 2 minutes. Add shallot and stir-fry for 1 minute. Add garlic and sesame oil and stir-fry until fragrant, 30 seconds to 1 minute. Remove from heat and stir in orange juice, lime juice and tamari, tossing well to coat. Sprinkle with sesame seeds and serve hot.

Tarragon tofu and chilled lemon zucchini rice

Baked tofu is sliced thin and served over an enticing salad of chilled rice, shredded zucchini, lemon zest, chervil and toasted pine nuts. The tarragon wine marinade is whisked with oil and lemon juice to become a lovely dressing. A perfect choice for a summer dinner on the deck.

✖ Variations

Rice salad and tofu may be rolled in lettuce leaves and served as lettuce wraps.

Or serve tofu hot. Toss shredded zucchini with hot rice, lemon zest, chervil, pine nuts, and 2 tbsp (30 mL) each lemon juice and olive oil.

✖ Baking sheet, lined with parchment paper, lightly oiled

Marinade

1 cup	white wine	250 mL
2 tbsp	vermouth	30 mL
1 tsp	freshly squeezed lemon juice	5 mL
1 tbsp	dried tarragon	15 mL
1/4 tsp	onion powder	1 mL
16 oz	extra-firm tofu, drained and pressed (see page 12)	500 g
4 cups	cooked and chilled white rice	1 L
1 cup	shredded zucchini	250 mL
	Zest and juice of 1 lemon	
3 tbsp	chopped chervil	45 mL
2 tbsp	toasted pine nuts	30 mL
3 tbsp	olive oil	45 mL
2 tsp	agave nectar	10 mL
Pinch	salt and freshly ground black pepper	Pinch
1	small head red leaf lettuce	1

1. *Marinade:* In a glass pie plate or baking dish, combine wine, vermouth, lemon juice, tarragon and onion powder, whisking well to incorporate. Cut tofu, crosswise into 4 pieces and place in pie plate. Cover and refrigerate for 1 hour, turning at least once.

2. Preheat oven to 375°F (190°C). Place tofu on prepared baking sheet. Reserve marinade and refrigerate. Bake tofu in preheated oven for 15 minutes. Remove from oven and let cool to room temperature.

3. In a bowl, toss together rice, zucchini, lemon zest, chervil and pine nuts and set aside. In a small bowl, whisk together 1/2 cup (125 mL) reserved marinade, oil, agave, 2 tbsp (30 mL) of lemon juice and salt and pepper. Pour 1/2 cup (125 mL) dressing over salad and toss to coat. Slice chilled tofu into 1/2-inch (1 cm) strips.

4. To serve, place 2 or 3 large lettuce leaves on each of 4 plates. Scoop a quarter of the rice salad onto each plate, top with sliced tofu and drizzle with a spoonful of dressing.

Cold buckwheat noodles with broccoli and sesame dressing

This enticing entrée with flavors of a traditional Japanese buckwheat noodle salad is ideal served on a warm summer day with chilled sake.

⊞ Tips

You can also toast sesame seeds in a 350°F (180°C) oven for 10 to 15 minutes.

Recipe can be made in advance and refrigerated in an airtight container for up to 4 hours. Bring to room temperature and add garnishes just before serving.

⊞ Blender
⊞ Steamer basket

6 tbsp	sesame seeds, divided (see Tips, left)	90 mL
1 tbsp	grated lemon zest	15 mL
2 tbsp	freshly squeezed lemon juice	30 mL
1 tbsp	grated gingerroot	15 mL
2 tbsp	agave nectar	30 mL
1/4 cup	rice wine vinegar	60 mL
1/3 cup	soy sauce	75 mL
2 tbsp	grapeseed oil	30 mL
2 tbsp	toasted sesame oil	30 mL
1/4 tsp	hot pepper flakes	1 mL
8 cups	water	2 L
1	package (12 oz/375 g) dried buckwheat soba noodles	1
5 cups	broccoli florets (about 2 bunches)	1.25 L
3 cups	ice	750 mL
6	green onions, thinly sliced	6
1/2 cup	finely chopped cilantro	125 mL
	Cilantro sprigs or fresh shiso leaves, optional	

1. In a heavy-bottomed skillet over medium heat, toast sesame seeds, shaking pan frequently, until golden, 4 to 6 minutes. Transfer to plate and let cool.

2. In blender, blend 2 tbsp (30 mL) of the sesame seeds, lemon zest, lemon juice, ginger, agave, vinegar, soy sauce, grapeseed oil, sesame oil and hot pepper flakes until smooth. Set dressing aside.

3. Pour water into stockpot and bring to a boil over high heat. Add noodles and boil, stirring occasionally to deter sticking, until al dente, about 5 minutes. Drain noodles and transfer to a large serving bowl. Add dressing and toss to coat. Let noodles cool to room temperature, stirring occasionally to recoat with dressing.

4. Place a steamer basket into same stockpot. Add water, making sure it is below bottom of steamer basket and bring to a boil. Add broccoli and steam until crisp and just tender, 4 to 5 minutes. Meanwhile, place ice in a large bowl. Transfer broccoli to ice bath and when cool, drain in colander. Add broccoli to noodles. Add green onions and chopped cilantro, tossing to combine. Taste and adjust seasoning with additional hot pepper flakes.

5. Serve at room temperature, garnished with remaining $\frac{1}{4}$ cup (60 mL) toasted sesame seeds and sprigs of cilantro or shiso leaves.

✛ Variations

Use asparagus or green beans in place of the broccoli.

For additional protein, add pan-fried tofu cubes.

Roasted red potato and green bean salad

Serves 4 to 6

Roasting the potatoes and green beans gives this salad a hearty savory flavor. Add baked tofu for a sumptuous and filling entrée. The best part is there are no big pots to wash!

❖ Tips

Salad with dressing will keep refrigerated in an airtight container for up to 3 days.

For a lower-fat version, place potatoes into stockpot and cover with water. Add salt and bring to a boil over high heat. Reduce heat to medium-high and boil for 6 minutes. Add green beans and boil until beans and potatoes are just tender, 3 to 4 minutes. Remove from heat and immediately transfer to a colander to drain and cool.

❖ Preheat oven to 400°F (200°C)
❖ 2 baking sheets, lined with parchment paper

6	red potatoes, peeled and cut into 1-inch (2.5 cm) cubes	6
4 tsp	olive oil, divided	20 mL
1 tsp	salt, divided	5 mL
1/2 tsp	freshly ground black pepper, divided	2 mL
1 lb	green beans, trimmed and halved	500 g

Dressing

1/3 cup	olive oil	75 mL
2 tbsp	freshly squeezed lemon juice	30 mL
2 tbsp	white wine	30 mL
1 tbsp	Dijon mustard	15 mL
3 tbsp	drained capers	45 mL
2 tbsp	chopped fresh tarragon	30 mL
1 tsp	freshly ground black pepper	5 mL

1. Place potatoes in a large bowl. Drizzle with 2 tsp (10 mL) oil and sprinkle with 1/2 tsp (2 mL) salt and 1/4 tsp (1 mL) pepper and toss to coat. Transfer to prepared baking sheet. Place in preheated oven for 15 minutes.

2. In same bowl, toss beans with 2 tsp (10 mL) oil, 1/4 tsp (1 mL) salt and 1/4 tsp (1 mL) pepper and toss to coat. Transfer to remaining prepared baking sheet. When potatoes have roasted for 15 minutes, place beans in oven. Roast potatoes and beans until tender and slightly browned, 15 to 25 minutes. Transfer to a large serving bowl and let cool.

3. *Dressing:* In a small bowl, whisk together oil, lemon juice, wine, mustard, capers, tarragon and pepper. Pour dressing over top of beans and potatoes. Gently toss to combine. Taste and adjust seasoning, adding additional salt and pepper if desired. Serve at room temperature or chilled.

> ## ❖ Variation
> Purple potatoes are a good substitute and create a beautiful presentation.

Black bean, white corn and nectarine salad

This delectable salad with few ingredients comes together in minutes and is a win-win recipe; a breeze for you and a hit with the family. A dazzling dish perfect for outdoor events and summer backyard barbecues.

✖ Tip

Canned black beans are a fine substitute but it is important to rinse them well and drain.

2 cups	cooked black beans (see Tip, left)	500 mL
2 cups	frozen roasted white corn, thawed and drained	500 mL
1/4 cup	minced red onion	60 mL
1/4 cup	minced green onion, white and green parts	60 mL
2 cups	sliced nectarines (3 to 4 medium)	500 mL
	Zest and juice of 1 lime	
1/4 cup	olive oil	60 mL
2 tsp	ground cumin	10 mL
1/4 tsp	ground New Mexico red chile powder	1 mL
	Salt and freshly ground black pepper	

1. In a large bowl, combine beans, corn, red onion, green onion, nectarines and lime zest. Whisk in $1\frac{1}{2}$ tbsp (22 mL) lime juice, oil, cumin, chile powder, $\frac{1}{2}$ tsp (2 mL) salt and $\frac{1}{2}$ tsp (2 mL) pepper. Taste and adjust seasonings. Let stand at room temperature for 30 minutes. Serve immediately or refrigerate for up to 2 days.

> ## ✖ Variation
> Substitute melons, plums, tomatillos or mango for the nectarines.

Cauliflower and zucchini slaw

Fresh and crisp green
and white fruit and
vegetables offer a
united and striking
presentation. Flecks
of almonds and black
poppy seeds with a
zippy dressing make
this salad a standout.

3	zucchini, grated	3
1	green apple, unpeeled and grated	1
1/2	head cauliflower, grated	1/2
2	green onions, white and green parts, chopped	2
1/2 cup	toasted slivered almonds	125 mL
1/4 cup	chopped fresh cilantro	60 mL

Dressing

1/4 cup	freshly squeezed lime juice	60 mL
1/4 cup	olive oil	60 mL
1/2 tsp	salt	2 mL
1/4 tsp	ground white pepper	1 mL
1 tbsp	poppy seeds	15 mL

1. In a large bowl, combine zucchini, apple, cauliflower, green onions, almonds and cilantro.

2. *Dressing:* In a small bowl, whisk together lime juice, oil, salt and white pepper. Taste and adjust seasonings. Pour dressing over salad. Add poppy seeds and toss to combine. Serve immediately or refrigerate in an airtight container for up to 2 days.

Cold curried rice and artichoke salad

This great salad is perfect for a crowd. It's easy to assemble and makes use of jarred ingredients. Once you have the rice cooked it is smooth sailing.

✖ Tips

To ensure rice is done, use a spoon to pull a small section away from side of pan and check that all liquid has cooked out. Taste rice to make sure it is tender. If rice is not tender but liquid has cooked out, add 2 to 4 tbsp (30 to 60 mL) of water, cover and continue cooking until done.

Salad keeps refrigerated in an airtight container for up to 3 days.

2 tsp	olive oil	10 mL
2 cups	long-grain white rice	500 mL
5 cups	Vegetable Broth (page 31) or store-bought	1.25 L
3	jars (each 6 oz/175 g) marinated artichoke hearts, drained, chopped, liquid reserved	3
5	green onions, white and green parts, chopped	5
1/4 cup	chopped fresh parsley	60 mL
1	jar (4 oz/125 g) garlic-stuffed green olives, sliced	1
1/2 cup	golden raisins	125 mL
1 1/2 cups	Creamy Mayonnaise (page 19) or store-bought vegan mayonnaise	375 mL
2 tsp	ground curry powder	10 mL
	Salt and freshly ground black pepper	

1. Place a medium heavy-bottomed saucepan over medium heat and let pan get hot. Add oil and tip pan to coat. Add rice, stir to coat with oil and cook, stirring constantly, until rice becomes opaque, 1 to 2 minutes. Add broth and bring to a boil. Reduce heat, cover pot and cook, without stirring, until rice is tender and water has cooked out, about 50 minutes (see Tips, left). Refrigerate rice until chilled.

2. Transfer chilled rice to a large bowl. Add artichoke hearts, reserved artichoke liquid, green onions, parsley, olives, raisins, mayonnaise and curry powder, tossing to combine. Season with salt and black pepper to taste. Cover and refrigerate for at least 6 hours. Taste and adjust seasonings before serving.

✖ Variation

Add chopped nuts, roasted red pepper or capers.

Fiesta pasta salad

Viva la fiesta! With its vibrant presentation and palate-pleasing flavors, this salad is a delightful addition to any meal.

✖ Tips

Check pasta package ingredients because many are made with eggs.

Refrigerate salad in an airtight container for up to 2 days.

10 oz	penne pasta (see Tips, left)	300 g
1/4 cup + 2 tbsp	olive oil, divided	90 mL
4	green onions, green parts only, chopped	4
1/2 cup	chopped dried apricots	125 mL
1/4 cup	toasted slivered almonds	60 mL
1 tsp	grated lemon zest	5 mL
1 cup	Salsa Verde (page 298) or store-bought	250 mL
1/4 cup	brown rice syrup	60 mL
1/4 cup	white wine vinegar	60 mL
1/4 cup	olive oil	60 mL
2	cloves garlic, finely minced	2
1 1/2 tsp	ground cumin	7 mL
1 tsp	freshly ground black pepper	5 mL
3/4 tsp	salt	3 mL
4	Roma (plum) tomatoes, seeded and chopped	4

1. In a large pot of boiling salted water, cook pasta according to package directions. Toss with 2 tbsp (30 mL) of the olive oil. Place in refrigerator to chill.

2. In a large bowl, combine pasta, green onions, apricots, almonds and lemon zest, tossing to combine.

3. In a small bowl, stir together salsa, brown rice syrup, vinegar, remaining 1/4 cup (60 mL) of oil, garlic, cumin, pepper and salt, mixing well to blend. Stir salsa mixture into pasta, mixing well to combine. Add tomatoes and gently toss. Taste and adjust seasoning. Serve at room temperature or chilled.

Hearts of palm and mushroom salad with lemon parsley vinaigrette

Serves 6

Look for white mushrooms to complement the creamy colors and flecks of vibrant green that swirl through this delightful salad.

✖ Tip

Walnuts add flavor and provide omega-3s and protein in every crunchy bite.

1 lb	white mushrooms, thinly sliced	500 g
1	can (14 oz/398 mL) hearts of palm, drained and sliced into bite-size pieces	1
³/₄ cup	chopped toasted walnuts (see Tip, left)	175 mL
3	green onions, white and green parts, finely chopped	3
²/₃ cup	olive oil	150 mL
¹/₂ cup	freshly squeezed lemon juice	125 mL
¹/₂ cup	finely chopped parsley	125 mL
¹/₂ tsp	salt	2 mL
¹/₂ tsp	freshly ground black pepper	2 mL

1. In a large serving bowl, gently toss together mushrooms, hearts of palm, walnuts and green onions.

2. In a pint jar or other jar with tight-fitting lid, place oil, lemon juice, parsley, salt and pepper and shake vigorously to blend. Pour over salad. Cover and refrigerate salad for 20 minutes. Toss to refresh and serve.

✖ Variation

If you are short on time or the local grocer is out of lemons, a good quality store-bought citrus dressing of your choice is a fine substitute.

Iceberg wedge with ranch dressing and tempehacon bits

Iceberg lettuce gets a bad rap as watery lettuce with a vapid taste. Not so! As few know how to select the perfect head (see Tip, below), a delicious lettuce is underutilized. Despite this unfortunate fact, this classic salad is back in vogue and sure to stick around.

✖ Tip

When shopping for iceberg lettuce, take the time to find a tight head, which indicates a dense and therefore flavorful heart. The perfect head will yield very little to a gentle squeeze and it will seem heavy for its size.

✖ 4 chilled salad plates

1	head iceberg lettuce, trimmed and cut into quarters	1
1	tomato, cored and cut into 8 wedges	1
1 cup	Ranch Dressing (page 306) or store-bought vegan alternative	250 mL
¼ cup	minced red onion	60 mL
1 cup	Crunchy Tempehacon Bits (page 22) or store-bought vegan alternative	250 mL
12 to 16	Giant Garlicky Croutons (page 119) or store-bought	12 to 16
	Freshly ground black pepper	

1. Place a lettuce wedge, turned on its side, in the center of each chilled plate. Set 2 tomato wedges next to it. Over each, pour ¼ cup (60 mL) of the dressing and top each with 1 tbsp (15 mL) of the red onion, ¼ cup (60 mL) of the bacon bits and 3 or 4 croutons. Top with a few grinds of fresh black pepper and serve.

Picnic macaroni salad

In this case less is definitely more. These few simple ingredients are perfectly balanced to produce a huge flavor.

✴ Tip

Blend vinegar with mayonnaise, salt and pepper for easy and even distribution.

1	package (1 lb/500 g salad or elbow macaroni, cooked according to package directions	1
1	small red onion, finely chopped	1
³/₄ cup	chopped fresh parsley	175 mL
1 cup	chopped black olives	250 mL
³/₄ cup	Creamy Mayonnaise (page 19) or store-bought vegan alternative	175 mL
¹/₄ cup	red wine vinegar	60 mL
¹/₂ tsp	salt	2 mL
¹/₂ tsp	freshly ground black pepper	2 mL

1. In a large bowl, combine macaroni, red onion, parsley, olives, mayonnaise, vinegar, salt and pepper, mixing well to blend. Cover and refrigerate for at least 1 hour. Salad will absorb moisture as it chills and additional mayonnaise, salt and pepper may be needed. Taste and adjust seasonings.

> ## ✴ Variation
> This salad is great just as it is, but if you want to add more ingredients, try capers, roasted red pepper or minced serrano chile.

Sweet mini peppers and broccoli slaw

Serves 6 to 8

A bright and healthy addition to any meal with most ingredients available year-round. Seasonal grapes can easily be replaced with raisins or dried cranberries.

✖ Tip

Salad keeps refrigerated in an airtight container for up to 2 days.

✖ Food processor

1	head broccoli, florets and stalk cut into 2-inch (5 cm) pieces	1
1 lb	sweet mini peppers, stemmed, seeded and halved	500 g
1	stalk celery with leaves, trimmed and cut into 1-inch (2.5 cm) pieces	1
1/2	bunch Italian flat-leaf parsley, trimmed	1/2
1/2 cup	Creamy Mayonnaise (page 19) or store-bought vegan alternative	125 mL
	Zest and juice of 1 lemon	
2 tbsp	agave nectar	30 mL
1/2 tsp	dry mustard powder	2 mL
1/2 tsp	salt	2 mL
1 cup	red seedless grapes, halved	250 mL

1. In food processor, pulse broccoli until coarsely chopped, 5 to 6 times. Transfer to a large bowl. Repeat with peppers and add to broccoli. Process celery and parsley together and add to bowl.

2. In a small bowl, thoroughly blend mayonnaise, lemon zest, lemon juice, agave, mustard powder and salt. Taste and adjust seasoning. Pour over slaw and mix well to combine. Add grapes and gently toss. Cover bowl and refrigerate until well chilled, about 1 hour and serve.

Middle eastern balela salad

This colorful bean salad makes use of canned beans and throws together in minutes. The next time you cook up a pot of chickpeas be sure to make extra with this recipe in mind.

✖ Tip

Tuck balela salad into a pita or wrap in a spinach tortilla for a quick lunch or dinner.

2	cans (each 14 to 19 oz/398 to 540 mL) chickpeas, drained and rinsed	2
1 cup	diced tomatoes	250 mL
1	small red onion, chopped	1
1/4 cup	minced fresh parsley	60 mL
2 tbsp	minced fresh mint	30 mL
1	clove garlic, minced	1
1/4 cup	olive oil	60 mL
1/2 cup	apple cider vinegar	125 mL
1/2 tsp	salt	2 mL
1/2 tsp	freshly ground black pepper	2 mL

1. In a serving bowl, toss together chickpeas, tomatoes, red onion, parsley, mint and garlic.

2. In a liquid measuring cup or small bowl, combine oil, vinegar, salt and pepper. Add to salad, tossing gently to combine. Taste and adjust seasonings. Let salad stand for at least 1 hour before serving to combine flavors.

✖ Variations

Use sun-dried tomatoes instead of fresh tomato.

Swap 1 can of the chickpeas with drained and rinsed black, kidney or cannellini beans.

Warm rainbow potato salad

Steaming a variety of potatoes and serving them warm creates a unique salad. Cooking in this manner maximizes the nutritional value and keeps the potatoes from getting soggy.

✖ Tip

Use any size potatoes, but it is important to cut cooked potatoes into approximately ½-inch (1 cm) size pieces. If using small potatoes, reduce cooking time to 10 to 15 minutes.

✖ Large stockpot with steamer basket

3 lbs	mixed red, purple, white and yellow potatoes (6 to 8 medium potatoes) fork pierced (see Tip, left)	1.5 kg

Dressing

1 cup	olive oil	250 mL
2 tbsp	freshly squeezed lemon juice	30 mL
2 tbsp	white wine vinegar	30 mL
2 tsp	dry mustard powder	10 mL
2 tsp	minced garlic	10 mL
1 tsp	Classic Pesto Sauce (page 286) or store-bought vegan basil pesto or 10 fresh basil leaves, minced	5 mL
½ tsp	salt	2 mL
¼ tsp	freshly ground black pepper	1 mL
⅓ cup	minced green onion	75 mL
¼ cup	white wine	60 mL
¼ cup	water	60 mL
¼ tsp	salt	1 mL
Pinch	black pepper	Pinch
1 cup	Crunchy Tempehacon Bits (page 22) or store-bought vegan alternative, optional	250 mL

1. Place 1-inch (2.5 cm) water into a large stockpot and insert steamer basket. Add potatoes and cover pot. Bring water to a boil over medium–high heat. Reduce heat to medium and steam at a gentle boil until a sharp knife is easily inserted, about 20 minutes.

2. *Dressing:* Meanwhile, whisk together oil, lemon juice, vinegar, mustard powder, garlic, pesto, salt and pepper. Set aside.

3. Transfer hot potatoes to a cutting board. Slice into ½-inch (1 cm) thick pieces and place in a large bowl. Add green onion, wine, water, salt and black pepper and toss. Let stand for 5 minutes to absorb liquids. Pour dressing over mixture and gently toss to combine. Sprinkle with Tempehacon Bits, if using, and serve warm.

Tuscan panzanella salad

Serves 4 to 6

This rustic and unfussy salad is made with fresh summer tomatoes and crusty Italian bread.

✖ Tip

During the winter months, freeze those bits and pieces of stale French or Italian bread. To make a delicious panzanella salad when tomatoes are ripe and plentiful, defrost the bread and crisp in a warm oven for 30 minutes.

✖ Preheat oven to 400°F (200°C)
✖ Baking sheet, lined with parchment paper

12 oz	coarse Italian bread, cut into 2-inch (5 cm) chunks	375 g
¾ cup	olive oil, divided	175 mL
3 tbsp	red wine vinegar	45 mL
2 tsp	white balsamic vinegar	10 mL
½ tsp	salt	2 mL
½ tsp	freshly ground black pepper	2 mL
1	red onion, finely chopped	1
4	large tomatoes, chopped	4
1	bunch basil, leaves torn into pieces	1

1. Place bread chunks in a large bowl. Toss with ¼ cup (60 mL) of the oil and spread on prepared baking sheet. Roast in preheated oven until edges are lightly toasted and golden, 5 to 10 minutes.

2. Meanwhile, in a large bowl, whisk together remaining ½ cup (125 mL) of oil, red wine and white balsamic vinegar, salt and pepper. Add red onion, tomatoes and basil, tossing to combine.

3. Transfer bread directly from oven to bowl and toss with vinaigrette to thoroughly combine. Let stand at room temperature, tossing occasionally, for at least 30 minutes before serving.

✖ Variations

Some prefer panzanella made with peeled and seeded tomatoes. If this is more to your liking, score an X in the bottom of tomatoes and drop whole into boiling water for 10 to 15 seconds. Remove with a slotted spoon, plunge into ice water and use a paring knife to easily remove skins.

Popular additions include capers, red and green bell peppers and peeled cucumbers.

Lemon cucumber tabbouleh

This gorgeous presentation with a palette of yellows and greens is a spicy version of the classic Middle Eastern salad.

❖ Tips

If lemon cucumbers are unavailable try Persian, English or American cucumbers.

Salad keeps refrigerated in an airtight container for up to 3 days.

1 cup	boiling water	250 mL
1/3 cup	freshly squeezed lemon juice (approx.), divided	75 mL
1 cup	coarse bulgur	250 mL
6	green onions, white and green parts, chopped	6
2	lemon cucumbers, peeled, cored and cut into large bite-size pieces (see Tips, left)	2
1	yellow heirloom tomato, seeded and chopped	1
1	clove garlic, finely minced	1
1	small serrano pepper, seeded and finely minced	1
1	bunch Italian flat-leaf parsley, chopped	1
1/4 cup	chopped mint leaves	60 mL
1/3 cup	olive oil	75 mL
1/2 tsp	salt	2 mL
1/2 tsp	freshly ground black pepper	2 mL

1. In a small bowl, combine boiling water and 1 tsp (5 mL) of the lemon juice. Place bulgur in a large bowl and pour boiling water mixture over bulgur. Stir and let stand until all liquid is absorbed, about 30 minutes. Transfer bulgur to a wire-mesh strainer set over a bowl and let bulgur drain any remaining liquid.

2. In a large bowl, toss together bulgur, green onions, cucumbers, tomato, garlic serrano, parsley and mint.

3. In a small bowl, whisk together oil, 1/3 cup (75 mL) of lemon juice, salt and pepper to blend. Pour over bulgur mixture, tossing gently to combine. Taste and adjust seasoning. Serve chilled or at room temperature.

> ## ❖ Variation
> For a milder salad, omit serrano pepper.

Kale quinoa tabbouleh

Serves 4

Serves 4

Halfway between a tabbouleh and a fresh vegetable slaw, this dish brightens all it shares a plate with. Serve it alongside a burger, a sandwich or as a breezy cool down to a spicy casserole.

1	bunch kale, stems removed, leaves finely chopped	1
2 cups	cooked quinoa	500 mL
2	tomatoes, seeded and finely chopped	2
4	green onions, white and light green parts only, chopped	4
2	cloves garlic, finely minced	2
1/2 cup	finely chopped parsley	125 mL
1/4 cup	finely chopped mint	60 mL
1/2 cup	freshly squeezed lemon juice	125 mL
1/4 cup	olive oil	60 mL
1 tsp	salt	5 mL
1/2 tsp	freshly ground black pepper	2 mL
Pinch	cayenne pepper	Pinch

1. In a large bowl, combine kale, quinoa, tomatoes, green onions, garlic, parsley and mint.

2. In a small bowl, whisk together lemon juice, oil, salt, pepper and cayenne and pour over vegetables. Gently toss to combine. Let stand for 10 minutes at room temperature before serving.

> ### ❖ Variation
> *Southwestern Tabbouleh:* Add 1 cup (250 mL) cooked black beans, 1/2 jalapeño, minced, and 3/4 tsp (3 mL) ground cumin.

Jicama, carrot and ginger salad

Fresh and oil free, this super-healthy salad brings color and zest to any table.

✖ Tip

To garner orange flesh, slice off both ends of orange. Use a sharp paring knife to remove the peel and pith. Slice into the orange along separating membrane and remove segments.

	Zest and juice of 2 limes	
½ tsp	cayenne pepper	2 mL
½ tsp	salt	2 mL
½	large jicama, peeled and cut into matchsticks	½
3	large carrots, peeled and grated	3
1	piece (1 inch/2.5 cm) gingerroot, peeled and cut into thin matchsticks	1
2	navel oranges, peeled and cut into segments (see Tip, left)	2

1. In a small bowl, whisk together lime zest, lime juice, cayenne pepper and salt.

2. In a large bowl, toss together jicama, carrots and ginger. Pour lime mixture over salad and toss to coat. Gently fold in orange segments. Taste and adjust seasonings and serve.

Green papaya salad

A favorite in Thailand, this exciting combination of flavors and textures create a tart, sweet, spicy, fresh and crunchy treat.

3 tbsp	freshly squeezed lime juice	45 mL
3 tbsp	brown sugar	45 mL
2 tbsp	tamari	30 mL
2	cloves garlic, finely minced	2
2	Thai bird's-eye chiles, minced	2
1 lb	green papaya, peeled and seeded	500 g
1	tomato, seeded and sliced	1
2	green onions, white and light green parts only, chopped	2
½ cup	chopped cilantro leaves	125 mL
½ cup	chopped roasted peanuts	125 mL

1. In a bowl, whisk together lime juice, brown sugar, tamari, garlic and chiles.

2. Using a julienne peeler, peel papaya into long strips and place in a large bowl. Add tomato, green onions and cilantro. Add dressing and toss to coat. Top with peanuts.

✖ Variation

Add 1 cup (250 mL) lightly steamed green beans.

Yellow tomato and three-melon salad

Serves 6 to 8

Beautifully ripe tomatoes and watermelon are plentiful and less expensive during the hottest days of summer. Together they provide a refreshing cooler, perfect for a party and easy on the pocketbook.

✖ Tip

Watermelons do not ripen further after picking. To ensure that a melon was ready for harvest, check to see that it is heavy for its size and the stem end is smooth, having separated cleanly from the vine.

4	yellow tomatoes, cut into 2-inch (5 cm) chunks	4
2 cups	red watermelon, seeded and cut into 2-inch (5 cm) chunks (see Tip, left)	500 mL
2 cups	cantaloupe, seeded and cut into 2-inch (5 cm) chunks	500 mL
2 cups	honeydew melon, seeded and cut into 2-inch (5 cm) chunks	500 mL
1/4 cup	olive oil	60 mL
2 tbsp	white balsamic vinegar	30 mL
2 tbsp	chopped mint leaves	30 mL
2 tbsp	chopped basil leaves	30 mL
3/4 tsp	freshly ground black pepper	3 mL
1/2 tsp	salt	2 mL

1. In a serving bowl, combine tomatoes, watermelon, cantaloupe and honeydew.

2. In a bowl, whisk together oil, vinegar, mint, basil, pepper and salt. Pour over tomato and melon mixture and toss to combine. Serve immediately or refrigerate for up to 4 hours.

Mandarin spinach salad with creamy poppy seed dressing

This salad is a welcome
classic of fresh baby
spinach, tangy red
onions, sweet and
succulent mandarin
oranges, creamy
avocado and Crunchy
Tempehacon Bits.
There will be no
leftovers.

✖ Tip
The dressing makes about
¾ cup (175 mL) and can be
made and refrigerated in
an airtight container for up
to 3 days. If refrigerated,
allow dressing to come
to room temperature
before using.

¼ cup	freshly squeezed orange juice	60 mL
2 tbsp	Creamy Mayonnaise (page 19) or store-bought vegan alternative	30 mL
2 tbsp	Champagne vinegar or white wine vinegar	30 mL
1 tbsp	minced shallot	15 mL
2 tsp	poppy seeds	10 mL
½ tsp	Dijon mustard	2 mL
½ tsp	salt	2 mL
Pinch	freshly ground black pepper	Pinch
½ cup	olive oil	125 mL
8 cups	baby spinach	2 L
½	small red onion, thinly sliced	½
4	mandarin oranges, peeled and sectioned	4
1	avocado, chopped	1
1 cup	Crunchy Tempehacon Bits (page 22) or store-bought vegan alternative	250 mL
2 cups	Giant Garlicky Croutons (page 119) or store-bought vegan alternative, optional	500 mL

1. In a small deep bowl, whisk together orange juice,
   mayonnaise, vinegar, shallot, poppy seeds, mustard, salt
   and pepper. Whisk in oil until dressing is thoroughly
   blended. Taste and adjust seasonings.

2. Place spinach in a large bowl. Add ¼ cup (60 mL) of
   the dressing and toss, adding more dressing if desired.
   Divide spinach among 4 salad plates, top with sliced
   red onion, orange wedges, avocado and Tempehacon
   bits. Scatter croutons over top, if using, and serve. Pass
   dressing at the table.

✖ Variation
In season, strawberries are a luscious substitute
for orange sections.

The Mains

Baked ginger-lime tofu with caramelized onions

Serves 4

Peanut oil adds a level of flavor to the caramelized onions, creating a rich and savory topping for the baked tofu steaks. The marinade is reduced to become a lovely sauce over steamed rice.

✖ Preheat oven to 400°F (200°C)
✖ 11-by 7-inch (28 by 18 cm) glass baking dish, lightly oiled
✖ Baking sheet, lined with lightly oiled parchment

2	onions, thinly sliced	2
2 tbsp	peanut oil	30 mL
1 tsp	salt	5 mL
3	cloves garlic, crushed	3
1	shallot, chopped	1
2/3 cup	tamari	150 mL
1/4 cup	freshly squeezed lime juice	60 mL
2 tbsp	grated fresh gingerroot	30 mL
2 tbsp	chopped fresh cilantro	30 mL
2 tsp	brown rice syrup	10 mL
1	package (16 oz/500 g) extra-firm tofu, drained, pressed (see page 12) and cut into 4 pieces	1
6 cups	hot steamed white rice	1.5 L

1. In prepared baking dish, toss onions with oil and salt. Cover with foil and roast in preheated oven, stirring occasionally, until golden brown and caramelized, 1 to 1½ hours. When done, cover with foil and set aside.

2. Meanwhile, in a blender, combine garlic, shallot, tamari, lime juice, ginger, cilantro and brown rice syrup and purée until smooth. Transfer to a shallow baking dish, add tofu and turn to coat. Cover dish and refrigerate, turning tofu at least once.

3. When onions have caramelized, reduce oven temperature to 375°F (190°C). Transfer tofu to prepared baking sheet. Pour marinade into a small saucepan and set aside. Bake tofu for 15 minutes. Flip tofu and bake for 10 minutes for moist tofu, or 15 to 20 minutes for dense and chewy tofu. During last 10 minutes of baking tofu, place saucepan with marinade over medium heat and bring to a boil. Reduce heat and simmer, stirring occasionally, until slightly thickened, 6 to 10 minutes.

4. Serve baked tofu topped with caramelized onions along with a generous serving of rice drizzled with reduced marinade.

Teriyaki tempeh satay with peanut sauce

Serves 4 to 6

Crispy teriyaki tempeh provides just the right crunch drizzled with a smooth and spicy peanut sauce. Super easy and very festive, this dish is perfect piled high on rice and served with bright sautéed pea greens and garlic.

Tip

Peanut sauce can be made ahead and refrigerated in an airtight container for up to 1 week. Bring to room temperature before using.

- Blender

Peanut Sauce

1 cup	natural unsweetened peanut butter	250 mL
2 tbsp	coconut milk	30 mL
2 tbsp	tamari	30 mL
2 tbsp	agave nectar	30 mL
1 tbsp	freshly squeezed lime juice	15 mL
1 tsp	garlic chile sauce	5 mL
1/4 to 1/2 cup	hot water	60 to 125 mL
2 cups	peanut oil	500 mL
2	packages (each 8 oz/250 g) teriyaki tempeh, cut lengthwise into 1/2-inch (1 cm) strips	2

1. *Peanut Sauce:* In blender, combine peanut butter, coconut milk, tamari, agave, lime juice and garlic chile sauce and purée until smooth, drizzling in hot water as needed to thin sauce. Set aside.
2. In a large heavy-bottomed saucepan, heat oil over high heat. When a small crumb of tempeh dropped into oil immediately sizzles, oil is ready. Working in batches, carefully place tempeh in hot oil and fry until light brown and crispy, 3 to 4 minutes. Using a slotted spoon remove from oil and transfer to a plate lined with paper towels. Serve hot with peanut sauce for dipping.

Classic tempehacon avocado burger

Hearty and toothsome ground seitan is held together with creamy and flavorful ground tempeh and mixed with finely chopped onion, a few spices and a dash of liquid smoke. Top this off with avocado and slices of Maple Bourbon Tempehacon for a sure winner.

✖ Tip

Tempeh is a delicious and versatile soy product with a nutty flavor and pleasing texture that is high in protein and low in fat. Cooked and fermented soy beans are formed into blocks or patties and sold in many grocery and natural food stores either plain or with added grains, flavorings and spices.

✖ Food processor

5½ oz	Old-School Seitan (page 28) or Quick Basic Seitan (page 29) or store-bought	165 g
3 oz	three-grain tempeh (see Tip, left)	90 g
⅓ cup	finely chopped onion	75 mL
1	clove garlic, minced	1
½ cup	chickpea flour, sifted, divided	125 mL
1 tbsp	dried parsley flakes	15 mL
½ tsp	smoked paprika	2 mL
½ tsp	dried thyme, crushed	2 mL
½ tsp	salt	2 mL
¼ tsp	freshly ground black pepper	1 mL
¾ tsp	liquid smoke	3 mL
2 tbsp	grapeseed oil	30 mL
4 tbsp	Creamy Mayonnaise (page 19) or store-bought vegan alternative	60 mL
4	sesame seed buns, halved and warmed	4
1	avocado, sliced	1
¼	red onion, very thinly sliced	¼
1	large very ripe tomato, thinly sliced	1
8 to 12	slices Maple Bourbon Tempehacon (page 27) or store-bought vegan alternative	8 to 12
4 to 8	red leaf lettuce	4 to 8

1. In food processor, pulse seitan until ground. Measure 1 cup (250 mL), reserving any extra for another use, and transfer to a bowl. Grind tempeh and measure ¾ cup (175 mL). Add to seitan in bowl. Add onion, garlic, ¼ cup (60 mL) of the chickpea flour, parsley, paprika, thyme, salt and pepper and mix with hands until well combined. Sprinkle liquid smoke over all and mix until well blended. Mixture should hold together when squeezed into a ball. If necessary, add additional liquid if too dry or chickpea flour if too wet.

✖ Tip

Patties may be formed up to 4 hours before using, covered and refrigerated. Do not dust with chickpea flour until just before cooking.

2. Divide burger mixture into four equal portions and form each into a ball, then carefully flatten into a patty, about ¾ inch (2 cm) thick, smoothing any rough edges (see Tip, left). Dust tops liberally with remaining ¼ cup (60 mL) of chickpea flour, carefully turn and dust bottoms.

3. Place a large heavy-bottomed skillet over medium-high heat and let pan get hot. Add oil and tip pan to coat. Using a spatula, carefully place patties into hot oil and cook until bottoms are well browned and slightly crisp, 2 to 4 minutes. Carefully flip and cook until second sides are browned and slightly crisp, 1 to 2 minutes. Transfer cooked burgers to a plate.

4. To serve, spread mayonnaise on cut side of bun halves. Place a burger on bottom half and layer with avocado slices, red onion slices, tomato slices, 2 to 3 slices of tempehacon and lettuce leaves. Set remaining bun halves on top and serve immediately.

Crispy tempeh pita with creamy tahini dressing

Serves 2

Hot crisp tempeh strips, cool crunchy vegetables, and a creamy savory dressing wrapped in a soft warm pita pocket makes a scrumptious meal destined to become a family favorite.

Tip

Garlic doesn't need to be chopped when adding to a mixture such as a marinade or to flavor oil. Crushing the garlic roughly once or twice with the side of a knife flattens and opens the clove, which allows the flavor to be incorporated into the marinade.

3 tbsp	tamari	45 mL
1 tbsp	grated fresh gingerroot	15 mL
1/2 tsp	dry mustard	2 mL
1 tsp	toasted sesame oil	5 mL
2	cloves garlic, crushed (see Tip, left)	2
8 oz	three-grain tempeh, cut lengthwise into 8 slices (see Tip, page 176)	250 g
2 to 3 tbsp	olive oil	30 to 45 mL
2	6-inch (15 cm) pitas, warmed	2
1/4 cup	Creamy Tahini Dressing (page 303) or store-bought vegan alternative	60 mL
1/2 cup	thinly sliced napa cabbage	125 mL
1/4	red bell pepper, thinly sliced	1/4
1/2	avocado, thinly sliced	1/2

1. In a shallow baking dish, whisk together tamari, ginger, mustard, sesame oil and garlic. Place tempeh slices in marinade and turn to coat. Cover and refrigerate, turning occasionally, for 2 hours.
2. Place a large skillet over medium-high heat and let pan get hot. Add 2 tbsp (30 mL) of the oil and tip pan to coat. Remove tempeh from marinade, draining well and discarding marinade. Carefully place tempeh into hot oil, in batches if necessary to avoid crowding pan, and fry, flipping once, until crispy and golden brown, about 2 minutes per side. If additional oil is needed between batches, allow oil to heat before adding tempeh. Transfer fried tempeh to a plate lined with paper towels.
3. Cut each pita in half, gently separate at opening to form a pocket. Spread 2 tbsp (30 mL) of the dressing inside pitas and fill each with half of the tempeh, cabbage, bell pepper and avocado. Serve immediately.

Variation

Spread uncut pitas with dressing and top with sandwich ingredients. Fold pita up like a gyro or taco.

Eggplant caponata with roasted potatoes

Serves 6	

Caponata is a Sicilian dish of eggplant and other vegetables with pine nuts cooked in olive oil and served at room temperature. Be sure to serve this with lots of rustic coarse bread.

⊞ Preheat oven to 450°F (230°C)
⊞ Baking sheet, lined with parchment paper

1	large eggplant, cut into 1/2-inch (1 cm) cubes	1
1 1/2 tsp	salt, divided	7 mL
2	medium Yukon gold potatoes, cut into 1/2-inch (1 cm) cubes	2
7 tbsp	olive oil, divided	105 mL
1/4 tsp	freshly ground black pepper, divided	1 mL
3	stalks celery, cut into matchsticks, or thinly sliced lengthwise, then cut into 1-inch (2.5 cm) pieces	3
6 oz	canned green olives, drained	175 g
3/4 cup	fresh or frozen corn kernels (thawed if frozen)	175 mL
1/2 cup	pine nuts	125 mL
3 tbsp	drained capers	45 mL
3 tbsp	white wine vinegar	45 mL

1. Place eggplant in a colander, toss with 1 tsp (5 mL) of the salt and set aside to drain for about 20 minutes. Rinse and pat dry.

2. In a bowl, toss potatoes with 1 tbsp (15 mL) of the oil, 1/4 tsp (1 mL) of salt and 1/8 tsp (0.5 mL) of black pepper. Spread potatoes on prepared baking sheet and bake in preheated oven until fork tender, about 15 minutes. Remove and set aside.

3. Place a large heavy-bottomed skillet over medium heat and let pan get hot. Add remaining 6 tbsp (90 mL) of oil and tip pan to coat. Add eggplant and cook, stirring frequently, until tender, 8 to 10 minutes. Using a slotted spoon transfer eggplant to a dish and set aside.

4. Return skillet to medium–high heat. Add roasted potatoes, celery, green olives, corn kernels, pine nuts and capers and cook, stirring frequently, until celery is tender, about 5 minutes. Add vinegar and cook, stirring frequently, until evaporated, 1 to 2 minutes. Add remaining 1/4 tsp (1 mL) of salt and 1/8 tsp (0.5 mL) of black pepper. Serve hot or at room temperature.

Korean BBQ

Serves 4 to 6

A sesame-soy marinade with a hint of sweetness glazes charred and crispy thinly sliced seitan. Once you taste this stove-top version of Korean BBQ, with a tender and savory center, it will be love at first bite. The marinade doubles as a sauce without the need to boil away any contaminates.

✂ Variation

For a traditional dipping sauce, try Daikon Dipping Sauce (page 287).

Marinade

1 cup	tamari	250 mL
1/4 cup	toasted sesame oil	60 mL
1/4 cup	granulated sugar	60 mL
10	green onions, white and green parts, thinly sliced	10
10	cloves garlic, minced	10
1 tbsp	grated fresh gingerroot	15 mL
1/4 cup	sesame seeds	60 mL
1 1/2 tbsp	freshly ground black pepper	22 mL
2 tsp	Asian hot sauce, such as sambal oelek	10 mL
1 1/2 lbs	Old-School Seitan (page 28) or Quick Basic Seitan (page 29) or store-bought, cut into 1/4-inch (0.5 cm) thick slices	750 g
1 tbsp	olive oil (approx.)	15 mL

1. *Marinade:* In a bowl, combine tamari, sesame oil, sugar, green onions, garlic, ginger, sesame seeds, pepper and hot sauce, mixing well to blend.

2. Place seitan in a large resealable storage bag and add marinade. Seal and lay bag flat in a baking dish, arranging so seitan slices are covered with marinade. Refrigerate for at least 4 hours or for up to 12 hours.

3. Preheat oven to 200°F (100°C).

4. Transfer seitan to a plate and pour marinade into a small pitcher. Place a large heavy-bottomed skillet over medium-high heat and let pan get hot. Add oil and tip pan to coat. Arrange seitan in pan, in batches if necessary to avoid crowding, taking care as dripping marinade will pop and spatter. Cook, flipping once, until edges are well browned and seitan is charred, 1 to 2 minutes per side. Transfer cooked seitan to an ovenproof platter, drizzle with a spoonful of marinade, loosely cover with foil and hold in warm oven. Add oil to coat bottom of pan, if necessary, and cook remaining slices. Serve and pass pitcher of marinade.

Laredo enchilada bake

Fresh ingredients are paired with a few store-bought items to make this a quick and satisfying supper. Serving this tasty entrée with a pre-packaged green salad makes this a great choice when a busy day spills into a busy night.

✖ Variations

Pinto or kidney beans may be added or substituted for black beans.

Vegan Monterey Jack cheese alternative can be substituted for Cheddar.

✖ Preheat oven to 375°F (190°C)
✖ 8-inch (20 cm) square glass baking dish, lightly oiled

3 tbsp	olive oil	45 mL
1/2	onion, chopped	1/2
2	cloves garlic, chopped	2
2 cups	diced potatoes	500 mL
2 cups	diced zucchini	500 mL
1 tsp	chili powder	5 mL
1 tsp	salt	5 mL
1/2 tsp	ground cumin	2 mL
1	can (14 to 19 oz/398 to 540 mL) black beans, drained and rinsed	1
1 cup	fresh or frozen corn kernels (thawed if frozen)	250 mL
1/2 cup	drained black olives, sliced	125 mL
1	can (4 oz/127 mL) chopped roasted mild green chiles	1
8	6-inch (15 cm) corn tortillas	8
4 oz	grated vegan Cheddar cheese alternative	125 g
1	jar or can (12 oz/375 mL) enchilada sauce	1
1/2 cup	Basic Sour Cream (page 21) or store-bought vegan alternative, optional	125 mL
1/2 cup	diced tomatoes, optional	125 mL

1. Place a large skillet over medium heat and let pan get hot. Add oil and tip pan to coat. Add onion and garlic and cook, stirring occasionally, until soft, 3 to 5 minutes. Add potatoes and cook, stirring frequently, about 5 minutes. Add zucchini, chili powder, salt and cumin and cook, stirring frequently, until potatoes are still slightly firm and not completely cooked, 4 to 5 minutes. Remove from heat, stir in black beans, corn, olives and green chiles.

2. Place 4 tortillas, overlapping, in bottom of prepared baking dish. Layer half of vegetable mixture, half of cheese and half of enchilada sauce on top. Repeat process, ending with enchilada sauce.

3. Cover with foil and bake in preheated oven until bubbly, 25 to 30 minutes. Uncover and bake until top is lightly browned and cheese is melted, 10 to 15 minutes more. Let cool for 10 minutes. Cut into squares and serve with a dollop of sour cream, if using, and a scattering of chopped tomatoes, if using.

Orange tequila sizzlin' fajitas

Fajitas are a great centerpiece for a party and everyone gets to join in the fun. While the heady aromas are wafting from the kitchen or the grill, serve Blended Top-Shelf Margaritas (page 325) and appetizers.

✖ Tip

Place platter of vegetables with tongs on the dining or buffet table along with the basket of tortillas and bowls of guacamole, salsa and lime wedges. Allow guests to assemble their own fajitas.

2 tbsp	each orange and lime juice	30 mL
2 tbsp	tequila	30 mL
2	cloves garlic, minced	2
1	small jalapeño, seeded and minced	1
2 tbsp	chopped fresh cilantro	30 mL
1 tsp	ground cumin	5 mL
2	portobello mushroom caps, sliced into $\frac{1}{2}$-inch (1 cm) strips	2
2 tbsp	olive oil (approx.)	30 mL
1	green bell pepper, seeded and sliced into $\frac{1}{2}$-inch (1 cm) strips	1
1	onion, sliced lengthwise into $\frac{1}{2}$-inch (1 cm) strips	1
$\frac{1}{2}$ tsp	salt	2 mL
12	6- to 10-inch (15 to 25 cm) flour tortillas	12
	Guacamole (page 50) or store-bought Year-Round Blender Tomato Salsa (page 300) Lime wedges	

1. In a shallow bowl, whisk together orange juice, lime juice, tequila, garlic, jalapeño, cilantro and cumin. Add mushrooms, turning to coat. Let marinate, turning occasionally, 20 to 30 minutes. Remove mushrooms from marinade, reserving marinade. Set aside.

2. Heat a large skillet over medium–high heat and let pan get hot. Add oil and tip pan to coat. Add mushrooms, bell pepper, onion and salt and cook, stirring frequently, for 2 minutes. Reduce heat to medium and cook, stirring occasionally, until vegetables are softened and mushrooms are golden brown, 6 to 8 minutes. Add additional oil, if necessary. Add marinade, increase heat to medium–high and cook, stirring frequently, until marinade is evaporated, 3 to 4 minutes. Transfer vegetables to a platter.

3. Meanwhile, heat tortillas in a large skillet over medium heat until hot and browned in a few areas, 1 to 2 minutes per side. Wrap tortillas in a clean kitchen towel placed in a basket to keep warm.

4. To make fajitas, spoon fajita mixture into a tortilla, top with a spoonful each of guacamole and salsa and a squeeze of lime and fold tortilla to enclose the filling.

Roasted beet tacos with marinated shredded kale

Serves 4 to 6

Jewel-toned beets topped with bright crisp greens combine to create a gorgeous and very healthy lunch or dinner entrée. This recipe saves time and energy by roasting the beets and oven caramelizing the onions at the same time. As long as you are heating up the oven, roast additional beets to use tomorrow in a roasted beet salad.

✖ Preheat oven to 400°F (200°C)
✖ 11- by 7-inch (28 by 18 cm) glass baking dish, lightly oiled
✖ Baking sheet, lined with parchment paper

2	large onions, thinly sliced	2
6 tbsp	olive oil, divided	90 mL
	Salt	
4	medium red or golden beets, with greens	4
1/2 tsp	freshly ground black pepper, divided	2 mL
	Grated zest and juice of 1 lemon	
6 cups	shredded kale (1/2 large bunch)	1.5 L
6 to 8	4-inch (10 cm) corn tortillas, warmed	6 to 8

1. Arrange racks in oven to accommodate both a baking sheet and shallow baking dish.

2. In prepared baking dish, combine onions, 2 tbsp (30 mL) of the oil and 1 tsp (5 mL) of salt. Cover with foil and roast in preheated oven, stirring occasionally, until golden brown and caramelized, 1 to 1 1/2 hours.

3. Meanwhile, trim greens from beets. Discard stems and chop greens. Set greens aside. Peel beets and cut into 1/4-inch (0.5 cm) dice. In a bowl, toss beets with 2 tbsp (30 mL) of olive oil, 1 tsp (5 mL) of salt and 1/4 tsp (1 mL) of black pepper. Spread beets onto prepared baking sheet and roast, stirring occasionally, until beets are fork-tender, 20 to 25 minutes.

4. Meanwhile, in a large bowl, whisk together lemon zest, 2 tbsp (30 mL) of the lemon juice, remaining 2 tbsp (30 mL) of oil, pinch of salt and remaining 1/4 tsp (1 mL) of black pepper. Add shredded kale and beet green tops and toss to coat. Cover and refrigerate until needed.

5. To serve, spoon a generous amount of caramelized onion down center of each warmed tortilla, top with roasted beets and marinated shredded kale and beet greens.

Roasted portobello sandwich with savory au jus

If you are craving a French dip sandwich look no further! The complex flavors of the rich Homemade Vegetable Bouillon create a hearty and delectable savory au jus dipping sauce.

✖ Tip

Worcestershire sauce is made with fish but there are very good substitutes on the market, such as Henderson's Relish. If a vegan substitute is not available, use tamari or liquid amino acids.

✖ Preheat oven to 400°F (200°C)
✖ 2 baking sheets, 1 sheet lined with parchment paper, 1 sheet lightly oiled

2	portobello mushroom caps, cut into $\frac{1}{4}$- to $\frac{1}{2}$-inch (0.5 to 1 cm) slices	2
2 tbsp	olive oil, divided	30 mL
$\frac{1}{2}$ tsp	salt, divided	2 mL
$\frac{1}{4}$ tsp	freshly ground black pepper, divided	1 mL
2	Japanese eggplants, cut into $\frac{1}{2}$-inch (1 cm) diagonal slices	2
2	red bell peppers, cut into $\frac{1}{2}$-inch (1 cm) rings	2
1	onion, cut into $\frac{1}{2}$-inch (1 cm) slices	1
$2\frac{1}{2}$ cups	water	625 mL
2 tsp	Homemade Vegetable Bouillon (page 32)	10 mL
2 tbsp	tomato paste	30 mL
1 tbsp	vegan Worcestershire sauce or tamari (see Tip, left)	15 mL
$\frac{1}{2}$ tsp	dried thyme	2 mL
$\frac{1}{2}$ tsp	finely chopped dried rosemary	2 mL
4	sandwich rolls, slit open	4

1. In a large bowl, gently toss portobello mushroom slices with 1 tbsp (15 mL) of the oil, $\frac{1}{4}$ tsp (1 mL) of salt and $\frac{1}{8}$ tsp (0.5 mL) of black pepper. Spread mushrooms evenly on oiled baking sheet and set aside. In same large bowl, toss eggplant, bell peppers and onion slices with remaining 1 tbsp (15 mL) of oil, $\frac{1}{4}$ tsp (1 mL) of salt and $\frac{1}{8}$ tsp (0.5 mL) of black pepper. Spread evenly on remaining baking sheet and place on bottom rack of oven. Place mushrooms on middle rack and bake for 10 minutes. Remove both sheets from oven, stir vegetables and mushrooms and return both sheets to oven. Bake until tender, about 10 minutes.

2. In a small saucepan over medium heat, combine water, vegetable bouillon, tomato paste, Worcestershire sauce, thyme and rosemary and bring to a boil. Reduce heat and simmer, stirring occasionally, until slightly reduced and thickened, about 10 minutes.

3. To serve, divide vegetables equally among split rolls. Ladle au jus into 4 individual bowls and serve with each sandwich.

Rustic beer-braised seitan and portobellos with macaroni

Serves 6 to 8

Tearing the seitan rather than cutting it creates an appealing uneven shape that helps to give this dish its rustic feel. For a more elegant dish, cut seitan into bite-size pieces and use flat cut pasta rather than shaped macaroni.

✖ Tip

Browning foods using high-heat cooking in a skillet or in the oven creates deep, rich flavors. Take full advantage of this by deglazing the pan. This is done by stirring in liquids while scraping the bottom of the pan to loosen and incorporate all of the browned bits. These flavors will be transferred into the cooking liquid and ultimately into the finished dish.

✖ Variation

Use 12 oz (375 g) fresh pasta and decrease cooking time to about 10 minutes.

✖ Preheat oven to 450°F (230°C)
✖ 14- by 11-inch (35 by 27.5 cm) roasting pan

1 lb	Old-School Seitan (page 28) or store-bought	500 g
2	onions, thinly sliced	2
4	large cloves garlic, coarsely chopped	4
3	large portobello mushroom caps, cut into large bite-size pieces	3
1/3 cup	olive oil	75 mL
2 tsp	dried thyme	10 mL
1 1/2 tsp	salt	7 mL
1 1/2 tsp	freshly ground black pepper	7 mL
2	bottles (each 12 oz/341 mL) sweet and nutty dark beer	2
4 cups	Vegetable Broth (page 31) or store-bought, divided	1 L
2 tbsp	tomato paste	30 mL
1 cup	drained oil-packed sun-dried tomatoes, sliced	250 mL
6 oz	dried macaroni	175 g
	Chopped parsley	

1. Form seitan into 12 pieces and place in roasting pan along with onions, garlic and mushrooms. Drizzle with oil, sprinkle with thyme, salt and pepper and toss to coat, breaking apart any seitan pieces that stick together. Bake in preheated oven, stirring once, for 25 minutes.

2. Stir in beer and 1 cup (250 mL) of the vegetable broth, scraping up all browned bits to deglaze pan. Stir in tomato paste and sun-dried tomatoes. Reduce oven temperature to 350°F (180°C) and braise, basting seitan occasionally with braising liquid as it browns, for 40 minutes.

3. Push seitan, mushrooms and onions to sides of pan, add remaining vegetable broth and return to oven until pan liquids begin to simmer. Stir in pasta, cover with foil and bake, stirring occasionally, until pasta is tender, but firm, about 20 minutes. Stir occasionally to ensure all pasta is immersed and cooking. Serve hot, garnished with chopped parsley.

Spicy adzuki futomaki with avocado and micro greens

Adzuki beans are
roughly mashed with
chile-garlic sauce and
sake to create a spicy
filling for fat rolls
called futomaki. Serve
with tamari sauce and
a dab of wasabi for
dipping and, of course,
cold Japanese beer.

✖ Tips

Fill a small bowl with water
and 2 tbsp (30 mL) rice
vinegar and wet hands
to prevent sticking while
rolling rolls.

Not all sake is vegan
friendly as some is filtered
with animal products.
Check websites such
as Barnivore for more
information or ask at your
local liquor store.

✖ Food processor
✖ Bamboo sushi rolling mat

Rice

2 cups	sushi or short-grain rice, rinsed until water runs clear	500 mL
2 cups	water	500 mL
3 tbsp	rice vinegar	45 mL
7 tsp	granulated sugar	35 mL
2 tsp	salt	10 mL

Filling

2 cups	cooked adzuki beans	500 mL
1 tbsp	vegan sake (see Tips, left)	15 mL
2 tsp	tamari	10 mL
2 tsp	grated fresh gingerroot	10 mL
$\frac{1}{2}$ tsp	chile-garlic sauce	2 mL
2 tsp	Creamy Mayonnaise (page 19) or store-bought vegan alternative	10 mL
4	sheets toasted nori	4
$\frac{1}{2}$ cup	chopped roasted peanuts	125 mL
1	avocado, thinly sliced	1
$\frac{1}{2}$ cup	micro greens	125 mL
2 tbsp	rice wine vinegar	30 mL
	Tamari, optional	
	Wasabi, optional	

1. *Rice:* Place rice in a medium saucepan, add water and bring to a boil over high heat. Reduce heat to low and cook, covered, for 15 minutes. Remove pan from heat and let stand, covered, without stirring, for 10 minutes.

2. Meanwhile, in a small microwave-safe bowl, combine vinegar, sugar and salt and microwave for 10 seconds. Stir to dissolve sugar. Let cool.

3. Fluff rice and transfer to a large bowl. Sprinkle vinegar mixture over rice while gently folding to combine and completely coat. Fan and fluff rice while cooling until just warm.

4. *Filling:* In a bowl, combine beans, sake, tamari, ginger, chile sauce and mayonnaise. Using a fork, roughly mash.

5. Place bamboo rolling mat on a work surface in front of you with bamboo strips running crosswise. Place a sheet of nori, shiny side down, on mat lined up with mat edge closest to you. Cover nori sheet with one-quarter of the rice, pressing to $\frac{1}{4}$-inch (0.5 cm) thickness and leaving a $1\frac{1}{2}$-inch (4 cm) border along edge farthest away from you.

6. Spoon one-quarter of the bean filling in a line on rice crosswise, about 1 inch (2.5 cm) from nearest edge. Sprinkle with one-quarter of the peanuts. Lay rows of one-quarter each of the avocado and micro greens crosswise along outer edge of filling row. Starting at edge closest to you, lift bamboo mat and fold over ingredients, rolling with a light but steady pressure and peeling mat back as you roll. Using fingers, moisten riceless nori border with vinegar and finish rolling. Using mat, press gently but firmly to close and seal roll. Repeat process with remaining ingredients to make 3 more rolls.

7. Cut roll crosswise into 6 or 8 slices. Serve with wasabi and tamari, if using, for dipping.

❖ Variation

Mash adzuki bean mixture with $\frac{1}{4}$ cup (60 mL) mashed cooked sweet potato, omit mayonnaise and substitute $\frac{1}{2}$ cup (125 mL) finely chopped blanched broccoli for avocado.

Spring vegetable pot pies

Makes 4

Celebrate the annual opening of your local farmer's market with this pot pie made with the first vegetables of spring. Delectable potatoes, asparagus and edamame are baked in an herbed sauce topped with a flaky golden crust. Perfect for a Sunday supper.

✖ Tip

For quick crackers, reroll dough scraps and cut to desired shapes and sizes. Prick with a fork and bake at 425°F (220°C) until golden brown, 5 to 10 minutes. Sprinkle with sesame seeds or salt and pepper while hot.

✖ Food processor
✖ Four 14-oz (425 mL) baking dishes or ramekins
✖ Baking sheet, lined with parchment paper

Crust

1¼ cups	all-purpose flour	300 mL
¼ cup	cornmeal	60 mL
½ tsp	salt	2 mL
3	sprigs fresh thyme, leaves stripped	3
¼ cup	vegan shortening, chilled	60 mL
¼ cup	vegan hard margarine, chilled, cut into 8 pieces (see Tips, right)	60 mL
3 to 4 tbsp	cold water	45 to 60 mL

Filling

2 cups	cubed yellow or red potatoes	500 mL
½ tsp	salt	2 mL
2 tbsp	vegan hard margarine	30 mL
1	small onion, chopped	1
1	small shallot, diced	1
8 oz	mushrooms, sliced	250 g
2 cups	shelled edamame, thawed if frozen	500 mL
½ cup	green peas	125 mL
½ cup	asparagus tips	125 mL
2 cups	packed baby spinach, chopped	500 mL
2 tbsp	all-purpose flour	30 mL
½ cup	Vegetable Broth (page 31) or store-bought	125 mL
2 tbsp	chopped Italian flat-leaf parsley	30 mL
½ tsp	salt	2 mL
½ tsp	freshly ground black pepper	2 mL
2 tsp	canola oil	10 mL
12	sprigs fresh thyme, optional	12

1. *Crust:* In food processor, combine flour, cornmeal and salt and pulse until combined. Add thyme leaves and pulse 2 times. Dot shortening and margarine around work bowl and pulse 10 times. Scrape down sides and pulse until mixture is combined, about 5 times more. Sprinkle in 3 tbsp (45 mL) of water and pulse 10 times until dough holds together when gently squeezed. If too dry, add water, 1 tbsp (15 mL) at a time, and pulse until

dough holds together. Gather dough into a ball, flatten into a disk, wrap in plastic wrap and refrigerate until chilled, for at least 30 minutes or for up to 24 hours.

2. *Filling:* In a large saucepan, cover potatoes with cold water, add salt and bring to a boil over high heat. Reduce heat and boil gently until tender when pierced with a fork, about 5 minutes. Drain, reserving cooking water. Set aside.

3. Place a large skillet with a lid or a Dutch oven over medium heat and let pan get hot. Add margarine and tip pan to coat. Add onion and shallot and cook, stirring occasionally, until translucent, 5 to 6 minutes. Add mushrooms, edamame and ½ cup (125 mL) reserved potato cooking water. Cover, reduce heat to medium and cook for 5 minutes. Add peas, asparagus tips and spinach and cook, covered, for 5 minutes. Stir in flour, while gently scraping bottom of pan. Gradually add vegetable broth, while constantly stirring. Simmer, stirring, until thickened, 3 to 5 minutes. Remove from heat and stir in potatoes, parsley, salt and pepper. Taste and adjust seasoning. Divide among baking dishes. Arrange on prepared baking sheet and set aside.

4. Preheat oven to 425°F (220°C).

5. Sprinkle work surface with a little flour. Cut dough into four equal pieces. Working with one piece at a time, roll into a rough circle, approximately 1 inch (2.5 cm) larger than baking dish. Arrange dough circle over ramekin, allowing edges to hang attractively over sides, pressing lightly to seal over edge. Cut three venting slashes in crust and brush with ½ tsp (2 mL) of oil. Repeat with remaining dough and pot pies.

6. Bake pot pies in preheated oven until edges are golden, 15 to 18 minutes. Place a few stems of thyme upright through vent slash of each pot pie, if using, and serve warm.

Variations

Substitute spring onions and leeks for onion and shallot or Swiss chard and snow peas for the spinach and asparagus. Use any combination of fresh vegetables in season.

Stacked green chile enchiladas

Stacked green chile enchiladas tops my long list of reasons for visiting Santa Fe, New Mexico. Stunning beauty, world-class art, historic culture and green chile. What more could you want?

✖ Tips

Save time by using store-bought soy chorizo instead of seasoned textured soy protein. Always read the label, and check the sodium content while you are at it, especially on simple items like vegetable juice, where the manufacturer is looking to heighten the flavors.

These enchiladas are created individually and baked right on the dinner plate. To avoid damage to a table, place each plate on another of equal size or serve on very thick place mats.

* Preheat oven to 350°F (180°C)
* Baking sheet, lined with parchment paper
* Food processor
* 4 ovenproof dinner plates

Seasoned Textured Soy Protein

¾ cup	tomato juice	175 mL
½ tsp	salt	2 mL
½ tsp	ground cumin	2 mL
½ tsp	onion powder	2 mL
½ tsp	granulated garlic	2 mL
½ tsp	New Mexico red chile powder (see Tips, page 195)	2 mL
1 cup	textured soy protein (TSP) flakes	250 mL

Filling

3 tbsp	olive oil, divided	45 mL
1	onion, chopped	1
3	cloves garlic, minced	3
1 tsp	New Mexico red chile powder	5 mL
1 tsp	ground cumin	5 mL
1½ tsp	freshly squeezed lime juice	7 mL
½ tsp	salt	2 mL
1	can (4 oz/127 mL) diced mild green chiles	1
2 tsp	sunflower oil, divided	10 mL
8	6-inch (15 cm) white corn tortillas	8
1	small onion, chopped	1
7 cups	Roasted Tomatillo Sauce (page 290) or store-bought	1.75 L
1½ cups	shredded vegan Monterey Jack cheese alternative	375 mL
¼ to ½ cup	Basic Sour Cream (page 21)	60 to 125 mL
¼ to ½ cup	tomato salsa	60 to 125 mL
2 cups	shredded lettuce	500 mL
2	tomatoes, diced	2
2	avocados, diced	2

1. *Seasoned Textured Soy Protein:* In a small saucepan, combine tomato juice, salt, cumin, onion powder, granulated garlic and chile powder and bring just to a boil over medium-high heat. Remove from heat and stir in TSP, making sure to dampen all flakes. Let stand until ready to use or refrigerate in an airtight container for up to 5 days.

2. *Filling:* Place a large skillet over medium heat and let pan get hot. Add 2 tbsp (30 mL) of the olive oil and tip pan to coat. Add onion, garlic, chile powder and ground cumin and cook, stirring occasionally, until onions are translucent, 4 to 6 minutes. Move onions to sides of pan, add remaining 1 tbsp (15 mL) of oil to center of pan and let oil get hot. Stir in reconstituted TSP, lime juice, salt and green chiles. Cook, stirring frequently, until slightly browned, 5 to 6 minutes. Remove from heat and set aside.

3. *Assembly:* Place a clean large skillet over medium heat and let pan get hot. Add 1 tsp (5 mL) of the sunflower oil and tip pan to coat. Arrange tortillas in pan in batches, as necessary, and cook for a few seconds on each side. Transfer to paper towels to drain and repeat with remaining tortillas, adding more oil as necessary. Place a heated tortilla in middle of an ovenproof dinner plate, spoon on 1/2 cup (125 mL) of filling, one-quarter of chopped onion, 3/4 cup (175 mL) of sauce and 2 tbsp (30 mL) shredded cheese. Top with another tortilla, spoon on 1 cup (250 mL) of sauce and scatter with 1/4 cup (60 mL) shredded cheese. Repeat process on three additional plates. Transfer plates to preheated oven and bake until sauce is bubbly and cheese is melted, about 10 minutes.

4. Carefully remove hot plates from oven and top each enchilada with dollops of sour cream and tomato salsa. Arrange one-quarter of the lettuce, chopped tomato and avocado slices on each plate to one side of the enchilada. Serve immediately.

> ## ✖ Variation
> Textured vegetable protein (TVP), may be substituted for the textured soy protein (TSP).

Three-pepper tamale pie

Just like Mom made, if Mom loved chiles that is. The flavor and texture of the cornmeal crust pairs perfectly with the spicy bean, chile and tomato filling. A real stick-to-your-ribs kind of dinner.

✖ Variation

For a spicier tamale pie, add 2 chopped chipotle chiles and 1 tbsp (15 mL) adobo sauce from canned chipotles when you add the green chiles.

✖ **8-cup (2 L) glass baking dish, lightly oiled**

2 tbsp	olive oil	30 mL
1	onion, chopped	1
1	red bell pepper, chopped	1
2	cloves garlic, minced	2
1½ cups	drained cooked pinto beans	375 mL
1 cup	drained cooked kidney beans	250 mL
1 cup	frozen roasted corn kernels	250 mL
1	can (4 oz/127 mL) diced roasted mild green chiles	1
1 cup	canned diced tomatoes with juice	250 mL
1 cup	tomato sauce	250 mL
2 tsp	New Mexico red chile powder	10 mL
2 tsp	ground cumin	10 mL
¾ tsp	salt	3 mL

Topping

¾ cup	cornmeal	175 mL
2 cups	water	500 mL
¾ tsp	salt	3 mL
¾ tsp	chipotle chile powder, optional	3 mL
2 tbsp	vegan hard margarine	30 mL
½ cup	pitted black olives	125 mL

1. Place a large heavy-bottomed skillet over medium heat and let pan get hot. Add oil and tip pan to coat. Add onion, bell pepper and garlic and cook, stirring, until softened and slightly browned, 6 to 8 minutes.

2. Increase heat to medium-high. Stir in pinto beans, kidney beans, corn, green chiles, tomatoes, tomato sauce, chile powder, cumin and salt and bring just to a boil. Reduce heat and simmer until thickened, 20 to 25 minutes. Transfer to baking dish. Preheat oven to 375°F (190°C).

3. *Topping:* In a small saucepan, whisk together cornmeal and water. Whisk in salt and chile powder, if using. Bring to a boil over medium-high heat. Reduce heat and simmer, stirring frequently, until thickened, 8 to 10 minutes. Whisk in margarine. Spread mixture evenly over filling and dot top with olives.

4. Bake in preheated oven until filling is bubbly and top is golden brown, 35 to 45 minutes. Let tamale pie cool slightly before cutting and serving.

Vegetable paella

With the colors of a Spanish landscape, this richly flavored one-pan meal is fun and festive. Dinner on the deck and a pitcher of sangria; now that's relaxing. As cooking with seasonal vegetables produces superior flavors, use green beans if asparagus is unavailable.

✶ Tips

When garlic is browned too quickly it will become bitter. If sautéing with other vegetables, add garlic toward the end of the browning process.

To ensure time with your guests, make the paella up to 1 day ahead. Refrigerate cooled paella in an airtight container for up to 2 days. Spread in paella pan, cover and reheat in a 350°F (180°C) oven for 25 to 30 minutes.

✶ Preheat oven to 350°F (180°C)
✶ Paella pan or large ovenproof skillet

3 tbsp	olive oil	45 mL
1	onion, diced	1
1	large fennel bulb, trimmed and cut into bite-size pieces	1
4	cloves garlic, chopped	4
2 cups	short- or medium-grain white rice	500 mL
2 cups	warm water	500 mL
1½ cups	dry white wine	375 mL
½ tsp	paprika	2 mL
¾ tsp	saffron threads or ground turmeric	3 mL
1 tsp	salt	5 mL
1	can (14 oz/400 mL) artichoke hearts in water, drained	1
¾ cup	sliced drained oil-packed sun-dried tomatoes	175 mL
8 oz	thin asparagus or green beans, trimmed and halved	250 g
⅓ cup	green olives	75 mL
3 tbsp	chopped Italian flat-leaf parsley	45 mL

1. Place paella pan over medium heat and let pan get hot. Add oil and tip pan to coat. Add onion and fennel and cook, stirring frequently, until vegetables begin to soften, 4 to 5 minutes. Add garlic and cook, stirring frequently, until onions and fennel are lightly browned, 3 to 5 minutes. Mix in rice, lightly coating all grains with oil. Stir in water, wine, paprika, saffron, salt, artichoke hearts and sun-dried tomatoes. Gently shake pan to distribute rice evenly. Reduce heat and simmer for 10 minutes.

2. Remove pan from heat and scatter asparagus and green olives over rice. Cover pan and bake in preheated oven until rice is tender with a slightly crusted bottom, about 30 minutes.

3. Scatter chopped parsley over top and serve hot.

Tofu tikka masala

Serves 4 to 6

Tikka means small bits, and here the marinated tofu steps in. Oven broiling and then roasting the tofu cubes adds depth to this sumptuous dish. Letting this stand awhile intensifies the flavor, making this a perfect do-ahead dinner party dish. Be sure to serve plenty of naan as you will want to sop up every drop.

Tip

For 2⅓ cups (575 mL) coconut milk, you need one 19-oz (540 mL) can or two 14-oz (400 mL) cans. Extra coconut milk can be transferred to an airtight container and refrigerated for up to 1 week or frozen for up to 6 months.

Baking sheet, lined with parchment paper

Marinade

½ cup	plain coconut or soy yogurt	125 mL
3 tbsp	mango chutney	45 mL
2 tsp	ground cumin	10 mL
2 tsp	ground turmeric	10 mL
1 lb	extra-firm tofu, cut into 1-inch (2.5 cm) cubes	500 g

Sauce

2 tbsp	olive oil	30 mL
1	small onion, diced	1
2	cloves garlic, minced	2
2 tbsp	grated fresh gingerroot	30 mL
2 tsp	garam masala	10 mL
2 tsp	ground coriander	10 mL
1 tsp	New Mexico red chile powder (see Tips, right)	5 mL
1 tsp	ground turmeric	5 mL
¾ tsp	salt	3 mL
⅛ tsp	ground cloves	0.5 mL
1 tbsp	tomato paste	15 mL
1 tbsp	mango chutney	15 mL
1	can (28 oz/796 mL) crushed tomatoes with juice	1
2⅓ cups	coconut milk (see Tip, left)	575 mL
¼ cup	water	60 mL
6 cups	hot cooked white basmati rice	1.5 L
¼ cup	chopped fresh cilantro	60 mL

1. *Marinade:* In a shallow glass dish, whisk together yogurt, chutney, cumin and turmeric. Gently mix in tofu cubes. Cover and refrigerate for 2 hours or up to overnight.
2. *Sauce:* Place a large heavy-bottomed saucepan over medium heat and let pan get hot. Add oil and tip pan to coat. Add onion and cook, stirring occasionally, until translucent and lightly browned, about 5 minutes. Reduce heat to medium. Add garlic, ginger, garam masala, coriander, chile powder, turmeric, salt and cloves

New Mexico red chile powder is ground from very flavorful dried chiles grown near Hatch, New Mexico. Look for ground powder or whole dried chiles in grocery stores and online as these chiles are well worth the effort. If New Mexico red chile powder is unavailable, substitute ½ to 1 tsp (2 to 5 mL) cayenne pepper.

If you don't have many of the spices called for or to save time, use a purchased curry powder or paste in place of individual spices in sauce. If you use a tikka masala paste, omit tomato paste in recipe. Many varieties of curry paste and powder are offered in most grocery stores and online. Read labels to discover which contain your favorite spice combinations.

and cook, stirring, for 1 minute. Add tomato paste, chutney, crushed tomatoes, coconut milk and water, stirring well to combine. Partially cover pan, reduce heat and gently simmer, stirring occasionally, until flavors are blended and sauce is thickened, about 20 minutes.

3. Meanwhile, preheat broiler. Transfer tofu cubes to prepared baking sheet, discarding excess marinade. Broil for 5 minutes. Set aside and preheat oven to 350°F (180°C). Bake tofu until firm and slightly browned on edges, about 12 minutes. Transfer tofu to simmering sauce, cover pan and continue to simmer for 15 minutes.

4. To serve, spoon a generous amount of sauce over rice and scatter cilantro over top.

Turkish chard bundles

Serves 4 to 6

Aleppo pepper is a Turkish spice with a moderate heat level. It is similar to New Mexico red chile powder with the added flavors of cumin, salt and a fruity touch of raisins and sun-dried tomatoes. It is available online or in specialty gourmet stores. Ancho chile powder is a fine substitute.

- **Preheat oven to 350°F (180°C)**
- **13- by 9-inch (33 by 23 cm) glass baking dish, lightly oiled**

Chard Bundles

1 tsp	apple cider vinegar	5 mL
2 cups	ice	500 mL
2	bunches Swiss chard (about 1 1/2 lbs/750 g)	2
1 1/2 cups	bulgur	375 mL
1/2 cup	Vegetable Broth (page 31) or store-bought, heated	125 mL
3 tbsp	chopped raisins	45 mL
1 1/2 cups	cooked lentils	375 mL
1	onion, finely chopped	1
2	cloves garlic, minced	2
1/4 cup	chopped fresh parsley	60 mL
2 tbsp	freshly squeezed lemon juice	30 mL
1 1/2 tsp	salt	7 mL
1 tsp	ground cumin	5 mL
1 tsp	ground allspice	5 mL
1 tsp	freshly ground black pepper	5 mL
1/2 cup	dry white wine	125 mL
2 tbsp	olive oil	30 mL

Sauce

2 tbsp	freshly squeezed lemon juice	30 mL
1/2 cup	chopped Italian flat-leaf parsley	125 mL
1/3 cup	finely chopped walnuts	75 mL
1/4 cup	chopped fresh mint	60 mL
1	clove garlic, minced	1
1/2 cup	plain soy yogurt	125 mL
2 tbsp	olive oil	30 mL
1/4 tsp	salt	1 mL
1/4 tsp	freshly ground black pepper	1 mL
Pinch	Aleppo pepper or ancho chile powder	Pinch

Tip

Refrigerate any unused sauce in an airtight container for up to 2 days.

1. *Chard Bundles:* Add vinegar to a large pot of water and bring to a boil over high heat. Fill a large bowl with ice and water and set aside. Hold chard by stems and plunge leaves into boiling water for 10 seconds. Immediately plunge chard into ice bath. Transfer to a colander to drain and let cool. When chard is cool, trim stems at bottom of leaves and flatten upper vein with spatula.

2. In a sieve, rinse bulgur and drain. Place in a bowl with heated vegetable broth. Add raisins and let soak until bulgur has absorbed broth, about 20 minutes. Add lentils, onion, garlic, parsley, lemon juice, salt, cumin, allspice and pepper and gently mix to combine.

3. Place a chard leaf on a work surface with large end closest to you, vein side up. Scoop 2 tbsp (30 mL) of bulgur mixture onto large end of leaf and roll over once. Fold both sides in, roll to end and carefully set finished bundle into prepared baking dish, seam side down. Repeat process, placing bundles close together. Pour wine over all and drizzle with oil. Cover baking dish loosely with foil and bake in preheated oven until tender, about 35 minutes, adding more wine or other liquid if needed.

4. *Sauce:* In a small bowl, combine lemon juice, parsley, walnuts, mint, garlic, yogurt, oil, salt, black pepper and Aleppo pepper. Or process in a blender for a smoother sauce. Serve bundles hot with a few spoonfuls of sauce.

Wild mushroom étouffée

A mirepoix is the classic French combination of chopped onion, celery and carrots used extensively in soups and stews. A Creole mirepoix replaces the carrots with green bell pepper and is often referred to as the Holy Trinity. When seasoning this dish, remember that purchased Creole seasoning contains salt, so taste, taste and taste again before adding more salt. Étouffée pairs well with cold frosty beer.

2 tbsp	olive oil	30 mL
1 lb	wild mushrooms, coarsely chopped (see Tip, right)	500 g
1	small shallot, thinly sliced	1
½ cup	grapeseed oil	125 mL
¾ cup	all-purpose flour	175 mL
1 cup	chopped onion	250 mL
1 cup	chopped celery	250 mL
½ cup	chopped green bell pepper	125 mL
2	cloves garlic, minced	2
1	bottle (12 oz/341 mL) dark beer	1
2 cups	Vegetable Broth (page 31) or store-bought	500 mL
1 tsp	dried thyme	5 mL
2	bay leaves	2
2 tbsp	Cajun Spice (page 310) or store-bought, divided	30 mL
1 tsp	hot pepper sauce	5 mL
1 cup	chopped fresh or drained canned tomatoes	250 mL
1 tsp	salt, or to taste	5 mL
6 cups	hot cooked white basmati rice	1.5 L
2	green onions, white and light green parts, minced	2

1. Place a large heavy-bottomed saucepan over medium heat and let pan get hot. Add olive oil and tip pan to coat. Add mushrooms and shallot and cook, stirring frequently, until softened and slightly browned around edges, 6 to 8 minutes. Remove mushrooms and shallot from pan and set aside.

2. In same pan, heat grapeseed oil over medium heat. When hot, gradually whisk in flour. Cook, whisking vigorously, until it forms a loose paste, 2 to 3 minutes. Reduce heat to low and cook, stirring, until roux turns a dark caramel color with a toasty aroma, 15 to 20 minutes. Add onion, celery, bell pepper and garlic and cook, stirring frequently, until vegetables are softened, 4 to 5 minutes. Remove pan from heat and

Tip

If fresh wild mushrooms are unavailable, 1½ oz (45 g) dried mushrooms reconstituted in ¾ cup (175 mL) hot water are a wonderful substitute and will give the dish a heartier texture. Follow package directions for reconstituting and straining grit.

quickly whisk in beer until mixture is smooth. Return pan to stove top and increase heat to medium–high. Add vegetable broth, thyme, bay leaves, Cajun Spice, hot pepper sauce and tomatoes and bring to a boil. Reduce heat to simmer and adjust seasonings. Stir in reserved mushrooms and any juices that have collected and simmer, stirring occasionally, until flavors have blended and sauce slightly thickens, 10 to 15 minutes.

3. Remove bay leaves and serve étouffée spooned over hot rice topped with green onions.

Stuffed sopapillas

Makes 16

With a flaky pastry texture, puffed sopapillas beg to be stuffed. Serve as an entrée for lunch or dinner or fry up small sopapillas, stuff and serve as appetizers. Perfect with an ice cold Mexican beer!

2 tbsp	olive oil	30 mL
¼	onion, chopped	¼
1	zucchini, diced	1
12 oz	soy chorizo sausage alternative	375 g
1 cup	frozen roasted corn kernels	250 mL
¼ cup	chopped fresh cilantro	60 mL
16	Sopapillas (page 120)	16
2 cups	Guacamole (page 50) or store-bought	500 mL

1. Place a large skillet over medium heat and let pan get hot. Add oil and tip pan to coat. Add onion and zucchini and cook, stirring frequently, until softened and slightly browned, 6 to 8 minutes. Stir in chorizo, corn and cilantro and cook, stirring, until chorizo is slightly browned, about 4 minutes.

2. Using a sharp knife, cut sopapillas along edge and fold top back without disconnecting. Spoon a very generous amount of filling into each sopapilla and top with a large dollop of guacamole. Gently fold top back over, to just rest on mound. Serve immediately.

Mushroom-topped polenta tart with mushroom sauce

Serves 6

Served piping hot, this savory polenta tart will warm you on a cold day. What could be better than guilt-free comfort food.

❖ Tip

This tart is delicious with any and all mushrooms. Try wild mushrooms such as chanterelle, porcini and morels or domesticated mushrooms such as cremini or button or a mixture of a few.

❖ **2 baking sheets, lined with parchment paper**

6 cups	Vegetable Broth (page 31) or store-bought, divided	1.5 L
1 cup	cornmeal	250 mL
4 tbsp + 1 tsp	olive oil, divided	65 mL
1½ lbs	mixed wild and domestic mushrooms, divided (see Tip, left)	750 g
1	red bell pepper, divided	1
½ cup	minced onion	125 mL
1 tsp	fresh thyme leaves	5 mL
1 tsp	minced fresh sage leaves	5 mL
⅛ tsp	freshly ground black pepper	0.5 mL
½ cup	dry white wine	125 mL
2 tbsp	cornstarch	30 mL
3 tbsp	water	45 mL
	Salt	

1. In a saucepan, bring 4 cups (1 L) vegetable broth to a boil over high heat. Gradually whisk in cornmeal and cook, stirring, for 2 minutes. Cover, reduce heat to low and simmer for 25 minutes, uncovering and stirring vigorously 2 or 3 times during cooking. Remove from heat. Brush one parchment-lined baking sheet with 1 tsp (5 mL) of the oil and pour polenta on prepared baking sheet, spreading to ½ inch (1 cm) thickness. Refrigerate for 1 hour and brush top with 1 tbsp (15 mL) of oil. You can cover polenta and refrigerate for up to 1 day.

2. Preheat oven to 450°F (230°C) with racks positioned in the middle and bottom of oven.

✖ Tip

No time for do-ahead tart? Serve the roasted mushrooms and sauce over soft polenta, skipping the step of spreading it on the baking sheet, chilling and baking.

3. Slice half of the mushrooms and half of the bell pepper into $\frac{1}{4}$-inch (0.5 cm) thick strips. Brush remaining baking sheet with 2 tbsp (30 mL) of oil. Spread sliced mushrooms and peppers evenly over baking sheet. Place baking sheet with vegetables on bottom rack and baking sheet with polenta on middle rack of oven. Bake for 20 minutes, turning vegetables halfway through cooking.

4. Coarsely chop remaining mushrooms and bell pepper. Place a large skillet over medium heat and let pan get hot. Add remaining 1 tbsp (15 mL) of oil and tip pan to coat. Add mushrooms, bell pepper, onion, thyme, sage and pepper and cook, stirring frequently, until softened, 4 to 6 minutes. Add wine and remaining 2 cups (500 mL) of vegetable broth and bring to boil. Reduce heat and simmer until flavors are combined and mixture is slightly reduced, 10 to 15 minutes. Whisk cornstarch into water and gradually drizzle into pan, adding enough to thicken. Add more wine or water to thin if necessary. Adjust seasoning, adding salt to taste.

5. To serve, top polenta tart with roasted mushrooms and peppers. Slice into squares and serve with sauce on the side.

Basic pizza dough

With a little forethought you can be enjoying homemade pizza in less time than it takes to have one delivered. Throw the dough together when you get up, let it rise until you leave for work and punch it down and let it ferment in the refrigerator, which only improves the flavor, until you arrive home from work. You will never order out again.

✖ Tip

To make dough ahead, let rise as directed in Step 2, then punch down dough and cut into three pieces. Wrap in plastic wrap and refrigerate for up to 4 days or freeze in resealable freezer bags for up to 3 months. Let thaw overnight in refrigerator.

✖ Food processor
✖ Pizza stone or pan

2 tsp	agave nectar	10 mL
1¼ cups	warm water	300 mL
1	package (¼ oz/8 g) active dry yeast	1
1½ cups	whole wheat flour	375 mL
2 cups	all-purpose flour	500 mL
½ tsp	salt	2 mL
1 tbsp	olive oil	15 mL

1. In a small bowl, dissolve agave in warm water. Gently stir in yeast and let stand until foamy, about 5 minutes.

2. In a food processor with dough blade, if available, combine whole wheat and all-purpose flours and salt and pulse to combine, 6 to 8 times. With motor running, drizzle in proofed yeast mixture and oil through the feed tube and process until dough forms a ball and pulls away from sides of bowl. Process for an additional 30 seconds and transfer dough to a large warm oiled bowl, flipping to coat with oil. Cover bowl with a clean kitchen towel and let rise in a warm, draft-free place until dough has doubled in size, 45 minutes to 1 hour.

3. Place pizza stone, if using, in center of oven. Preheat oven to 450°F (230°C).

4. Punch down dough. Cut dough into three pieces (see Tip, left) Working with one piece of dough at a time, place on a lightly floured work surface and scatter a little flour on top. Shape dough into a disk by stretching outward from center. Roll dough to a circle about ¼ inch (0.5 cm) thick. Using fork tines, dot dough with small holes.

5. Place dough on pizza pan, if using. Cover pizza with desired sauce and toppings. Place on stone in preheated oven (or place pan in oven). Bake until crust is lightly browned, 15 to 25 minutes. Transfer pizza to a cutting board and let cool for a few minutes before cutting.

> ## ✖ Variations
>
> Omit whole wheat flour and use 3½ cups (875 mL) all-purpose flour.
>
> Replace ½ cup (125 mL) of the all-purpose flour or whole wheat flour with amaranth, teff or buckwheat flour.

Quick cherry tomato and pesto pizza

There is no better way to use those fabulous summertime sparklers, cherry tomatoes.

✷ Tip

Pre-roasting tomatoes intensifies their flavor and reduces the amount of liquid, thus no soggy pizza.

✷ Rimmed baking sheet, lined with parchment paper
✷ Pizza stone or pan

1¹/₂ cups	cherry tomatoes, halved	375 mL
2¹/₂ tbsp	olive oil, divided	37 mL
¹/₄ tsp	salt	1 mL
¹/₈ tsp	freshly ground black pepper	0.5 mL
¹/₃	recipe Basic Pizza Dough (page 202) or vegan store-bought	¹/₃
2 tbsp	all-purpose flour	30 mL
1 tbsp	Classic Pesto Sauce (page 286) or vegan store-bought	15 mL
3 tbsp	pine nuts	45 mL
2	cloves garlic, slivered	2

1. Place pizza stone, if using, on middle rack of cold oven and heat oven to 450°F (230°C). In a bowl, toss tomatoes with 2 tsp (10 mL) of the oil, salt and pepper. Transfer to prepared baking sheet and roast in preheated oven until softened and slightly browned, about 12 minutes. Remove from oven and set aside.

2. Place dough on a lightly floured work surface and scatter with flour. Shape dough into a disk by stretching outward from center. Roll dough to about ¹/₄-inch (0.5 cm) thick circle. Using fork tines, dot dough with small holes. Place on pizza pan, if using.

3. In a small bowl, combine remaining oil with pesto sauce and spread over pizza crust. Top with pine nuts, garlic, and roasted tomatoes. Place pizza on stone, if using. Bake in preheated oven until crust is lightly browned, 15 to 20 minutes. Transfer pizza to a cutting board and let cool for 3 to 4 minutes before cutting.

Caramelized shallot and mushroom pizza with arugula pesto

Tangy arugula pesto is a fresh contrast to sweet caramelized shallots and earthy mushrooms in this contemporary pizza.

⠿ Food processor
⠿ Pizza stone or pan

Pesto

2	cloves garlic, crushed	1
2 cups	arugula	500 mL
2 cups	basil leaves	500 mL
1/4 cup	toasted walnuts	60 mL
1/2 tsp	freshly ground black pepper	2 mL
1/4 tsp	salt	1 mL
3/4 to 1 cup	olive oil	175 to 250 mL

Topping

4 tbsp	olive oil, divided	60 mL
6	shallots, thinly sliced	6
2	cloves garlic, minced	2
1 lb	cremini mushrooms, sliced	500 g
3 tbsp	brandy	45 mL
1/2 tsp	salt	2 mL
1/2 tsp	freshly ground black pepper	2 mL
2/3	recipe Basic Pizza Dough (page 202) or 1 1/2 lbs (750 g) vegan store-bought	2/3

1. Place pizza stone in oven, if using. Preheat oven to 450°F (230°C).

2. *Pesto:* In food processor, with motor running, drop garlic through feed tube and process until finely chopped. Scrape sides and add arugula and basil. Pulse until chopped. Add walnuts, salt and pepper and pulse to combine. Stop to scrape sides as necessary. With motor running, drizzle enough of the oil through feed tube until a rough but smooth paste is formed. Set aside.

3. *Topping:* Place a large heavy-bottomed skillet over medium heat and let pan get hot. Add 2 tbsp (30 mL) of the oil and tip pan to coat. Add shallots and cook, stirring occasionally, until softened and starting to brown, 8 to 10 minutes. Push shallots to sides and add 2 tbsp (30 mL) of oil to center of pan. Add garlic and mushrooms and stir in shallots. Cook, stirring occasionally, until mushrooms and shallots are golden and slightly browned, about 10 minutes. Stir in brandy, salt and pepper and cook until liquid is evaporated, 3 to 5 minutes. Remove from heat and set aside.

4. Place dough on a lightly floured work surface and scatter a little flour on top. Divide dough in half and shape each half into a disk by stretching outward from center. Roll each disk to about a $\frac{1}{4}$-inch (0.5 cm) thick circle. Using fork tines, dot dough with small holes. Place on pizza pan, if using.

5. Spread half of the pesto on each pizza. Arrange shallots and mushrooms over top. Carefully slide one pizza onto stone and bake until golden brown, 15 to 25 minutes. Remove from oven, slide in second pizza and repeat cooking process. Let pizza cool for 3 to 5 minutes before cutting.

⁇ Variation

Use a store-bought vegan basil pesto and add $\frac{1}{2}$ cup (125 mL) sun-dried tomatoes packed in oil to mushroom and shallot topping.

Carolina barbecued seitan sandwich with vinegar coleslaw

This vinegar-based slaw includes a touch of mayonnaise, which creates a delicious yet light and creamy dressing for the vegetables and strikes a balance with the tangy barbecued seitan. Serve with crisp dill pickles for a Carolina experience.

❖ Tip

You should have about 2 cups (500 mL) each of green and red cabbage.

Slaw

1/4 cup	freshly squeezed lemon juice	60 mL
2 tbsp	apple cider vinegar	30 mL
2 tbsp	vegetable oil	30 mL
2 tbsp	Creamy Mayonnaise (page 19) or store-bought vegan alternative	30 mL
3/4 tsp	Dijon mustard	3 mL
1 tbsp	granulated sugar	15 mL
1 tsp	salt	5 mL
1/4 tsp	celery seeds	1 mL
1/4 tsp	freshly ground black pepper	1 mL
1/4	medium head green cabbage, shredded (see Tip, left)	1/4
1/4	medium head red cabbage, shredded	1/4
1	carrot, shredded	1
1	green onion, white and light green part only, chopped	1
2 tbsp	finely chopped fresh parsley	30 mL
2 cups	Homemade Barbecue Sauce (page 288) or store-bought vegan alternative	500 mL
1 tbsp	yellow mustard	15 mL
2 tsp	liquid smoke, optional	10 mL
12 oz	Old-School Seitan (page 28) or Quick Basic Seitan (page 29) or store-bought, sliced	375 g
4	buns, halved and warmed	4

1. *Slaw:* In a large bowl, combine lemon juice, vinegar, oil, mayonnaise, Dijon mustard, sugar, salt, celery seeds and black pepper and whisk to incorporate. Toss in green and red cabbage, carrot, green onion and parsley to coat. Cover and refrigerate for 2 hours.

2. In a saucepan, combine barbecue sauce, yellow mustard and liquid smoke, if using. Bring to a boil over medium heat, stirring occasionally. Reduce heat and simmer for 2 minutes. Add seitan and simmer, gently turning, until heated through, 8 to 10 minutes.

3. Divide seitan among bottom buns, reserving any sauce left in pan. Top seitan with a generous helping of slaw, replace bun tops and serve. Pass reserved sauce.

Roasted potatoes and tofu

Serves 4

This amazingly simple dish is so versatile and delicious no matter how you serve it! Serve it warm, serve it at room temperature or serve it chilled. Any way you slice it, you are sure to be delighted by the wonderful flavors. For a real treat, dress it up with Caper and Pine Nut Vinaigrette.

✖ Tip

To serve chilled, refrigerate potatoes and tofu for at least 2 hours and toss with vinaigrette. Store any unused in an airtight container and refrigerate for up to 3 days.

✖ Preheat oven to 450°F (230°C)
✖ Baking sheet, lined with parchment paper

8 oz	extra-firm tofu	250 g
1½ lbs	Yukon gold potatoes, cut into ½-inch (1 cm) cubes	750 g
1 tbsp	olive oil	15 mL
½ tsp	salt	2 mL
¼ tsp	freshly ground black pepper	1 mL
	Caper and Pine Nut Vinaigrette (page 302), optional	

1. Drain tofu, wrap in a clean thick kitchen towel or paper towels and place on a dinner plate. Place a second dinner plate on top, place a heavy can on top and set aside for 1 hour. Cut pressed tofu into ½-inch (1 cm) cubes.

2. In a bowl, toss together potatoes, tofu, oil, salt and pepper. Spread evenly on prepared baking sheet. Bake in preheated oven, stirring once, until potatoes are golden and tender, about 20 minutes. Let cool slightly. Serve immediately as is or toss with vinaigrette, if desired.

✖ Variation

Toss with vinaigrette and serve over a handful of fresh arugula or shredded lettuce.

Spelt-stuffed eggplant with indian spices

Serves 4		

Eggplant is native to India and has been cultivated in eastern Asia since prehistory. This spicy Indian-inspired dish is made heartier with the addition of nutty spelt berries.

✛ **8-inch (20 cm) glass baking dish, lightly oiled**

1/2 cup	spelt berries, rinsed, soaked 6 hours or overnight	125 mL
1 1/2 cups	Vegetable Broth (page 31) or store-bought	375 mL
2	small eggplants (each about 12 oz/375 g)	2
2 1/2 tsp	salt, divided	12 mL
2 tbsp	olive oil	30 mL
1/2 cup	chopped onion	125 mL
1 tbsp	minced fresh gingerroot	15 mL
2 tsp	minced garlic	10 mL
2 tsp	ground turmeric	10 mL
1 tsp	ground cumin	5 mL
1/8 tsp	hot pepper flakes	0.5 mL
1/8 tsp	freshly ground black pepper	0.5 mL
1/2 cup	water	125 mL
1 1/2 cups	seeded and chopped tomatoes	375 mL

1. Drain spelt. In a saucepan, combine spelt and vegetable broth and bring to a boil over high heat. Cover, reduce heat to low and simmer until spelt is tender and most of the liquid is absorbed, about 1 1/2 hours. Drain and set aside. This may be done up to 2 days ahead of time.

2. Cut eggplants in half, lengthwise. Run a small knife 1/4- to 1/2-inch (0.5 to 1 cm) from the outer edge of eggplant skin. Then make two lengthwise cuts through eggplant halves, being careful not to cut through bottom. Gently pull and cut lengthwise sections away from shell to hollow out, leaving the 1/4- to 1/2-inch (0.5 to 1 cm) thick walls, reserving flesh. Place hollowed out shells in prepared baking dish and set aside.

3. Coarsely chop reserved eggplant flesh and place in colander. Toss with 2 tsp (10 mL) of the salt and let stand for 20 minutes to sweat. Rinse thoroughly, drain and pat dry with a clean kitchen towel.

4. Preheat oven to 350°F (180°C).

5. Place a large skillet over medium heat and let pan get hot. Add oil and tip pan to coat. Add onion, ginger and garlic and cook, stirring, until softened, 6 to 8 minutes. Stir in chopped eggplant, turmeric, cumin, $\frac{1}{2}$ tsp (2 mL) of salt, hot pepper flakes, black pepper and water. Reduce heat to low, cover and cook, stirring occasionally, until eggplant is soft, about 10 minutes. Remove from heat, stir in cooked spelt and tomatoes.

6. Fill eggplant shells with spelt mixture. Cover with foil and bake until filling is hot and eggplant shells are tender, 40 to 50 minutes. Serve immediately.

> ### ✖ Variation
> Add diced zucchini or carrots to the vegetable sauté mixture with the chopped eggplant.

Horseradish mustard and panko-encrusted tofu

Crunch down through the tangy, crispy golden brown panko crust and bite into the velvety soft tofu center of these absolutely fabulous dinner delights. The zesty flavors of horseradish and mustard add just the right touch of snap hidden in a middle layer between crunchy and creamy.

◆ Baking sheet, lined with parchment paper
◆ Immersion blender or upright blender

1 lb	firm tofu	500 g
½ cup	dry white wine	125 mL
4 oz	firm or extra-firm silken tofu	125 g
¼ cup	plain soy milk	60 mL
5 tsp	Dijon mustard	25 mL
1 tbsp	prepared horseradish	15 mL
1 tbsp	freshly squeezed lemon juice	15 mL
½ cup	all-purpose flour	125 mL
2 tbsp	tapioca flour or cornstarch	30 mL
½ tsp	salt	2 mL
3 cups	panko bread crumbs	750 mL
¼ cup	canola oil, divided	60 mL

1. Drain tofu, wrap in a clean thick kitchen towel or paper towels and place on a dinner plate. Place a second dinner plate on top, place a heavy can on top and set aside for 1 hour.

2. Cut pressed firm tofu in half crosswise. Set each half on one narrow side and cut into two 1-inch (2.5 cm) thick pieces. Pour wine into a shallow bowl and lay tofu slices in wine.

3. In a 2-cup (500 mL) glass measuring cup, using an immersion blender or in an upright blender, combine silken tofu, soy milk, mustard, horseradish and lemon juice and purée into a very smooth sauce. Pour mixture into another shallow bowl and set aside.

4. In a third shallow bowl, whisk together flour, tapioca and salt. Pour panko into fourth shallow bowl.

5. Working in batches, flip tofu in wine to dampen both sides, then remove from wine. Dredge tofu in flour mixture, turning to coat all sides and transfer to mustard mixture. Using fork and fingers, turn tofu to generously coat all sides. Using fork and fingers lift and transfer tofu to panko and turn to coat all sides. Transfer coated tofu to prepared baking sheet.

Tip

Any leftover tofu can be cooled and stored in an airtight container in the refrigerator for up to 2 days. Reheat in a 400°F (200°C) oven for 20 minutes to heat and crisp and serve atop a green salad.

6. Place a heavy-bottomed skillet over medium-high heat and let pan get hot. Add 3 tbsp (45 mL) of the oil and heat until it shimmers. Carefully place 1 or 2 tofu pieces at a time into hot oil and cook until bottom is golden brown and crusty, 1 to 1½ minutes. Flip tofu and cook until bottom is crispy, about 1 minute. If feeling clever, tip tofu up onto sides and cook until crispy. Transfer to a platter lined with paper towels to drain. Continue with remaining tofu, adding oil and adjusting heat as necessary between batches. Serve hot.

County fair corn chip pie

Serves 2

This recipe is inspired by the traditional Frito's recipe with a vegan twist. In Texas this classic is served at every public gathering of more than three people and with good reason — it's incredible. Crunchy and salty topped with saucy and savory; it just doesn't get any better! It must be served in the bag or you have missed the entire point.

2 cups	Boy Howdy Texas Chili and Beans (page 279) or store-bought vegan bean chili	500 mL
2	bags (each 2 oz/56 g) corn chips	2
1 cup	shredded non-dairy Cheddar cheese alternative	250 mL
¼ cup	chopped white onions	60 mL

1. In a small saucepan, heat chili over low heat, stirring occasionally, until hot and bubbly, about 5 minutes. Cut one chip bag open along one side and spoon half of the hot chili on top of chips. Immediately scatter cheese over top and sprinkle with chopped onions. Repeat with remaining bag, chili and toppings and serve immediately.

Variation
Top with shredded lettuce and chopped tomatoes.

Louisiana red beans and rice dinner loaf

Serves 6 to 8

Cajun spices, a classic mirepoix of celery, onion and bell pepper, and Louisiana red beans and rice blend into a sassy dinner loaf. If there happens to be any leftover, it makes a great sandwich on crusty French bread with Cajun-spiced mayonnaise and fresh tomato slices.

✖ Tip

Liquid aminos are an excellent and tasty substitute for tamari. Made from soy beans and purified water, I like to use Braggs brand, which is not fermented and is gluten-free.

✖ Food processor
✖ 9- by 5-inch (23 by 12.5 cm) glass loaf pan, lightly oiled

¼ cup	olive oil, divided	60 mL
2	stalks celery, finely chopped	2
1	onion, finely chopped	1
½	green bell pepper, seeded and chopped	½
½	red bell pepper, seeded and chopped	½
3	cloves garlic, chopped	3
1 tsp	salt	5 mL
¾ tsp	smoked paprika	3 mL
½ tsp	freshly ground black pepper	2 mL
½ tsp	cayenne pepper	2 mL
½ tsp	ground cumin	2 mL
¼ tsp	ground nutmeg	1 mL
6 oz	firm or extra-firm silken tofu	175 g
3 tbsp	tomato paste, divided	45 mL
2 tbsp	liquid amino acids, divided (see Tip, left)	30 mL
2 cups	cooked red beans	500 mL
2 cups	cooked brown rice	500 mL
1 cup	panko bread crumbs, divided	250 mL

1. Place a large skillet over medium heat and let pan get hot. Add 2 tbsp (30 mL) of the oil and tip pan to coat. Add celery, onion, red and green bell peppers and cook, stirring occasionally, until softened, 5 to 6 minutes. Stir in garlic and cook, stirring, until softened, 1 to 2 minutes. Set aside.

2. In a small bowl, combine salt, paprika, black pepper, cayenne pepper, cumin and nutmeg and set aside.

3. In food processor, combine tofu, 2 tbsp (30 mL) of the tomato paste, 1 tbsp (15 mL) of the liquid amino acids, 1 tbsp (15 mL) of oil and spice mixture and pulse until smooth. Add beans and pulse into a very chunky purée. Transfer to a bowl. Add rice, $\frac{1}{2}$ cup (125 mL) of the panko and all but $\frac{1}{2}$ cup (125 mL) of cooked vegetables and gently mix to incorporate. Transfer mixture to prepared loaf pan, smoothing top.

4. In a small bowl, whisk together remaining 1 tbsp (15 mL) of tomato paste, 1 tbsp (15 mL) of liquid amino acids and 1 tbsp (15 mL) of oil and brush over top of loaf. In another small bowl, combine reserved vegetables and remaining panko and scatter over top. Cover with foil and refrigerate for 30 minutes.

5. Preheat oven to 350°F (180°C). Bake, covered with foil, for 30 minutes. Remove foil and bake until center is hot and top is crunchy, about 30 minutes. Let loaf stand for 10 minutes before cutting.

> ## ▓ Variation
> You can substitute 1 tbsp (15 mL) prepared Cajun spice blend for salt, paprika, black pepper, cayenne pepper, cumin and nutmeg.

Northwest passage cedar-planked tofu

Tender on the inside with a glistening glaze, tofu steaks are char grilled on cedar planks for a fabulous flavor and a fun presentation. Great with Grilled Artichokes with Jalapeño Mignonette Sauce (page 142).

✖ Tip

Plan ahead. This dish requires freezing and thawing tofu as well as soaking the cedar planks overnight.

✖ Four 6-inch (15 cm) square food grade cedar planks
✖ 13- by 9-inch (33 by 23 cm) glass baking dish
✖ Barbecue grill

2	blocks (each 14 to 16 oz/400 to 500 g) extra-firm tofu	2
	Hot water	
1/4 cup	olive oil, divided	60 mL
3	shallots, finely chopped	3
3/4 cup	tamari	175 mL
1/2 cup	orange juice	125 mL
1/2 cup	Dijon mustard	125 mL
1/4 cup	packed brown sugar	60 mL
1/4 cup	pure maple syrup	60 mL
2 tbsp	brown rice syrup	30 mL
1/4 tsp	liquid smoke	1 mL

1. Drain tofu, wrap in a clean thick kitchen towel or paper towels and place on a dinner plate. Place a second dinner plate on top, place a heavy can on top and set aside for 1 hour. Transfer to a resealable freezer bag and freeze for at least 12 hours. Let tofu thaw to room temperature before using.

2. In a large pan, immerse cedar planks in hot water. Weigh planks down with a water–filled jar or heavy mug to keep them immersed and let soak overnight.

3. Meanwhile, place a skillet over medium heat and let pan get hot. Add 2 tbsp (30 mL) of the oil and tip pan to coat. Add shallots and cook, stirring occasionally, until just starting to brown, 4 to 6 minutes. Stir in tamari and orange juice and deglaze, stirring up all the browned bits on the bottom of pan. Whisk in mustard, brown sugar, maple syrup, brown rice syrup and liquid smoke, stirring well to dissolve mustard and sugar. Reduce heat to low and simmer, stirring occasionally, until thoroughly combined, 3 to 4 minutes. Remove sauce from heat, transfer to baking dish and let cool thoroughly.

4. Place tofu blocks with the narrow-side down on a cutting board and cut in half lengthwise to form 1- to 1½-inch (2.5 to 4 cm) thick steaks. Immerse in marinade and turn to coat. Cover and refrigerate for at least 4 hours or overnight.

5. Preheat barbecue grill to high heat (400° to 450°/ 200° to 230°C).

6. Remove tofu from marinade, reserving marinade and set tofu aside. Pour marinade into a small saucepan and bring to a boil over medium heat. Reduce heat and simmer until sauce thickens and reduces by one-quarter, stirring occasionally, 6 to 8 minutes.

7. Drain cedar planks and pat dry. Lightly spread 2 tbsp (30 mL) of oil over top side of planks and place on hot grill, oiled side up. Preheat for 5 to 6 minutes to allow cedar flavor to absorb into the oil. Transfer planks to a baking sheet and place tofu steaks on planks. Coat top and all sides of tofu generously with sauce.

8. Return planks to grill, close lid and cook until tofu is very hot in the center and encrusted by a caramelized glaze, checking occasionally to ensure planks are not burning, 15 to 20 minutes. Remove planks from heat and drizzle tofu with additional sauce. Either remove tofu from planks and serve or for a festive presentation, place cedar planks on a platter and serve, allowing guests to serve themselves.

✖ Variation

Add apple cider, white wine or rosemary branches to the soaking water to enhance the flavor imparted during cooking.

Panko-crusted tofu sandwich with apple and celery rémoulade slaw

Serves 4

Sweet, savory, creamy and crunchy are balanced and piled high on a delightful potato roll, creating a memorable sandwich that is high on everyone's list of classic comfort foods.

❖ Immersion blender or upright blender
❖ Baking sheet, lined with parchment paper

Apple and Celery Rémoulade Slaw

¼ cup	Creamy Mayonnaise (page 19) or store-bought vegan alternative	60 mL
2 tbsp	freshly squeezed lemon juice	30 mL
1 tbsp	Dijon mustard	15 mL
2 tbsp	chopped fresh tarragon	30 mL
½ tsp	salt	2 mL
¼ tsp	ground black pepper	1 mL
3	stalks celery with leaves, thinly sliced	1
1	Granny Smith apple, grated	1
1 lb	firm tofu, drained and pressed (see page 12)	500 g
¼ cup	dry white wine	60 mL
4 oz	firm or extra-firm silken tofu	125 g
6 tbsp	plain soy milk	90 mL
¾ tsp	salt, divided	3 mL
½ cup	all-purpose flour	125 mL
2 tbsp	cornstarch	30 mL
1 tsp	freshly ground black pepper	5 mL
3 cups	panko bread crumbs	750 mL
¼ cup	canola oil, divided	60 mL
4	Potato Rolls (page 123) or vegan store-bought sandwich rolls, split and warmed	4
¼ cup	Creamy Mayonnaise (page 19) or store-bought vegan alternative	60 mL
1	tomato, sliced	1
2 cups	baby arugula	500 mL

1. *Apple and Celery Rémoulade Slaw:* In a bowl, whisk together mayonnaise, lemon juice, mustard, tarragon, salt and pepper. Stir in celery and apples, mixing well to combine. Taste and season with additional salt and pepper, if needed. Set aside.

2. Cut pressed firm tofu in half crosswise. Set each half on one narrow side and cut each into two 1-inch (2.5 cm) pieces. Pour wine into a shallow bowl and lay tofu slices in wine.

3. In a 2-cup (500 mL) glass measuring cup, using immersion blender or in upright blender, combine silken tofu, soy milk and $\frac{1}{4}$ tsp (1 mL) of the salt and purée into a very smooth sauce. Pour mixture into a shallow bowl and set aside. In a third shallow bowl, whisk together flour, cornstarch, black pepper and remaining $\frac{1}{2}$ tsp (2 mL) salt. Place bread crumbs in fourth shallow bowl.

4. Working in batches, flip tofu in wine to dampen both sides, then remove from wine. Dredge tofu in flour mixture, turning to coat all sides and transfer to milk mixture. Using a fork and fingers, turn tofu to generously coat all sides. Using fork and fingers, lift and transfer tofu to bread crumbs and coat all sides, pressing lightly to help crumbs adhere. Transfer coated tofu to prepared baking sheet.

5. Place a large heavy-bottomed skillet over medium-high heat and let pan get hot. Add 3 tbsp (45 mL) of the oil and heat until it shimmers. Carefully place 1 or 2 tofu pieces at a time into hot oil and cook until bottom is golden brown and crusty, 1 to $1\frac{1}{2}$ minutes. Flip tofu and cook until bottom is crispy, about 1 minute. Transfer to a platter lined with paper towels to drain. Continue with remaining tofu, adding more oil and adjusting heat as necessary between batches.

6. Spread roll halves with mayonnaise. Layer bottom half of roll with rémoulade slaw, crispy tofu, tomato slices and arugula. Top with other roll half and press lightly. Cut each sandwich on the diagonal and serve.

Grilled vegetable sandwich with garlic aïoli

Savory charred vegetables are delicious between grilled rustic olive bread slices spread with roasted garlic herbed aïoli. Serve with a crisp salad and a cold glass of white wine.

✖ Tip

Roasted garlic is a simple matter. *To roast garlic:* Trim the top of the head just enough to expose the cloves. Place on a large square of foil, drizzle with olive oil and sprinkle with herbs such as thyme, basil, oregano and/or rosemary. Wrap the foil up to enfold the garlic and bake in a 350°F (180°C) oven until tender, about 45 minutes.

✖ Two 12-inch (30 cm) metal skewers
✖ Barbecue grill preheated to medium-high heat

Aïoli

1/2 cup	Creamy Mayonnaise (page 19) or store-bought vegan alternative	125 mL
1	head garlic, roasted (see Tip, left)	1
3 tbsp	finely chopped fresh basil	45 mL
2 tsp	finely chopped fresh chives	10 mL
1/4 tsp	salt	1 mL
1/4 tsp	freshly ground black pepper	1 mL
1	eggplant, peeled	1
2 tbsp	salt	30 mL
1	white onion, cut crosswise into 1-inch (2.5 cm) thick slices	1
2	portobello mushroom caps	2
2	yellow crookneck squash, cut lengthwise into 1/2-inch (1 cm) thick slices	2
2	red bell peppers, seeded, quartered lengthwise and smashed flat	2
1/2 cup	olive oil, divided	125 mL
1/2 tsp	salt	2 mL
1/4 tsp	freshly ground black pepper	1 mL
8	thick slices Rosemary and Olive Bread (page 114) or vegan store-bought bread	8

1. *Aïoli:* In a small bowl, whisk together mayonnaise, roasted garlic, basil, chives, salt and black pepper until smooth. Set aside.

2. Cut eggplant crosswise into 1/2-inch (1 cm) thick slices. Generously salt slices and place in a colander over sink. Let eggplant sweat for at least 30 minutes. Rinse eggplant and pat dry.

Refrigerate any unused aïoli in an airtight container for up to 2 days.

Aïoli can be thinned with a little water or vinegar and used as a salad dressing.

3. Insert skewers crosswise through onion slices to secure rings together. Brush onions, eggplant, mushrooms caps, squash and bell peppers with ¼ cup (60 mL) of the oil. Sprinkle with salt and black pepper. Place on preheated grill, working in batches, as necessary. Grill vegetables, flipping once, until tender and lightly charred, 8 to 10 minutes per side. Cut each mushroom into 6 slices. Transfer grilled vegetables to a platter and lightly tent with foil to keep warm.

4. Place bread slices on grill and toast, flipping once, until warmed and golden, 2 to 3 minutes per side.

5. Spread one side of each grilled bread slice with aïoli. Pile each of 4 slices with one-quarter of grilled vegetables. Top with remaining 4 bread slices, aïoli side down. Cut each sandwich in half on the diagonal and serve immediately.

Cilantro black bean burgers

Just the thing when summer heats up and evening al fresco dining is tops on the schedule. Invite the neighbors for a potluck and let them bring the salad and dessert. Serve Guacamole with Blue Corn Chips (page 50) as an appetizer.

✳ Food processor

1/3 cup	rolled spelt flakes	75 mL
1 tsp	ground cumin	5 mL
1 tsp	dried oregano	5 mL
1 tsp	each salt and freshly ground black pepper	5 mL
1/2 tsp	chipotle pepper powder	2 mL
1/2 tsp	garlic powder	2 mL
2 cups	cooked black beans	500 mL
2 tbsp	grated onion	30 mL
2 tbsp	finely chopped cilantro	30 mL
1/4 cup	cooked short-grain rice	60 mL
2 to 4 tbsp	olive oil	30 to 60 mL
1	large tomato, sliced into 6 slices	1
1	avocado, sliced	1
1	small red onion, thinly sliced	1
6 to 12	romaine lettuce leaves	6 to 12
1/2 cup	Chipotle Lime Mayonnaise (page 293) or store-bought vegan mayonnaise alternative	125 mL
6	burger buns, split and warmed	6

1. In food processor, combine spelt, cumin, oregano, salt, pepper, chipotle powder and garlic powder and pulse to combine, 3 or 4 times. Add beans, onion and cilantro and process until mixture is blended but still chunky, 10 to 20 seconds.

2. Transfer mixture to a bowl and using your hands, mix in rice. Using clean wet hands, form mixture into 6 patties, about 1 inch (2.5 cm) thick. Place on a plate and let stand for 5 minutes.

3. Place a large heavy-bottomed skillet over medium heat and let pan get hot. Add 2 tsp (10 mL) of the oil and tip pan to coat. Using a spatula, carefully place patties into hot oil, in batches as necessary, and cook until bottoms are well-browned and slightly crisp, 3 to 4 minutes. Carefully flip burgers and cook until bottoms are browned and burgers are heated through, 2 to 3 minutes. Transfer cooked burgers to plate. Repeat with remaining patties, adding oil and adjusting heat between batches, as necessary.

4. Place tomato, avocado, red onion and lettuce leaves on a large platter. Scoop chipotle mayonnaise into a small bowl. Serve burgers along with warm buns and pass condiments and spread.

Asian tempeh tacos

Small, Baja-style tacos are filled with a sensational combination of crispy, sweet-hot tempeh and luscious stir-fried Asian-style vegetables for a truly international taco. Delish topped with the contrasting cool of Avocado Cilantro Dip. Set ingredients out buffet-style and let everyone help themselves.

1 tbsp	toasted sesame oil, divided	15 mL
2 tbsp	canola oil, divided	30 mL
1	package (14 oz/400 g) tempeh, cubed	1
1 tbsp	sweet Asian hot sauce	15 mL
1	white onion, cut in half and thinly sliced	1
1	red bell pepper, seeded and thinly sliced	1
3/4 cup	snow peas	175 mL
1/4	head purple cabbage, thinly shredded	1/4
1 tsp	minced fresh gingerroot	5 mL
2 tbsp	rice wine vinegar	30 mL
1 tbsp	tamari	15 mL
1/4 cup	toasted sesame seeds	60 mL
1/2 cup	Avocado Cilantro Dip (page 291) or store-bought vegan sour cream alternative	125 mL
	Grated zest and juice of 1 lime	
8 to 12	3 1/2-inch (8 cm) corn tortillas, warmed	8 to 12
1/4 cup	coarsely chopped toasted peanuts	60 mL
2	green onions, white and light green parts only, finely chopped	2

1. Place large heavy-bottomed skillet over medium-high heat and let pan get hot. Add 2 tsp (10 mL) of the sesame oil and 1 tbsp (15 mL) of the canola oil and tip pan to coat. Add tempeh and cook, stirring frequently, until crisp, 5 to 6 minutes. Transfer to a bowl. Add sweet Asian hot sauce and toss to coat. Set aside.

2. Return pan to medium-high heat. Add 1 tsp (5 mL) of sesame oil and 1 tbsp (15 mL) of canola oil and tip pan to coat. Add onion and cook, stirring occasionally, until translucent, 4 to 6 minutes. Add bell pepper and snow peas and cook, stirring frequently, until peppers are softened and start to brown, 4 to 6 minutes. Add cabbage and ginger and cook, stirring frequently, until cabbage is wilted, 3 to 4 minutes. Add vinegar, tamari and sesame seeds, stirring well to combine. Cook, stirring frequently, until liquid evaporates, 2 to 3 minutes. Stir tempeh into vegetables to combine.

3. In a small bowl, whisk together Avocado Cilantro Dip with lime zest and juice until smooth. Spoon tempeh mixture into warm tortillas, add a dollop of avocado sauce and top with peanuts and green onions.

Pad thai with crispy tofu

Now that you know the
secret to a traditional
Pad Thai you won't
have to trudge through
the sleeting rain to
enjoy this international
favorite. Find tamarind
in the ethnic food aisle
at your local grocery
store or at Asian
grocery stores.

❖ Small food processor

10 oz	extra-firm tofu	300 g
1	piece (1 inch/2.5 cm) tamarind pulp	1
1 cup	hot water, divided	250 mL
4	dried red chiles	4
8 oz	wide rice noodles	250 g
6 tbsp	peanut oil, divided	90 mL
3	shallots, finely minced	3
3 tbsp	tamari	45 mL
1 tbsp	Thai palm sugar or brown sugar	15 mL
1 tsp	freshly squeezed lime juice	5 mL
3 tbsp	peanut oil	45 mL
1 cup	bean sprouts	250 mL
2	green onions, white and green parts, chopped	2
¼ cup	chopped roasted peanuts	60 mL
1	lime, cut into wedges	1

1. Drain tofu, wrap in a clean thick kitchen towel or paper
   towels and place on a dinner plate. Place a second dinner
   plate on top, place a heavy can on top and set aside for
   1 hour. Drain and cut into cubes.

2. Meanwhile, in a small bowl, soak tamarind pulp in
   ½ cup (125 mL) of the hot water until softened, 10 to
   20 minutes. In another small bowl, soak dried red chiles
   in ½ cup (125 mL) of hot water until softened, 20 to
   30 minutes. In a large bowl, soak rice noodles in cold
   water to cover by at least 1 inch (2.5 cm) until softened,
   about 30 minutes.

3. Place a skillet over medium-high heat and let pan get
   hot. Add 2 tbsp (30 mL) of the peanut oil and tip pan to
   coat. Add tofu and fry, turning frequently, until browned
   and crispy on all sides, 6 to 8 minutes. Transfer to a plate
   lined with paper towels. Set aside.

4. In same skillet over medium heat, let pan get hot.
   Add 1 tbsp (15 mL) of peanut oil and tip pan to coat.
   Add shallots and cook, stirring constantly, until lightly
   browned, about 3 minutes.

5. Strain soaked tamarind through a fine-mesh sieve, pressing as necessary to push pulp into a bowl, reserving liquid. Discard solids. Drain chile peppers, discarding soaking liquid.

6. In food processor, combine cooled shallots, strained tamarind pulp, softened chiles, tamari, palm sugar, lime juice and 3 tbsp (45 mL) tamarind soaking water and process into a smooth paste, adding additional tamarind soaking water if necessary.

7. Drain noodles. Place same skillet over medium-high heat and let pan get hot. Add 3 tbsp (45 mL) of peanut oil and chile paste, stirring to combine. Add noodles and toss to coat, adding 1 to 2 tbsp (15 to 30 mL) of water to loosen paste, if necessary. Cook, stirring frequently, until noodles are further softened but not mushy, about 5 minutes. Stir in bean sprouts and crispy tofu. Top with green onions and peanuts and garnish with lime wedges. Serve immediately.

Curried lime crispy tempeh

Serve fried tempeh over rice or steamed vegetables with a few drizzles of pungent Pantry Ponzu Sauce (page 288) or a cooling Lime Sour Cream Dipping Sauce (page 289).

1/2 cup	water	125 mL
1/4 cup	tamari	60 mL
2 tbsp	freshly squeezed lime juice	30 mL
2 tbsp	agave nectar	30 mL
1 tbsp	minced fresh gingerroot	15 mL
1 tbsp	Curry Powder (page 311) or store-bought	15 mL
2 lbs	tempeh, cut into 32 pieces	1 kg
2 cups	peanut oil	500 mL

1. In a baking dish, whisk together water, tamari, lime juice, agave, ginger and curry powder. Add tempeh and gently toss to coat with marinade. Cover and refrigerate overnight, gently stirring once or twice.

2. Pour oil into a large saucepan and heat over high heat. When a small crumb of tempeh dropped into oil immediately sizzles, oil is ready. Remove tempeh from marinade, gently tapping to remove excess liquid to avoid splattering while frying. Discard marinade. Working in batches, carefully place in hot oil and fry, carefully turning with slotted spoon, until light brown and crispy, 3 to 4 minutes. Using a slotted spoon, remove from oil and transfer to a plate lined with paper towels to drain. Serve hot.

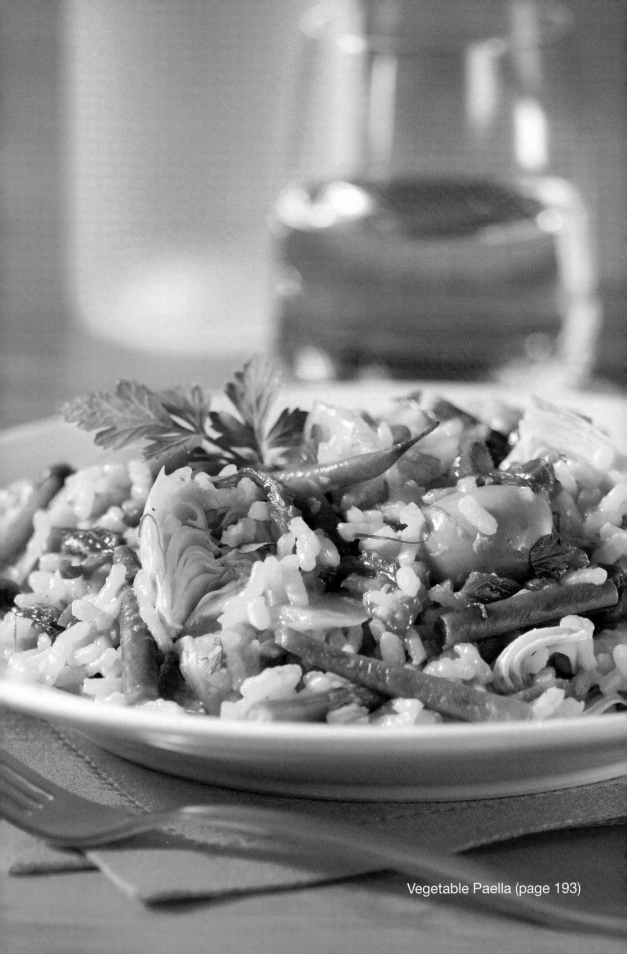

Vegetable Paella (page 193)

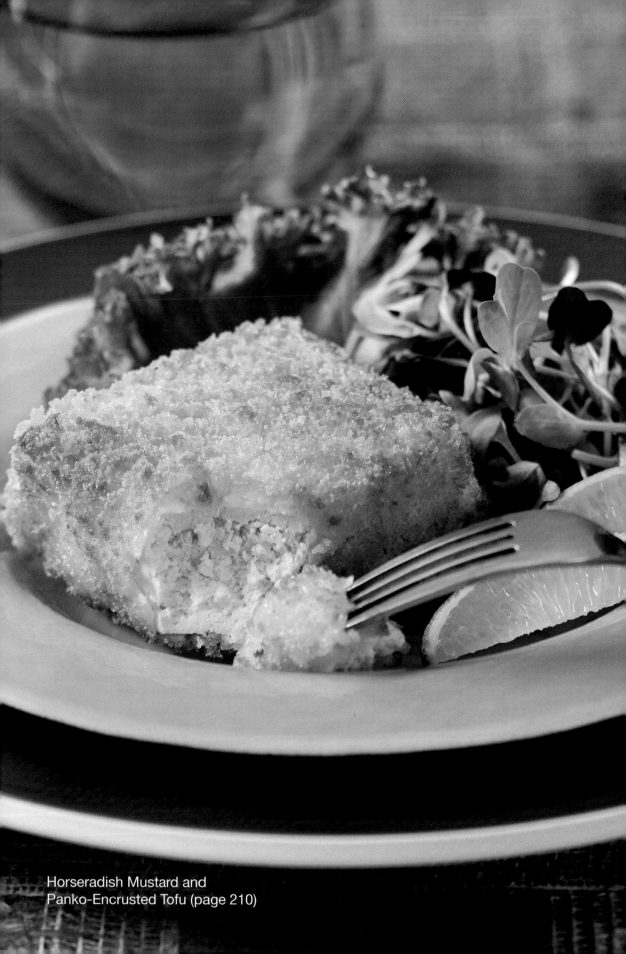

Horseradish Mustard and
Panko-Encrusted Tofu (page 210)

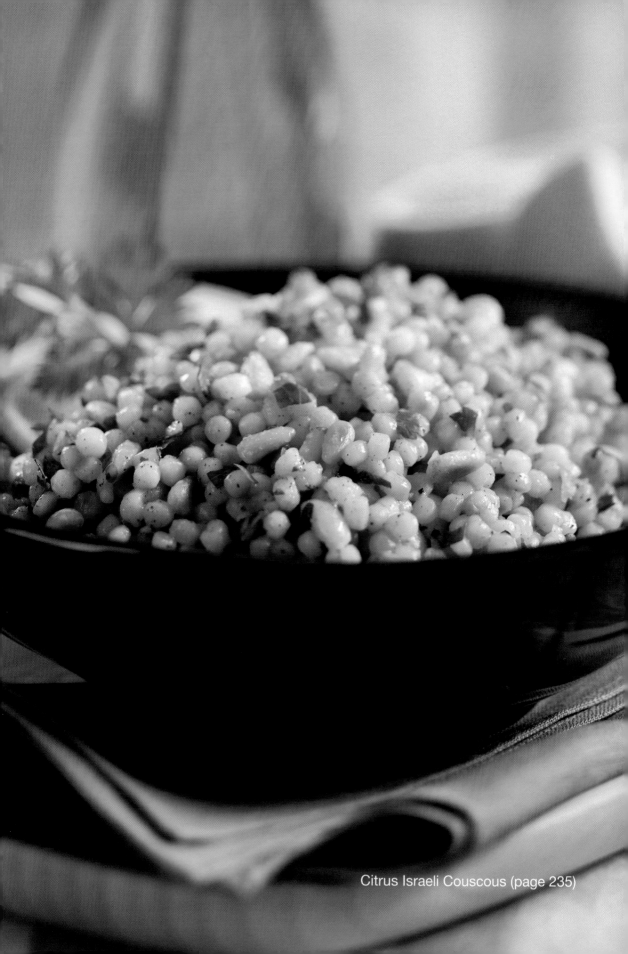

Citrus Israeli Couscous (page 235)

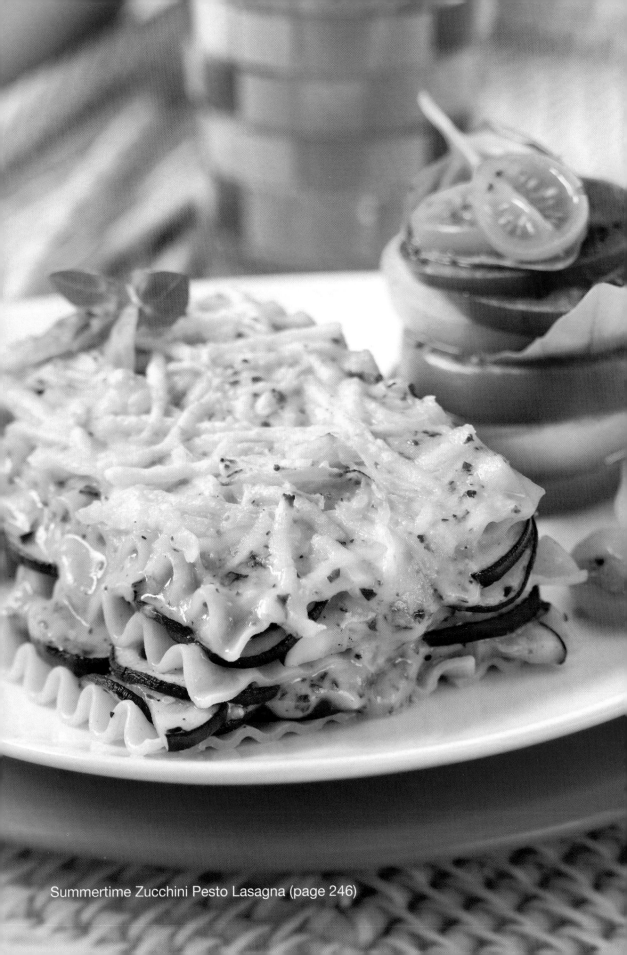

Summertime Zucchini Pesto Lasagna (page 246)

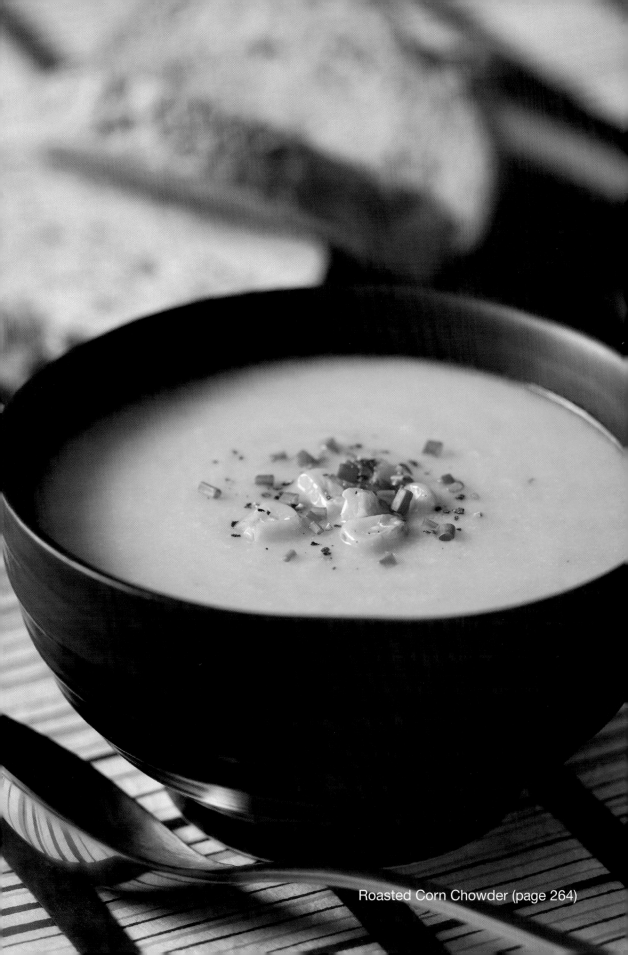

Roasted Corn Chowder (page 264)

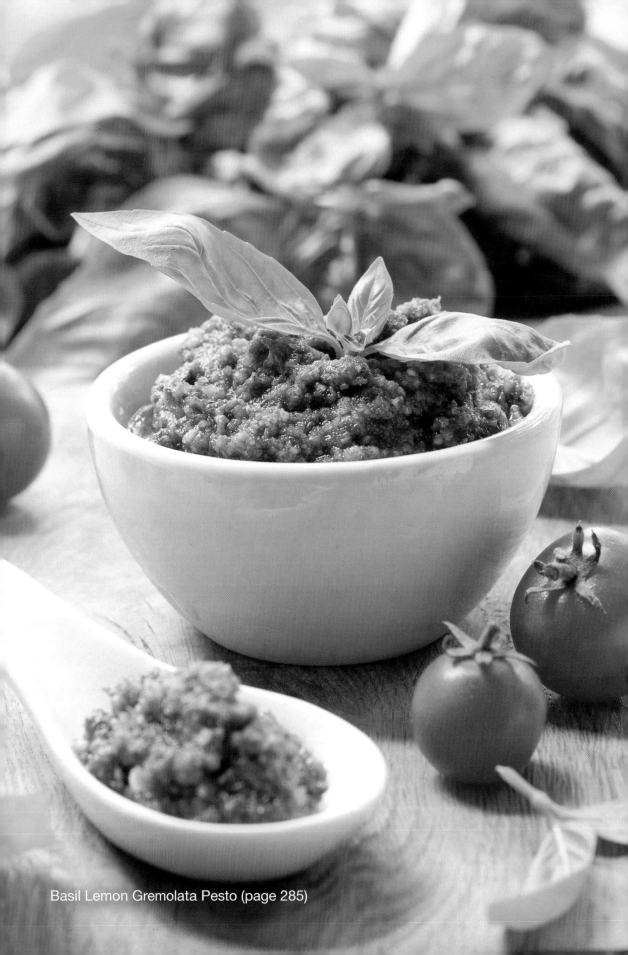

Basil Lemon Gremolata Pesto (page 285)

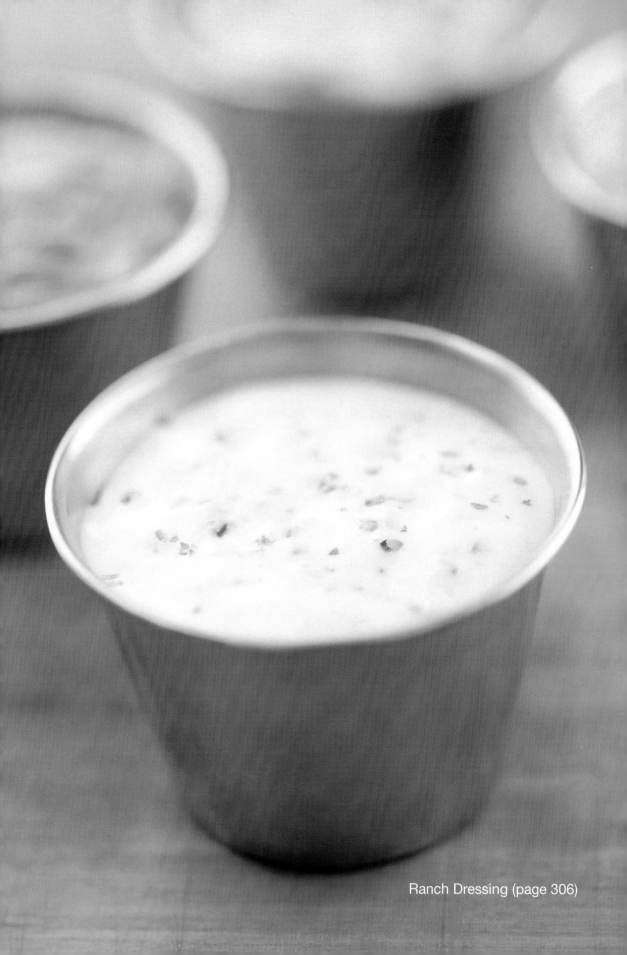

Ranch Dressing (page 306)

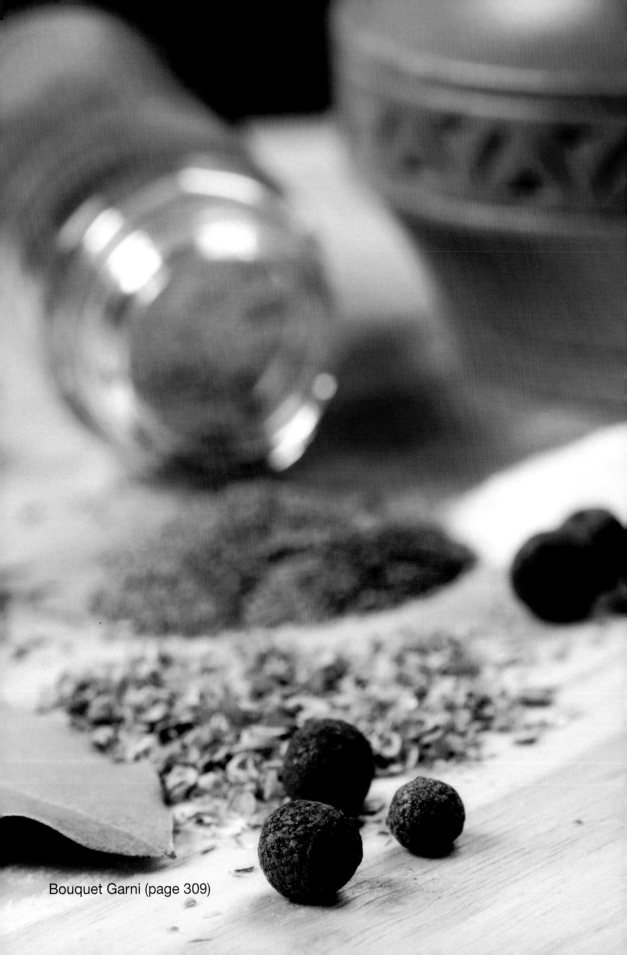

Bouquet Garni (page 309)

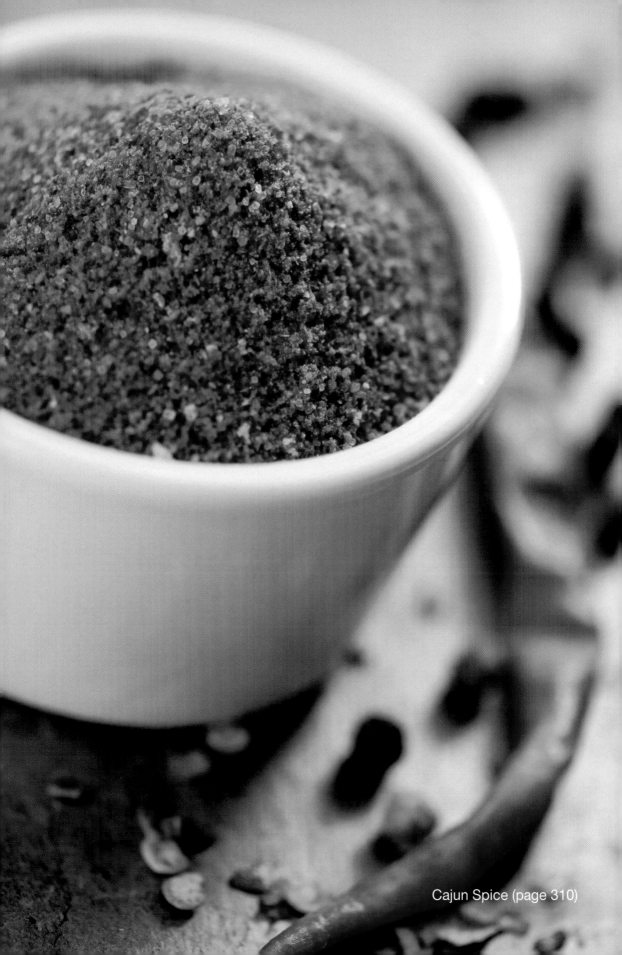

Cajun Spice (page 310)

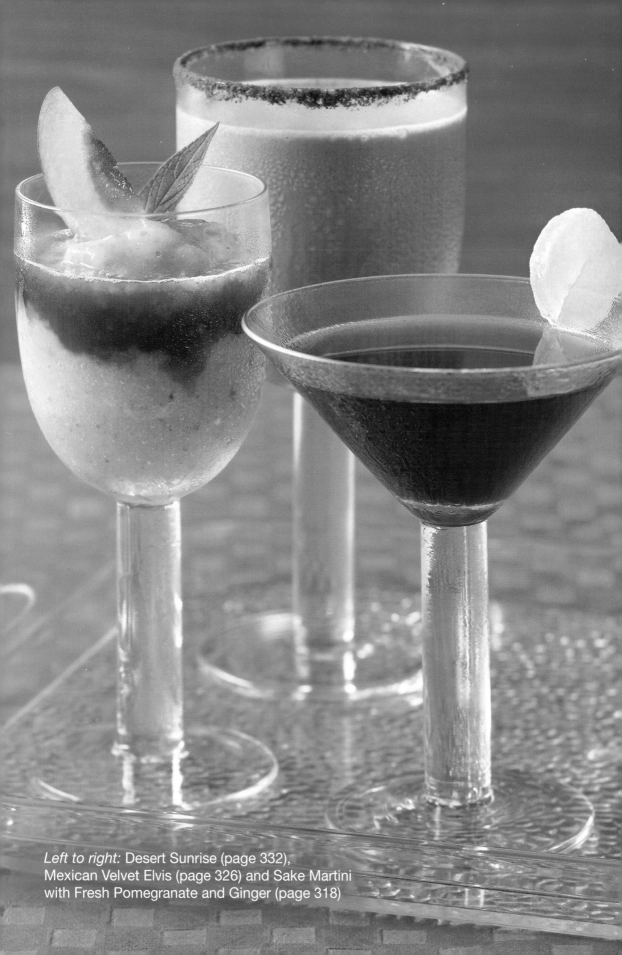

Left to right: Desert Sunrise (page 332),
Mexican Velvet Elvis (page 326) and Sake Martini
with Fresh Pomegranate and Ginger (page 318)

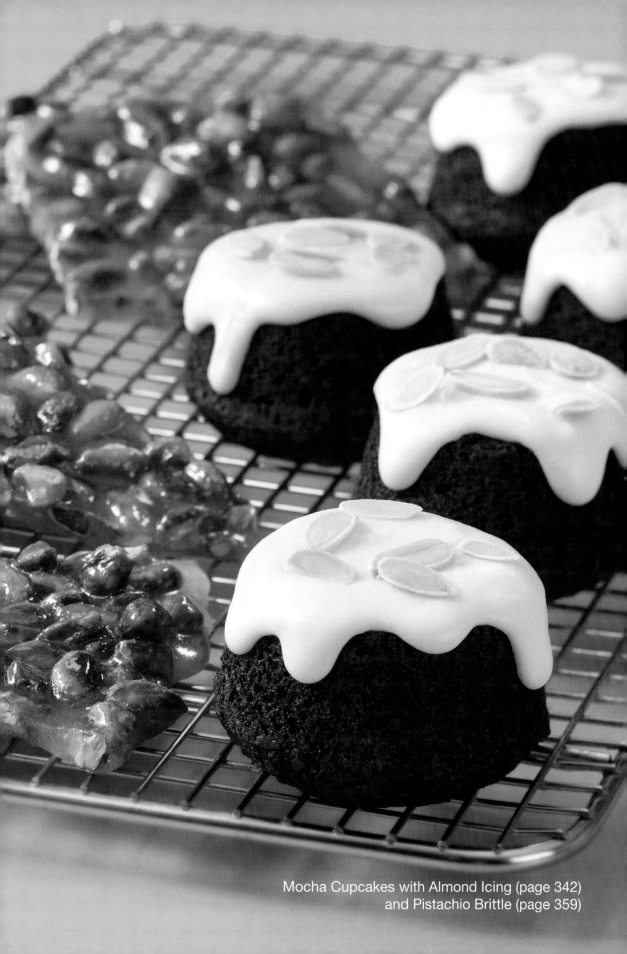

Mocha Cupcakes with Almond Icing (page 342)
and Pistachio Brittle (page 359)

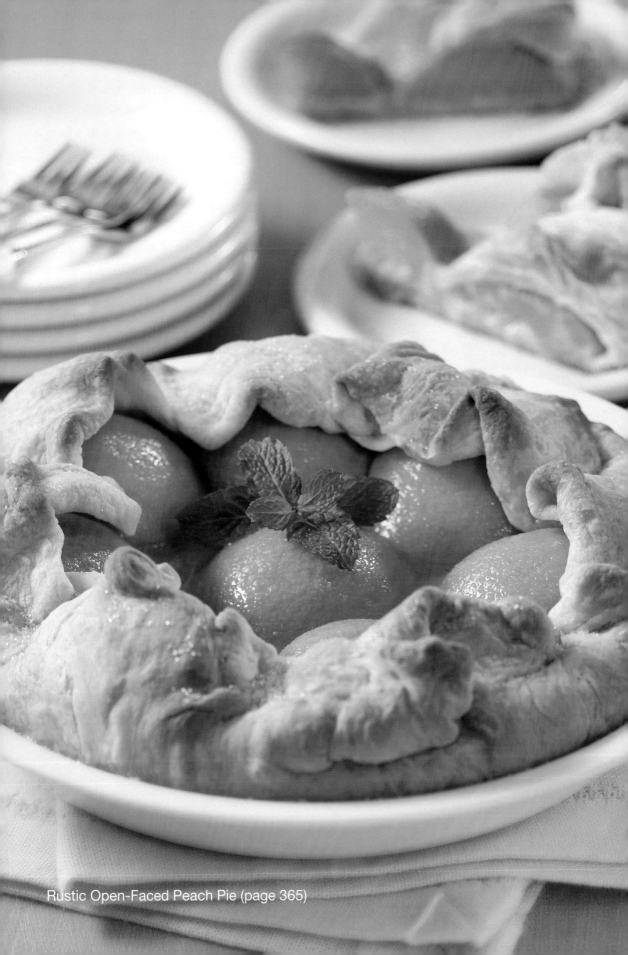

Rustic Open-Faced Peach Pie (page 365)

Beans, Pasta and Grains

✖—✖—✖—✖—✖—✖—✖—✖—✖—✖—✖—✖—✖

Boston baked beans

Serves 8 to 10

Old-fashioned flavors and tantalizing aromas make this dish a double winner. This is a good choice for a cold winter day because the beans are baked in the oven for several hours, heating the house and hinting at what is to come. Serve with Serrano and Roasted Pepper Cornbread (page 117).

✖ Tip

Refrigerate beans in an airtight container for up to 4 days. Beans will thicken as they cool and liquid may need to be added while reheating. Beans may be frozen for up to 1 month.

✖ **Dutch oven or ovenproof heavy bottomed saucepan**

2 cups	dried navy beans (see Beans, page 231)	500 mL
2 tbsp	olive oil	30 mL
1	onion, chopped	1
2	cloves garlic, minced	2
2	chipotle peppers, chopped	2
1/4 cup	blackstrap molasses	60 mL
1/4 cup	pure maple syrup	60 mL
1/4 cup	bourbon	60 mL
1/4 cup	tomato paste	60 mL
1 tbsp	liquid amino acids (see Tip, page 212)	15 mL
2 tsp	smoked paprika	10 mL
1 1/2 tsp	dry mustard powder	7 mL
1/2 tsp	freshly ground black pepper	2 mL
2 to 4 cups	Vegetable Broth (page 31) or store-bought	500 mL to 1 L
1 tsp	salt	5 mL

1. Pick through beans and discard any pebbles or beans that are shriveled or discolored. Rinse beans well under running water. Soak in water to cover for 8 hours or overnight.

2. Pour beans and their soaking water into a large stockpot and cover with water by 2 inches (5 cm). Bring to a full boil over medium–high heat. Reduce heat and simmer, covered, until almost tender, 45 minutes to 1 hour. Drain beans, reserving liquid.

3. Place a Dutch oven or ovenproof saucepan over medium heat and let pan get hot. Add oil and tip pan to coat. Add onion and garlic and cook, stirring occasionally, until softened, about 5 minutes. Add chipotle, molasses, maple syrup, bourbon, tomato paste, amino acids, paprika, mustard and pepper, stirring well to combine. Stir in beans and enough reserved liquid to cover, adding Vegetable Broth, if necessary. Increase heat to high, bring to a boil and remove from heat. Stir in salt.

4. Preheat oven to 325°F (160°C). Cover pan and bake in preheated oven until beans are tender, 3 to 4 hours. Check beans occasionally, adding heated reserved liquid or Vegetable Broth during cooking if beans become dry. Taste and adjust seasoning, as necessary. Remove lid during the last 45 minutes of cooking to thicken beans and develop a slight top crust. Serve hot.

Chana masala

Serves 6 to 8

This tantalizing blend of exotic flavors transform into this hearty and satisfying dish. Served over fragrant basmati rice, this is a fun make-ahead dish that is just right for buffet-style party.

Tip

Canned chickpeas are a quick substitute, but remember canned beans must be well rinsed and drained before use.

2 tbsp	olive oil	30 mL
1	onion, chopped	1
3	cloves garlic, minced	3
1	serrano chile, seeded and minced	2
1 tbsp	minced fresh gingerroot	15 mL
3 tbsp	Curry Powder (page 311) or store-bought	45 mL
2	cans (each 28 oz/796 mL) diced tomatoes with juice	2
3 cups	cooked chickpeas (see Tip, left)	750 mL
1/4 cup	finely chopped fresh parsley, divided	60 mL
3 tbsp	finely chopped fresh cilantro, divided	45 mL
1 tsp	salt	5 mL
1 tsp	freshly ground black pepper	5 mL
8 cups	cooked white basmati rice	2 L

1. Place a large deep heavy-bottomed saucepan over medium-high heat and let pan get hot. Add oil and tip pan to coat. Add onion and cook, stirring frequently, until well browned, 6 to 8 minutes. Stir in garlic, serrano, ginger and curry powder and cook, stirring constantly, until garlic is softened, 1 to 2 minutes. Stir in tomatoes with juice, chickpeas, 3 tbsp (45 mL) of the parsley, 2 tbsp (30 mL) of the cilantro, salt and pepper.
2. Cover pan and bring to a boil. Reduce heat and simmer for 10 minutes. Remove lid and simmer until thickened, 10 to 15 minutes.
3. To serve, place a few scoops of rice in a bowl and top with a generous serving of Chana Masala. Sprinkle with remaining chopped cilantro and parsley.

Creamy polenta with braised beans

Serves 6		

This is pure comfort food perfection on a crisp autumn day. Making the beans from scratch takes a little overnight planning, but is worth the effort.

✖ Tip

Beans can be prepared 1 or 2 days ahead and refrigerated in an airtight container.

Beans

1½ cups	dried cannellini beans (see Beans, page 231)	375 mL
2 tbsp	olive oil, divided	30 mL
¼ cup	chopped onion	60 mL
¼ cup	chopped celery	60 mL
¼ cup	chopped carrot	60 mL
4 tsp	minced garlic, divided	20 mL
1	bay leaf	1
1½ tsp	salt, divided	7 mL

Polenta

4 cups	Vegetable Broth (page 31) or store-bought	1 L
1 cup	cornmeal	250 mL
1 cup	coarsely chopped stemmed kale	250 mL
	Grated zest of 1 lemon	
¼ cup	freshly squeezed lemon juice	60 mL
¼ tsp	freshly ground black pepper	1 mL

1. *Beans:* Pick through beans and discard any pebbles or beans that are shriveled or discolored. Rinse beans well under running water. Soak in water to cover for 8 hours or overnight. Do not drain.

2. Place a skillet over medium heat and let pan get hot. Add 1 tbsp (15 mL) of the oil and tip pan to coat. Add onion, celery and carrot and cook, stirring occasionally, for 3 minutes. Add 2 tsp (10 mL) of the minced garlic and cook, stirring occasionally, until vegetables are softened, about 2 minutes. Transfer soaked beans with soaking liquid to vegetables, adding more water to cover, if necessary. Add bay leaf and bring mixture to a full boil over medium-high heat. Reduce heat, cover and simmer until beans are just tender but firm, about 45 minutes. Remove from heat, stir in 1 tsp (5 mL) of the salt and set aside.

3. *Polenta:* In a saucepan, bring vegetable broth to a boil over high heat. Gradually whisk in cornmeal, stirring constantly to eliminate lumps, for 2 minutes. Reduce heat to low, cover and simmer, stirring vigorously 2 or 3 times, until thickened, about 25 minutes. Remove from heat, cover and keep warm until beans are ready.

4. Meanwhile, place a large skillet over medium heat and let pan get hot. Add remaining 1 tbsp (15 mL) of oil and tip pan to coat. Add remaining 2 tsp (10 mL) of minced garlic and 1/2 tsp (2 mL) salt and cook, stirring, for 1 minute, being careful not to burn. Add kale, lemon zest, lemon juice and pepper and cook, stirring frequently, until kale is wilted, 6 to 8 minutes. Using a slotted spoon, transfer cooked beans to skillet with wilted kale, adding just enough of the cooking liquid to pan to keep mixture slightly moist. Spoon polenta into bowls and top with bean mixture. Serve immediately.

Giant christmas limas in herbed tomato jam

The Christmas lima is a large flat bean of a light cream color with deep maroon swirls and speckles that retain their beautiful markings during cooking. Their nut-like flavor and hearty texture make them the star of any dish. You might want to make extra as these beans taste even better a day or two later. Worth searching out, these fabulous heirloom beans are available from many online sources.

1 1/2 cups	dried Christmas Lima beans (see Beans, page 231)	375 mL
2 tbsp	olive oil, divided	30 mL
3/4 cup	chopped onion, divided	175 mL
1/4 cup	chopped carrot	60 mL
1/4 cup	chopped celery	60 mL
2	cloves garlic, minced	2
1	bay leaf	1
1 1/2 tsp	salt, divided	7 mL
3	cloves garlic, thinly sliced	3
2 1/2 cups	Roasted Roma Tomato Jam (page 297) or store-bought vegan alternative pasta sauce	625 mL
1/2 cup	torn fresh basil leaves	125 mL
2 tbsp	chopped fresh parsley	30 mL
1 tsp	fresh thyme leaves	5 mL
1/4 tsp	hot pepper flakes	1 mL
1/8 tsp	freshly ground black pepper	0.5 mL

1. *Beans:* Pick through beans and discard any pebbles or beans that are shriveled or discolored. Rinse beans well under running water. Soak in water to cover for 8 hours or overnight. Do not drain.

2. Place a large saucepan over medium heat and let pan get hot. Add 1 tbsp (15 mL) of the oil and tip pan to coat. Add 1/4 cup (60 mL) of the onion, carrot and celery and cook, stirring occasionally, for 3 minutes. Add minced garlic and cook until vegetables are softened, about 2 minutes. Add soaked beans with soaking liquid, adding more water to cover, if necessary. Add bay leaf and bring to a full boil over medium–high heat. Reduce heat to low, cover and simmer until beans are just cooked but still firm, about 45 minutes. Remove from heat, add 1 tsp (5 mL) of salt and set aside.

✂ Tip

Both beans and Roasted Roma Tomato Jam can be made ahead and refrigerated in an airtight container for up to 4 days.

✂ Variation

For a heartier meal, serve over brown rice or your favorite cooked grain.

3. Place another skillet over medium heat and let pan get hot. Add 1 tbsp (15 mL) of oil and tip pan to coat. Add ½ cup (125 mL) of onion and cook, stirring occasionally, until softened, 3 to 5 minutes. Reduce heat slightly, add sliced garlic cloves and cook until softened, about 2 minutes. Drain beans and add to pan. Stir in tomato jam, basil, parsley, thyme, hot pepper flakes, ½ tsp (2 mL) of salt and pepper. Increase heat to medium–high and when mixture begins to boil, reduce heat and simmer, partially covered, for 20 minutes. Stir and check beans often for doneness, making sure not to overcook. Beans should be firm, like a baked potato, not crunchy. Serve hot.

✂ Beans

To soak and cook dried beans: Pick through beans discarding any debris or dried and discolored beans. Cover dried beans with at least 4 inches (10 cm) of cold water and let soak for 8 hours or overnight. Check beans and add additional water, if necessary. When ready to cook, transfer beans and soaking liquid to an appropriate size pot. Do not drain beans as soaking water holds flavor and nutrients. Add additional water if necessary to cover beans by at least 3 inches (7.5 cm). Bring to a full boil over medium-high heat. Reduce to very lowest possible heat to keep beans at a gentle simmer until beans are just barely tender, 1½ to 2½ hours. Salt beans about 10 minutes before beans are finished cooking. Refrigerate beans in cooking liquid in an airtight container for up to 4 days. Beans may be frozen for up to 1 month.

Chile verde pinto beans

Serve up a piping hot bowl of Chile Verde Pinto Beans with warmed flour tortillas for a meal that will satisfy and warm your bones. Add protein and a Southwestern flavor to tacos, enchiladas or incorporate them into your favorite burger recipe.

✛ Tip

If you prefer fresh chiles, roast 5 to 6 medium-size Hatch or Anaheim chiles under your broiler. Use tongs to turn chiles until all sides are blackened. Wrap chiles in a damp clean kitchen towel to loosen skins. Peel charred skins from chiles before using.

2 cups	pinto beans	500 mL
1 tbsp	olive oil	15 mL
1	onion, chopped	1
3	cloves garlic, chopped	3
2	cans (each 4 oz/127 mL) chopped roasted mild green chile (see Tip, left)	2
1 tsp	sea salt	5 mL
1¼ tsp	ground cumin	6 mL
1 tsp	dried oregano	5 mL

1. Pick through beans and discard any that are shriveled or discolored. In a large stockpot, cover beans with water and soak for 8 hours or overnight.

2. Place a skillet over medium–high heat and let pan get hot. Add oil and tip pan to coat. Stir in onion and sauté until onion just begins to brown, 4 to 5 minutes. Stir in garlic and green chile and sauté for 3 to 4 minutes.

3. When beans are soaked, do not drain. Place pot on the stovetop, add water to cover beans by at least 2 inches (5 cm) and bring to a full boil over medium–high heat. Reduce heat to low, stir in sautéed vegetables, cover pot and simmer beans until tender, about 1½ hours. Add additional heated water if necessary to keep beans covered. Add salt, cumin and oregano about 10 minutes before beans are finished cooking. Taste and adjust seasoning, adding additional salt or cumin, if desired.

> ## ✛ Variation
> If you desire more heat in your beans, add jalapeño or serrano chiles.

Red chile posole

This recipe is easily doubled to serve a larger gathering. In New Mexico this would be called Christmas Posole as it is cooked with both red and green chiles.

✖ Tip

Look for ground New Mexico red chile in the Mexican section of your grocery store. If ground chile is unavailable, purchase the whole chiles and grind in a spice or coffee grinder, choosing mild, hot or a combination to suit your heat preference.

Posole

8 oz	dried posole	250 g
6 cups	water	1.5 L
1	onion, chopped	1
1	poblano pepper, stem and seeds removed	1
3	cloves garlic, coarsely chopped	3
1 tsp	dried oregano	5 mL
1 tsp	freshly squeezed lime juice	5 mL

Red Chile Sauce

1 tbsp	canola oil	15 mL
1 tbsp	all-purpose flour	15 mL
2 tbsp	New Mexico ground red chile powder	30 mL
1 cup	water	250 mL
1/4 tsp	sea salt	1 mL
1/4 tsp	ground cumin	1 mL
4 to 6	flour tortillas, any size, warmed	4 to 6
1	small onion, diced	1
1	avocado, cut into bite-size pieces	1
6	sprigs fresh cilantro, leaves minced	6

1. *Posole:* Rinse posole well under running water. Soak in water to cover for 8 hours or overnight.

2. In a large heavy-bottomed pot, combine soaked posole, water, onion, poblano pepper, garlic, oregano and lime juice and bring to a boil over medium–high heat. Reduce heat and simmer until posole is tender and most have popped open, 2 to 3 hours.

3. *Red Chile Sauce:* Meanwhile, in a small saucepan, heat oil over medium heat. Whisk in flour and cook, stirring constantly, for 1 minute. Whisk in chile powder to form a thick roux. Cook, stirring constantly, for 1 minute. Gradually whisk in water, stirring constantly, taking care that no lumps form. Reduce heat, add sea salt and cumin and simmer, stirring occasionally, until flavors are developed and sauce is slightly thickened, for 15 minutes.

4. When posole is tender and most have popped open, stir in half of the red chile sauce into posole. Mix well and taste, adding more sauce, if desired. Place any remaining sauce in a small serving bowl.

5. Serve posole hot with tortillas and pass bowls of onion, avocado, cilantro and any remaining red chile sauce.

Artichoke ravioli

The tried and true pairing of artichoke with white wine produces a tantalizing filling for homemade ravioli. A drizzle of your best olive oil, a few toasted pine nuts, a handful of Italian parsley and freshly ground black pepper only enhance the delicate flavors inside.

✖ Tips

While sealing ravioli it is important to push out any air because trapped air will cause ravioli to burst while cooking. After sealing with fingertips, press ravioli edges firmly together with tines of a fork to ensure a strong seal.

Recipes that use floating ravioli as an indication that they are done can be misleading because many ravioli float from the second they touch the water. The best indicator is pasta that is just tender to the bite.

✖ **Food processor**
✖ **Rolling pin or pasta machine**

Filling

2 tbsp	olive oil	30 mL
1	shallot, chopped	1
1 cup	canned or frozen artichoke hearts, thawed and chopped	250 mL
2 tbsp	dry white wine	30 mL
1 cup	Basic Ricotta (page 21) or store-bought vegan alternative	250 mL
	Salt and freshly ground black pepper	
¼ tsp	ground nutmeg	1 mL
1	Basic Homemade Pasta Dough recipe (page 236) or 1 lb (500 g) store-bought vegan fresh pasta noodles	1
	Flour	
¼ cup	olive oil	60 mL
¼ cup	toasted pine nuts	60 mL
¼ cup	chopped Italian flat-leaf parsley	60 mL

1. *Filling:* Place a skillet over medium heat and let pan get hot. Add oil and tip pan to coat. Add shallot and cook, stirring, until softened, 2 to 3 minutes. Add artichoke hearts and wine and cook, stirring, to combine flavors, about 1 minute. Remove from heat and let cool.

2. Transfer cooled mixture to food processor. Add ricotta, ½ tsp (2 mL) salt, ½ tsp (2 mL) black pepper and nutmeg and pulse until coarsely chopped, 4 to 6 times.

3. Place pasta dough on a lightly floured work surface. Divide into quarters and cover with a clean kitchen towel. Working with one piece of dough at a time, roll pasta into ⅛-inch (3 mm) thick sheets. Cut pasta sheets into 48 1-inch (2.5 cm) squares or 32 2-inch (5 cm) squares. Spoon 1 tsp (5 mL) of the filling for small squares or 1½ tsp (7 mL) for large squares in the center of each square, taking care not to overfill. Moisten around filling with water and top with another square. Press down to seal, pushing out any air. Lightly dust ravioli with flour and cover with a clean kitchen towel while rolling and filling remaining pasta dough.

4. Bring a large pot of salted water to a boil over medium–high heat. Gently place 8 to 12 ravioli at a time into boiling water without overcrowding. Adjust heat to keep water at a gentle boil and cook ravioli until just tender, 6 to 10 minutes, depending on size and thickness. With a slotted spoon, transfer cooked ravioli to a warmed serving platter, drizzle with olive oil and loosely cover while cooking remaining ravioli. Before serving, scatter with pine nuts, parsley and black pepper to taste. Serve immediately.

Citrus israeli couscous

Serves 4

Big beautiful pearls of Israeli couscous are cooked with lime and orange juice, cinnamon and black pepper. Tossed with pine nuts and parsley, this colorful dish looks as good as it tastes.

2 tbsp	olive oil	30 mL
1 cup	Israeli couscous	250 mL
1/2 tsp	ground cinnamon	2 mL
	Salt and freshly ground black pepper	
1/4 cup	freshly squeezed lime juice	60 mL
1/4 cup	freshly squeezed orange juice	60 mL
1 1/2 cups	water	375 mL
2 tbsp	chopped Italian flat-leaf parsley	30 mL
1/2 cup	toasted pine nuts	125 mL

1. Place a saucepan over medium–high heat and let pan get hot. Add oil and tip pan to coat. Stir in couscous, cinnamon, 1/2 tsp (2 mL) salt and 1/2 tsp (2 mL) pepper and cook, stirring occasionally, until lightly browned, 3 to 4 minutes. Stir in lime juice and orange juice and deglaze pan, stirring up all the browned bits on the bottom. Add water and bring to a boil. Reduce heat and simmer, stirring occasionally, until all liquid is absorbed, 10 to 12 minutes. Stir in parsley, pine nuts and salt and pepper to taste and serve.

Basic homemade pasta dough

Makes 1 lb (500 g)

Why spend a fortune at the grocery store for fresh pasta when it is so easy to make at home from flour and water? Fresh pasta elevates any dish and is fabulous with just a splash of nut oil and a sprinkle of salt and pepper.

✖ Tips

To knead the pasta dough: Using palms of your hands, push dough down and away from you. Grab furthest edge of dough and fold toward you to form a ball. Turn ball a quarter-turn and repeat process. Place a clean kitchen towel over back of a chair, drape cut pasta over it and let dry for 20 to 30 minutes for easier handling and storage.

Rolled and cut fresh pasta may be frozen in a resealable freezer bag for up to 3 months. If freezing, defrost dough on a floured work surface before cooking.

1 1/2 cups	all-purpose flour	375 mL
1 cup	semolina flour	250 mL
	Salt	
1/2 to 1 cup	water	125 to 250 mL

1. On a work surface, combine all-purpose flour, semolina flour and 1/2 tsp (2 mL) salt and form a mound. Create a well in center and add 1/4 cup (60 mL) of the water. With your hands, mix water into flour until a rough dough begins to form. Pull flour in from sides and push outer flour up to maintain a well while adding water, 1 tbsp (15 mL) at a time, until all flour is incorporated into a stiff dough. Knead dough, lightly flouring your hands, work surface or dough as needed, until elastic and slightly sticky, 8 to 10 minutes. Cover dough with a kitchen towel and let rest for 15 minutes.

2. Roll dough out and cut pasta according to recipe or wrap tightly in plastic wrap and refrigerate for up to 3 days.

3. To cook fresh pasta, bring a large stockpot of salted water to a boil over medium-high heat. Add pasta and adjust heat to keep water at a gentle boil. Cook pasta, stirring occasionally to prevent sticking, until just tender, 1 to 2 minutes for very thin pasta and 10 to 14 minutes for shaped, filled and thicker pasta.

> ## ✖ Variations
> Substitute 1/4 cup (60 mL) wine for an equal amount of water. Add 1 tbsp (15 mL) pumpkin purée, tomato paste, olive paste, olive or flavored oils or finely minced fresh herbs.

Capellini with sun-dried tomatoes and gremolata

Serves 4 to 6

Parsley provides the herby freshness in a bright and beautiful gremolata. Fresh pasta is tossed with this gorgeous and fragrant pairing dotted with ruby red sun-dried tomatoes.

Gremolata

	Zest of 2 lemons (about 4 tsp/20 mL)	
4	cloves garlic, finely chopped	4
1 cup	finely chopped fresh parsley	250 mL
½ cup	olive oil	125 mL
¾ cup	chopped sun-dried tomatoes in oil, drained	175 mL
2 tbsp	freshly squeezed lemon juice	30 mL
2 tsp	hot pepper flakes	10 mL
1 lb	fresh capellini pasta	500 g
¾ cup	toasted pine nuts	175 mL
	Salt and freshly ground black pepper	

1. *Gremolata:* In a small bowl, combine lemon zest, garlic and parsley, mixing well. Set aside.

2. In another small bowl, whisk together oil, sun-dried tomatoes, lemon juice and hot pepper flakes. Set aside.

3. Bring a large pot of salted water to a boil over medium-high heat. Add capellini and boil, stirring occasionally, until cooked al dente, 3 to 5 minutes. Drain, reserving ½ cup (125 mL) water and transfer pasta to a large serving bowl. Pour sun-dried tomato mixture over pasta and toss to coat. Add 2 tbsp (30 mL) hot pasta water, gremolata and pine nuts and toss to combine. Add salt and pepper to taste and serve hot.

> ## ❖ Variation
> Substitute fresh basil for parsley or use ½ cup (125 mL) Basil Lemon Gremolata Pesto (page 285) or store-bought non-dairy basil pesto.

Caramelized eggplant with fettuccini and roasted red pepper sauce

Sweet almonds, charred red peppers and aromatic Hungarian paprika blend into a sumptuous sauce ladled over fresh pasta and topped with crispy sautéed eggplant. Serve this with a simple mix of greens, a drizzle of olive oil and a rustic loaf of bread.

✴ **Food processor**

Eggplant

1	large eggplant, peeled, cut into 1-inch (2.5 cm) cubes	1
	Salt	
2 tbsp	olive oil	30 mL
1 tbsp	chopped fresh oregano	15 mL
1/4 tsp	freshly ground black pepper	1 mL

Roasted Red Pepper Sauce

1	can (15 oz/425 mL) crushed tomatoes	1
2 cups	roasted red bell peppers (about 3)	500 mL
1 cup	almond butter	250 mL
3	cloves garlic, crushed	3
1/2 cup	dry white wine	125 mL
1/4 to	water	60 to
1/2 cup		125 mL
1 tbsp	smoked Hungarian paprika	15 mL
1 tsp	hot pepper sauce	5 mL
1 tsp	salt	5 mL
3/4 tsp	freshly ground black pepper	3 mL

1 1/2 lbs	vegan store-bought fresh fettucini, cooked	750 g
1/4 cup	chopped parsley	60 mL
1/4 cup	Sprinkle (page 30) or store-bought grated vegan Parmesan cheese alternative, optional	60 mL

1. Place eggplant in a colander, toss with 1 tsp (5 mL) salt and set aside to drain for about 20 minutes. Rinse and pat dry (see Tip, right).

2. *Roasted Red Pepper Sauce:* Meanwhile, in food processor, combine tomatoes, red peppers, almond butter and garlic and process until smooth. Add wine, $\frac{1}{4}$ cup (60 mL) of the water, paprika, hot pepper sauce, salt and pepper and process until smooth, adding additional water if needed to make a smooth pouring sauce.

3. Transfer sauce to a saucepan and bring to a boil over medium heat, stirring occasionally. Reduce heat to low, cover and simmer, stirring occasionally, until slightly thickened, 10 to 15 minutes. Taste and adjust seasoning.

4. *Eggplant:* Place a large skillet over medium-high heat and let pan get hot. Add oil and tip pan to coat. Add eggplant, oregano, $\frac{1}{4}$ tsp (1 mL) salt and pepper and cook, stirring frequently, until softened with caramelized edges, 6 to 8 minutes. Remove from heat.

5. Divide fettuccini among 4 serving bowls, top with a generous ladle of sauce and one-quarter of caramelized eggplant. Top with parsley and Sprinkle, if using.

Rice noodle bowl with lime-arugula pesto

Rice noodles are a pleasant change from wheat pasta. They are delicious tossed with this Asian-inspired pesto, and are kind to those looking for gluten-free options.

✖ Tip

Soak rice stick noodles according to package directions, checking frequently because noodles are easily over "cooked" and become mushy.

✖ Variations

Use angel hair or favorite pasta in place of rice noodles. Stir in 2 cups (500 mL) sautéed vegetables such as red bell pepper and yellow summer squash. Add hot vegetable broth to make a quick noodle soup.

✖ **Food processor**

Lime-Arugula Pesto

2 cups	packed fresh arugula	500 mL
	Zest and juice of 1 lime	
¾ cup	toasted almonds	175 mL
2 tbsp	rice wine vinegar	30 mL
1 tbsp	toasted sesame oil	15 mL
1 tbsp	white miso	15 mL
½ cup	almond or olive oil	125 mL
	Salt and freshly ground black pepper	
1	package (8 oz /250 g) rice noodles (see Tip, left)	1
1 tsp	olive oil	5 mL
2	cloves garlic, chopped	2
2 tsp	grated gingerroot	10 mL
2 tbsp	toasted sesame seeds, optional	30 mL

1. *Lime-Arugula Pesto:* In food processor, combine arugula, lime zest, lime juice, almonds, rice wine vinegar, sesame oil and miso and pulse until coarsely chopped, 30 to 45 seconds. Scrape sides and, with machine running, drizzle in almond oil through feed tube while processing mixture into a smooth pesto. Scrape sides, add salt and pepper to taste, pulse to combine and set aside.

2. Place rice noodles in a large bowl. Cover with warm water and soak until softened, depending on thickness of noodles. Drain noodles, reserving ½ cup (125 mL) of soaking water.

3. Place a large skillet over medium heat and let pan get hot. Add olive oil and tip pan to coat. Add garlic and ginger and cook, stirring frequently, for 30 seconds. Stir in pesto and ¼ cup (60 mL) reserved noodle water to slightly loosen pesto, adding more water, if needed. Add rice noodles and toss to coat with pesto. Serve noodles hot in bowls garnished with sesame seeds, if using.

Hearty seitan tomato sauce with linguine

Serves 8 to 10

This is a real stick to your ribs, satisfying meal guaranteed to take the chill off a cold winter's night. The recipe makes enough for a crowd and is a great make-ahead dish because it actually benefits from a couple of days in the refrigerator. Serve with thick slices of hot garlic bread to scoop up every last bit.

Tips

Store-bought vegetable bouillons can be salty so if using, add salt only after tasting sauce.

Sauce can be served with pasta immediately or refrigerate in an airtight container for up to 5 days.

4 tbsp	olive oil, divided	60 mL
1	onion, chopped	1
4	cloves garlic, chopped	4
2	cans (each 28 oz/796 mL) crushed tomatoes	2
2 tbsp	tomato paste	30 mL
1/2 cup	dry red wine	125 mL
2 2/3 cups	ground seitan	650 mL
1 tbsp	Homemade Vegetable Bouillon (page 32) or store-bought (see Tips, left)	15 mL
2 tsp	vegan browning sauce, such as Kitchen Bouquet (see page 10)	10 mL
2	bay leaves	2
1 tbsp	dried basil	15 mL
3/4 tsp	granulated sugar	3 mL
1/2 tsp	salt	2 mL
1/4 tsp	freshly ground black pepper	1 mL
1 to 2 lbs	linguine, cooked	500 g to 1 kg
1/4 cup	chopped fresh parsley	60 mL

1. Place a large high-sided skillet over medium-high heat and let pan get hot. Add 2 tbsp (30 mL) of the oil and tip pan to coat. Add onion and cook, stirring occasionally, until browned and softened, 4 to 5 minutes. Reduce heat, add garlic and cook until garlic begins to soften, 1 to 2 minutes.
2. Add tomatoes and tomato paste, mixing well to combine. Stir in wine, seitan, bouillon, browning sauce, bay leaves, basil, sugar, salt, pepper and 2 tbsp (30 mL) of oil and cook, stirring occasionally, for 20 minutes. Reduce heat to low, taste and adjust seasoning, adding more salt, if necessary. Cook sauce until thick and rich, about 1 hour.
3. Place cooked pasta in a large pasta serving bowl, pour sauce over all and scatter with parsley. Serve hot.

Orecchiette pasta with eggplant garlic sauce

Orecchiette, loosely translated is Italian for "little ear," which its shape definitely resembles. It is absolutely the perfect little pasta for scooping up this beautiful thick sauce.

✖ Tip

Although fresh is always best, in this recipe 1 tsp (5 mL) dried herbs could easily be substituted for fresh herbs.

✖ Variations

Substitute penne pasta for orecchiette pasta.

Stir in 2 cups (500 mL) fresh chopped tomatoes at the very end, just before serving.

1½ lbs	eggplant, unpeeled, cut into ½-inch (1 cm) cubes	750 g
3 tsp	salt, divided	15 mL
½ cup	olive oil	125 mL
¼ cup	chopped onion	60 mL
6	cloves garlic, chopped	6
¼ cup	chopped fresh parsley	60 mL
¼ cup	chopped fresh basil	60 mL
2 tsp	fresh thyme leaves	10 mL
½ tsp	freshly ground black pepper	2 mL
¼ cup	freshly squeezed lemon juice	60 mL
½ cup	white wine	125 mL
½ cup	Vegetable Broth (page 31) or store-bought	125 mL
8 oz	orecchiette pasta	250 g
¼ cup	toasted pine nuts	60 mL

1. Place eggplant in a colander, toss with 2 tsp (10 mL) of the salt and stir to coat cubes and set aside to drain for 20 minutes. Rinse and pat dry (see Tip, page 239).

2. Place a large skillet over medium–low heat and let pan get hot. Add oil and tip pan to coat. Add onion and garlic and cook, stirring occasionally, adjusting heat to keep from burning garlic, until softened, 6 to 8 minutes. Add eggplant, parsley, basil, thyme, remaining 1 tsp (5 mL) of salt and pepper, stirring to combine. Cover, reduce heat to low and cook, stirring occasionally, until eggplant is soft, about 20 minutes. Add lemon juice, wine and broth and continue cooking, stirring occasionally, until sauce is thick but not dry, about 5 minutes.

3. Bring a large pot of salted water to a boil over high heat. Add pasta and cook, stirring occasionally, until al dente, 10 to 12 minutes. Using a slotted spoon, add pasta to sauce, allowing a little of pasta water to splash into sauce if it needs thinning. Combine well, stir in pine nuts and serve.

Manicotti florentine

This rich dish is perfect for a little dinner party and is easily made ahead to the baking stage. Refrigerate and bake as your guests arrive. The tantalizing aroma will hint at what's to come. Open a bottle of wine and allow guests to "help" make the salad.

✖ Tip

To remove grit from fresh spinach: Fill clean sink with water, stir in 2 tbsp (30 mL) vinegar and add spinach. Swish spinach through water and let stand, swishing once or twice, for 5 minutes. Vinegar will loosen grit on leaves allowing it to fall. Carefully transfer spinach to a colander set over a bowl, avoiding contact with bottom of sink. Drain water, place colander in sink and rinse spinach.

✖ Preheat oven to 350°F (180°C)
✖ Pastry bag with tip or resealable large plastic bag
✖ 13- by 9-inch (33 by 23 cm) glass baking dish

	Salt	
1 lb	spinach (see Tip, left)	500 g
10	manicotti shells	10
1 lb	Basic Ricotta (page 21) or store-bought vegan alternative	500 g
½ cup	grated vegan Parmesan cheese alternative	125 mL
2 tbsp	nutritional yeast powder	30 mL
¾ tsp	ground nutmeg	3 mL
½ tsp	freshly ground black pepper	2 mL
½ cup	packed chopped basil	125 mL
6 cups	Fresh Pomodoro Sauce (page 287) or store-bought marinara sauce	1.5 L
12	basil leaves, torn	12

1. Bring a large pot of salted water to a boil over medium–high heat. Prepare ice bath by filling a large bowl three-quarter full of ice and set aside. Add spinach to boiling water and cook until tender, 3 to 5 minutes. Using a slotted spoon, transfer spinach to ice bath, leaving water in pot to use for cooking pasta. Drain spinach and squeeze out excess water. Chop and set aside.

2. Bring spinach water back to a boil. Add pasta and cook, stirring occasionally, until tender but still firm to the bite, 10 to 12 minutes or according to package directions. Drain pasta and set aside to dry.

3. In a large bowl, combine ricotta, Parmesan, nutritional yeast, nutmeg, pepper and ¼ tsp (1 mL) salt, mixing well to blend. Stir in basil and spinach.

4. Spread 1 cup (250 mL) of the sauce over bottom of baking dish. Spoon ricotta filling into pastry bag. Fill cooked and dried noodles with ricotta mixture and arrange in prepared baking dish. Spoon remaining sauce over noodles covering edges to ensure moist pasta. Bake in preheated oven until manicotti is heated through and sauce is bubbly, 30 to 35 minutes. Remove from oven and let stand for about 5 minutes. Top with basil leaves and serve.

Savory porcini lasagna

The intense and earthy flavors of dried porcini mushrooms are the centerpiece of this hearty lasagna. Serve with a glass of bold red wine, a few simply tossed garden fresh greens and a loaf of warm crusty bread and you have a feast fit for your favorite land baron.

✖ Tip

Make an extra effort to clean dried mushrooms well even if the packaging states "clean no-sand." One bite containing grit can spoil the dish.

✖ Fine-mesh sieve, lined with coffee filter or triple layer of cheesecloth
✖ Food processor
✖ 13- by 9-inch (33 by 23 cm) glass baking dish, lightly oiled

3 oz	dried porcini mushrooms	90 g
1 cup	water	250 mL
1/2 cup	dry red wine	125 mL
1 tbsp	olive oil	30 mL
1/3 cup	sliced drained oil-packed sun-dried tomatoes	75 mL
3	cloves garlic, chopped	3
1 1/2 tsp	chopped fresh thyme	7 mL

Sauce

1 tbsp	olive oil	30 mL
1	large onion, chopped	1
1 1/2	cans (28 oz/796 mL) crushed tomatoes	1 1/2
2 tbsp	tomato paste	30 mL
1 tbsp	chopped fresh rosemary	15 mL
1 tsp	salt	5 mL
1 tsp	freshly ground black pepper	5 mL

Filling

2 cups	Basic Ricotta (page 21) or store-bought vegan alternative	500 mL
1 cup	packed fresh basil	250 mL
2 tsp	nutritional yeast powder	10 mL
1 tsp	onion powder	5 mL
1 tsp	freshly ground black pepper	5 mL
1/4 tsp	ground nutmeg	1 mL
9	vegan oven-ready lasagna noodles	9
8 oz	grated vegan Parmesan cheese alternative	250 g

1. Rinse dried mushrooms under running water while opening crevices to expose trapped grit. In a small saucepan, heat water and wine over low heat until steaming but do not boil. Remove pan from heat, add mushrooms and let soak for 30 minutes to reconstitute.

Substitute 1 lb (500 g)
fresh mushrooms, sliced,
for 3 oz (90 g) dried, skip
Step 1 and add 1 cup
(250 mL) vegetable broth
and ½ cup (125 mL) red
wine to the sauce.

Using a slotted spoon, remove mushrooms from soaking liquid and transfer to a colander (reserving soaking liquid). Rinse mushrooms well under running water and set aside to drain. Strain soaking liquid through prepared sieve into a small bowl and set aside.

2. *Sauce:* Place a large saucepan over medium heat and let pan get hot. Add oil and tip pan to coat. Add onion and cook, stirring occasionally, until softened, 4 to 5 minutes. Stir in reserved mushroom liquid, tomatoes, tomato paste, rosemary, salt and pepper and bring to a boil. Partially cover pan, reduce heat to low and cook, stirring occasionally, until sauce is thickened, about 30 minutes.

3. Place a skillet over medium heat and let pan get hot. Add 1 tbsp (15 mL) oil and tip pan to coat. Add reserved mushrooms and cook, stirring, until slightly browned, 4 to 6 minutes. Stir in sun-dried tomatoes, garlic and thyme and cook, stirring, until garlic is softened, 1 to 2 minutes. Set aside.

4. *Filling:* In food processor, pulse ricotta, basil, nutritional yeast, onion powder, black pepper and nutmeg until roughly blended, 8 to 10 times.

5. Preheat oven to 350°F (180°C).

6. Spread 2 cups (500 mL) sauce over bottom of prepared baking dish and layer with 3 lasagna noodles. Spread one-third of ricotta filling over noodles and top with one-third of mushroom mixture. Cover with one-third of the remaining sauce. Layer 3 noodles over sauce, spread noodles with half of remaining ricotta filling and top with half of remaining mushrooms. Spoon half of remaining sauce over mushrooms and top with last layer of noodles. Spread remaining ricotta filling over noodles and top with remaining mushrooms. Spoon remaining sauce over mushrooms and sprinkle cheese alternative over top. Loosely cover dish with foil, avoiding contact with lasagna. With oven-ready noodles, it is best to let assembled lasagna rest for about 30 minutes, allowing noodles to absorb liquid before baking.

7. Bake in preheated oven for 30 minutes. Remove foil and bake until lasagna is bubbly, noodles are tender and cheese is golden brown, about 10 minutes. Let stand until firm, about 20 minutes.

Summertime zucchini pesto lasagna

In the summertime, zucchini and basil abound in backyard gardens and farmer's markets. This magnificent dish stars two summertime favorites in this tasty lasagna.

> ✖ Preheat oven to 450°F (230°C)
> ✖ Baking sheet, lined with parchment paper
> ✖ 13- by 9-inch (33 by 23 cm) glass baking dish, lightly oiled

2 lbs	zucchini, sliced into $\frac{1}{4}$-inch (0.5 cm) rounds	1 kg
$3\frac{1}{2}$ tbsp	olive oil, divided	52 mL
$\frac{3}{4}$ tsp	salt, divided	3 mL
$\frac{1}{2}$ tsp	freshly ground black pepper, divided	2 mL
$\frac{1}{3}$ cup	all-purpose flour	75 mL
$3\frac{1}{2}$ cups	soy, nut or hemp milk	875 mL
$\frac{1}{2}$ cup	Classic Pesto Sauce (page 286) or vegan store-bought pesto	125 mL
12	vegan oven-ready lasagna noodles	12
6 oz	vegan mozzarella cheese alternative, grated and divided	175 g

1. In a large bowl, combine zucchini, $1\frac{1}{2}$ tbsp (22 mL) of the oil, $\frac{1}{4}$ tsp (1 mL) of the salt and $\frac{1}{4}$ tsp (1 mL) of the black pepper. Spread zucchini onto prepared baking sheet in a single layer. Roast in preheated oven until softened and slightly browned, 10 to 12 minutes. Remove from oven and set aside. Reduce oven temperature to 350°F (180°C).

2. Place a saucepan over medium heat and let pan get hot. Add 2 tbsp (30 mL) of oil and tip pan to coat. Gradually whisk in flour and cook, whisking vigorously, until a loose paste forms, 2 to 3 minutes. Gradually add milk, whisking to incorporate before adding more milk to avoid lumps. Bring to a gentle boil, whisking, until sauce is thickened, about 1 minute. Remove from heat and stir in pesto, $\frac{1}{2}$ tsp (2 mL) of salt and $\frac{1}{4}$ tsp (1 mL) of black pepper.

3. Place 4 lasagna noodles in bottom of prepared baking dish, overlapping slightly. Layer with one-third of roasted zucchini followed by one-third of cheese alternative and one-third of pesto sauce. Repeat layering with 4 noodles, half of remaining roasted zucchini, half of cheese and half of pesto sauce. Top with remaining 4 noodles. Pour remaining pesto sauce over noodles, scatter remaining cheese over sauce and top with

remaining zucchini. With oven-ready noodles, it is best to let assembled lasagna rest for about 30 minutes, allowing noodles to absorb liquid before baking.

4. Bake in preheated oven until noodles are tender, sauce is bubbly and top is browned, 35 to 40 minutes. Remove from oven and let stand until firm, 10 to 15 minutes before serving.

Spicy soba and chinese broccoli stir-fry

Serves 2 to 4

Bottled Asian garlic and chile sauce packs a punch, adding heat and flavor to this tasty stir-fry. Chinese broccoli, portobello mushrooms and baked tofu make this sumptuous meal a healthy one.

❌ Tip

Find Chinese broccoli at your local Asian grocery store or well-stocked supermarkets.

2 tbsp	canola oil	30 mL
2 cups	chopped Chinese broccoli (see Tip, left)	500 mL
2	cloves garlic, minced	2
2 tbsp	grated gingerroot	30 mL
1	Japanese eggplant, trimmed and cubed	1
1	baby bok choy, trimmed and thinly sliced	1
1	portobello mushroom cap, halved and thinly sliced	1
2 tbsp	rice wine vinegar	30 mL
1 to 2 tsp	Asian garlic-chile sauce	5 to 10 mL
8 oz	soba noodles, cooked	250 g
6	green onions, white and light green parts only, sliced	6
2 cups	cubed Hearty Savory Baked Tofu (page 25) or store-bought baked tofu	500 mL

1. Place a large heavy-bottomed skillet over medium-high heat and let pan get hot. Add oil and tip pan to coat. Add Chinese broccoli and cook, stirring frequently, until slightly softened, 2 to 3 minutes. Add garlic, ginger, eggplant, bok choy and mushrooms and cook, stirring frequently, until softened and fragrant, about 6 minutes. Stir in vinegar and chile sauce and cook, stirring constantly to combine, about 1 minute.

2. Toss in soba noodles, green onions and tofu, gently stirring to combine. Taste and add additional chile sauce, if desired.

Swiss chard ravioli

Serves 8

Using ready-made vegan wonton wrappers makes this a simple dish to accomplish. The rewards will be great as you savor the delicate flavors of the ravioli topped with Fresh Pomodoro Sauce.

- Baking sheet, lined with parchment paper

1	bunch Swiss chard, stems removed	1
10 oz	firm tofu, drained	300 g
1/4 cup	almond milk	60 mL
	Zest of 1 orange	
	Zest of 1 lemon	
1 tbsp	freshly squeezed orange juice	15 mL
1 tbsp	freshly squeezed lemon juice	15 mL
1 tsp	cornstarch	5 mL
1 tsp	granulated sugar	5 mL
1 tsp	salt	5 mL
1/4 tsp	ground black pepper	1 mL
40	vegan wonton wrappers	40
4 to 6 tsp	olive oil	20 to 30 mL
	Fresh Pomodoro Sauce (page 287) or store-bought vegan marinara sauce	
16 to 24	basil leaves	16 to 24

1. Place chard in a large pot with about 1 inch (2.5 cm) of water. Turn heat to high and bring water to a boil. Reduce heat to low, cover pan and steam chard until completely wilted, about 5 minutes. Transfer to a colander to drain. When cool enough to handle, using hands, squeeze out all liquid. Finely dice chard and set aside.
2. In a large bowl, mash together tofu and almond milk. In a small bowl, whisk together orange juice, lemon juice and cornstarch. Add to tofu mixture along with chopped chard, orange and lemon zest, sugar, salt and pepper and gently mix to incorporate.

3. Place a small bowl of water near work area. Working in batches, lay a few wonton wrappers on a clean work surface and, using fingertips, brush edges with water. Place 1 tsp (5 mL) of filling in center of each wrapper, taking care not to overfill. Fold wrapper in half, diagonally to form a half triangle. Press down to seal, pushing out any air. Transfer ravioli to prepared baking sheet and repeat until all are assembled.

4. Place a large serving platter in oven and set oven to 200°F (100°C). Bring a large pot of salted water to a boil over medium-high heat. Gently place 8 to 12 ravioli into boiling water without overcrowding. Adjust heat to keep water at a gentle boil and cook ravioli until just tender, 6 to 10 minutes, depending on size and thickness. With a slotted spoon, transfer cooked ravioli to warmed platter and drizzle with about 1 tsp (5 mL) oil. Loosely cover and return platter to oven until all ravioli are cooked.

5. To serve, arrange a few ravioli on a plate and top with Fresh Pomodoro Sauce and 2 or 3 torn fresh basil leaves.

Potato gnocchi with lemon herb sauce

Serves 4

Simple flavors of lemon zest and fresh parsley create a light and fresh sauce that tosses beautifully with potato gnocchi.

✖ Tip

To bake large potatoes: Rinse potatoes well. Cut a sliver from each end and bake in a 350°F (180°C) oven until tender, 45 to 55 minutes.

Potato Gnocchi

2	large russet (Idaho) potatoes, baked, skins removed (about 2 lbs/1 kg) (see Tip, left)	2
1 tbsp	olive oil	15 mL
	Salt	
1¾ cups	all purpose flour	425 mL
8 cups	water	2 L

Sauce

2 tbsp	olive oil	30 mL
2 tbsp	vegan hard margarine	30 mL
½ cup	white wine	125 mL
1 tbsp	grated lemon zest	15 mL
3 tbsp	freshly squeezed lemon juice	45 mL
¼ cup	finely chopped parsley	60 mL
2 tbsp	chopped chives	30 mL
¾ tsp	freshly ground black pepper	3 mL

1. *Potato Gnocchi:* Place hot and skinned baked potatoes in a bowl. Add oil and ½ tsp (2 mL) salt and mash. Gradually mix in flour, ½ cup (125 mL) at a time, until dough is sticky but workable. Turn out onto a floured work surface and knead for 2 to 3 minutes. Break off pieces of dough and using palm, roll out into 1-inch (2.5 cm) thick ropes and cut into ¾-inch (2 cm) pieces. Using thumb, press each piece against floured fork tines to form imprinted gnocchi.

2. Bring a large pot of salted water to a boil over medium-high heat. Working in batches, gently place gnocchi into boiling water without overcrowding. Adjust heat to keep water at a gentle boil and cook gnocchi until just tender, 5 to 6 minutes, depending on size and thickness. With a slotted spoon, drain and transfer cooked gnocchi to a baking sheet and loosely cover with foil while cooking remaining gnocchi.

3. *Sauce:* Place a heavy-bottomed skillet over medium-high heat and let pan get hot. Add olive oil and tip pan to coat. Add margarine to melt. Whisk in wine, lemon zest and lemon juice. Reduce heat and simmer until reduced by one-quarter, 3 to 4 minutes. Stir in parsley, chives, pepper and ½ tsp (2 mL) salt to combine. Remove sauce from heat and stir in gnocchi, tossing gently to coat. Serve hot.

Ouzo orzo with fresh oregano

A symphony of
Mediterranean flavors
tumbles into a rustic
dish that is likely to be
found in a waterside
taverna in a small
Greek village.

1 cup	orzo	250 mL
2 tbsp	olive oil	30 mL
1 cup	thinly sliced fennel bulb	250 mL
1	shallot, finely chopped	1
2	clove garlic, minced	2
1	medium tomato, seeded and chopped	1
1/4 cup	toasted pine nuts	60 mL
1/4 cup	ouzo	60 mL
1/4 cup	dry white wine	60 mL
2 tbsp	freshly squeezed lemon juice	30 mL
2 tbsp	chopped fresh oregano	30 mL
1 tbsp	chopped fresh dill	15 mL

1. Bring a large saucepan of salted water to a boil over medium-high heat. Add orzo and boil, stirring often, until al dente, 8 to 10 minutes. Drain orzo, reserving 1/2 cup (125 mL) of the cooking water and set aside.

2. Meanwhile, place a skillet over medium heat. Add oil and tip pan to coat. Add fennel, shallot and garlic and cook, stirring frequently, until slightly softened, 3 to 4 minutes. Add tomato, pine nuts, ouzo, white wine, lemon juice and reserved pasta water and cook, stirring occasionally, until liquid is reduced by half, about 6 minutes. Stir in cooked orzo, oregano and dill and serve hot.

▓ Variations

Substitute any anise-flavored liquor for orzo.

Chopped almonds and marjoram can be used in place of oregano and dill.

Lemongrass soba noodles

Serves 2 to 4

This robust dish is full of color and flavor. Serve as an entrée or alongside baked or broiled tofu or tempeh.

✖ Tips

Fresh lemongrass can be found in the produce section of most ethnic food store and many grocery stores. Look for tight stalks that color from ivory at the bulb to bright green on the upper leave ends. Peel away the tough outer leaves to expose the tender stalk and slice off the tough bulb. Use only tender lower and light-colored end of the stalk, cut crosswise into rings and then finely mince. A food processor does a great job of mincing lemongrass. The upper stalk is woody and not suitable for eating, however the stalk is commonly used to flavor soups and curries but is removed before serving. Dried lemongrass may be substituted for fresh, using 1 tbsp (15 mL) of dried for every fresh stalk called for, but dried must be or soaked in warm water for at least 10 minutes before using.

Refrigerate unused portion in an airtight container for up to 2 days. Serve chilled.

Sauce

1/4 cup	tamari	60 mL
1 tsp	grated lime zest	5 mL
2 tbsp	freshly squeezed lime juice	30 mL
1 tbsp	green curry paste	15 mL
1 tbsp	Thai palm sugar or brown sugar	15 mL
2 tsp	toasted sesame oil	10 mL

Vegetables

2 tbsp	peanut oil, divided	30 mL
1/2	red onion, thinly sliced	1/2
1	red bell pepper, thinly sliced	1
1	carrot, thinly sliced	1
1	head broccoli, trimmed into florets (about 4 cups/1 L)	1
2	cloves garlic, finely minced	2 mL
1	piece (2 inches/5 cm) gingerroot, peeled and cut into thin matchsticks	1
1	stalk fresh lemongrass, finely minced (see Tips, left)	1
3 tbsp	chopped basil leaves	45 mL
2 tbsp	chopped fresh mint	30 mL
2 tbsp	chopped fresh cilantro	30 mL
1	package (8 oz/250 g) buckwheat soba noodles, cooked	1

1. *Sauce:* In a small bowl, whisk together tamari, lime zest, lime juice, curry paste, sugar and sesame oil. Set aside.

2. *Vegetables:* Place a large skillet over medium–high heat and let pan get hot. Add 1 tbsp (15 mL) of the oil and tip pan to coat. When oil is hot, add red onion and cook, stirring frequently, until soft, about 3 minutes. Add bell pepper, carrot, broccoli, garlic, ginger and lemongrass and cook, stirring frequently, until just softened, 4 to 5 minutes. Add basil, mint and cilantro, tossing well to combine and cook, until lightly browned, 3 to 4 minutes. Add noodles and sauce, tossing well to combine. Serve immediately.

Greek rice casserole

The addition of cinnamon and nutmeg, traditionally used in many Greek dishes, adds an aromatic bonus to an already flavorful casserole. Serve with Braised Baby Artichokes with Wine and Herbs (page 143) and a bottle of chilled Retsina, a delicious pine-scented Greek wine.

❖ Preheat oven to 350°F (180°C)
❖ 13- by 9-inch (33 by 23 cm) glass baking dish, lightly oiled

2 tbsp	olive oil	30 mL
1	large onion, chopped	1
½	green bell pepper, chopped	½
3	cloves garlic, minced	3
2	cans (each 28 oz/796 mL) diced tomatoes with juice	2
2 cup	Old-School Seitan (page 28) or Quick Basic Seitan, ground (page 29) or store-bought	500 mL
2 tsp	dried oregano	10 mL
2 tsp	ground nutmeg	10 mL
1½ tsp	ground cinnamon	7 mL
2 tsp	vegan browning sauce, such as Kitchen Bouquet (see page 10)	10 mL
2 tsp	Angostura bitters	10 mL
	Salt and freshly ground black pepper	
3 cups	cooked white rice	750 mL
1 cup	grated vegan Parmesan cheese alternative	250 mL
½ cup	Crunch (page 31), optional	125 mL
12	pitted kalamata olives	12

1. Place a large skillet over medium–high heat and let pan get hot. Add oil and tip pan to coat. Add onion and bell pepper. Reduce heat to medium and cook, stirring frequently, until well browned, 6 to 8 minutes. Add garlic and cook, stirring, until garlic is softened, 1 to 2 minutes. Stir in tomatoes with juice, seitan, oregano, nutmeg, cinnamon, browning sauce and bitters. Add salt and pepper to taste. Reduce heat and simmer, stirring occasionally, until slightly thickened, 40 to 50 minutes. Taste and adjust seasonings, adding additional spices or bitters, if necessary.

2. In prepared baking dish, layer rice, sauce and ½ cup (125 mL) cheese alternative and gently mix to partially combine. Scatter remaining cheese over mixture, top with Crunch, if using, and dot with kalamata olives.

3. Bake in preheated oven until top is slightly crisp and casserole is heated through, 20 to 30 minutes.

Shallot and strawberry risotto

A beautiful dish, popular in Northern Italy, is easily adapted to this delightful non-dairy version. The delicate color and flavors pair nicely with sparkling Italian Prosecco and a warm summer evening.

✦ Tip

Perfect risotto is simple to achieve if you stir constantly while ensuring that added liquid is almost completely absorbed before adding more.

✦ Variations

Soak strawberries in 1 cup (250 mL) champagne overnight. Use soaking liquid in place of wine.

Try stirring in 2 tbsp (30 mL) toasted pine nuts just before serving.

✦ Food processor

1¼ cups	strawberries, divided	300 mL
2 tbsp	balsamic vinegar	30 mL
4 cups	Vegetable Broth (page 31) or store-bought	1 L
2 cups	water	500 mL
3 tbsp	vegan hard margarine	45 mL
1	shallot, sliced	1
½ cup	chopped white onion	125 mL
1½ cups	Arborio rice	375 mL
1 cup	white wine	250 mL
½ tsp	salt	2 mL
3 tbsp	slivered basil	45 mL
¼ tsp	freshly ground black pepper	1 mL

1. In food processor, combine 1 cup (250 mL) of the strawberries and balsamic vinegar and pulse into a thick purée, 3 or 4 times. Coarsely chop remaining strawberries and add to purée. Set aside.

2. In a small saucepan over medium-heat, bring vegetable broth and water just to a simmer. Reduce heat to low and keep liquid hot.

3. Place a heavy-bottomed saucepan over medium heat and let pan get hot. Add margarine and tip pan to coat. Stir in shallot and onion and cook, stirring occasionally, until softened, 3 to 4 minutes. Reduce heat to low, add rice and stir well to coat grains. Add wine and stir constantly until rice has absorbed liquid. Stir in salt and ¼ cup (60 mL) of strawberry mixture. Add 1 cup (250 mL) hot broth, stirring constantly until liquid is absorbed. Continue adding broth, ½ cup (125 mL) at a time, stirring constantly with each addition until liquid is absorbed before adding more. Cook until rice is softened and creamy with a slightly firm center, 15 to 20 minutes. Stir in remaining strawberry mixture, basil and black pepper. Taste and adjust seasoning, adding additional salt and pepper, if necessary. Let risotto cool slightly before serving.

Chanterelle and sage risotto

Elegant yet earthy, this creamy and rich risotto is a savory blend of chanterelles, shallots and fresh sage.

6 cups	Vegetable Broth (page 31) or store-bought	1.5 L
2 tbsp	olive oil, divided	30 mL
8 oz	chanterelle mushrooms, coarsely chopped	250 g
1	shallot, finely chopped	1
1 tsp	dried thyme	5 mL
3/4 tsp	salt	3 mL
Pinch	freshly ground black pepper	Pinch
1 1/2 cups	Arborio rice	375 mL
1/2 cup	dry white wine	125 mL
2 tbsp	marsala wine	30 mL
1/2 cup	coarsely chopped toasted walnuts	125 mL
2 tbsp	chopped fresh sage	30 mL

1. In a large saucepan, heat vegetable broth over medium heat until steaming. Reduce heat to low and keep hot.

2. Place a large saucepan over medium heat and let pan get hot. Add oil and tip pan to coat. Stir in mushrooms, shallot, thyme, salt and pepper and cook, stirring occasionally, until softened, 6 to 8 minutes.

3. Reduce heat to maintain a simmer. Add rice and stir well to coat grains. Add white wine and marsala and stir constantly until rice has absorbed liquid. Add 1 cup (250 mL) hot broth and simmer, stirring constantly until liquid is absorbed. Continue adding broth, 1/2 cup (125 mL) at a time, stirring constantly with each addition until liquid is absorbed before adding more and adjusting heat as necessary to maintain a simmer. After 15 to 20 minutes rice will become softened and creamy with a slightly firm center. Stir in walnuts and fresh sage. Taste and adjust seasoning, adding additional salt and pepper, if necessary. Serve hot.

Fragrant rice-stuffed peppers

Peppers roasted and served with their tops lend a festive air to lunch or dinner. Serve with a crisp green salad and crusty bread.

✛ Tip

Leaves and tender top stems of beets are often trimmed and tossed away. These leaves, also referred to as beet greens, are delicious and a source of nutritious antioxidants.

✛ Preheat oven to 425°F (220°C)
✛ Baking sheet, lined with parchment paper
✛ 13- by 9-inch (33 by 23 cm) baking dish, lightly oiled

Filling

1 cup	brown jasmine rice	250 mL
1¾ cups	Vegetable Broth (page 31) or store-bought	425 mL
8	beets, trimmed and peeled, beet greens reserved	8
5 tbsp	olive oil, divided	75 mL
3½ tsp	balsamic vinegar, divided	17 mL
½ tsp	salt, divided	2 mL
½ tsp	freshly ground black pepper, divided	2 mL
2	green onions, white and green parts, thinly sliced	2
2	cloves garlic, minced	2
¾ cup	coarsely chopped toasted walnuts	175 mL
4	yellow or red bell peppers	4

1. *Filling:* In a small saucepan over medium-high heat, combine rice and vegetable broth and bring to a boil. Reduce heat, cover and simmer for 50 minutes.

2. Cut beets into ¼-inch (0.5 cm) pieces and toss with 1 tbsp (15 mL) of the olive oil, 3 tsp (15 mL) of the balsamic vinegar, ¼ tsp (1 mL) of the salt and ¼ tsp (1 mL) of the black pepper. Spread beets onto prepared baking sheet and roast in preheated oven until softened and slightly browned, 20 to 25 minutes.

3. Remove and discard tough stems from beet greens, coarsely chop greens and set aside. Place a large skillet over medium-high heat and let pan get hot. Add 2 tbsp (30 mL) of oil and tip pan to coat. Add green onions and garlic and cook, stirring frequently, until softened, about 1 minute. Add beet greens, ½ tsp (2 mL) of balsamic vinegar, ¼ tsp (1 mL) of salt and ¼ tsp (1 mL) of black pepper and cook until most of liquid has evaporated, 2 to 3 minutes. Remove from heat and stir in cooked rice, roasted beets and toasted walnuts, mixing to incorporate. Taste and adjust seasonings.

4. Cut tops off peppers and reserve. Remove and discard seeds and membranes and slice a thin strip off pepper bottoms to level. Arrange peppers in prepared baking dish and spoon in filling. Replace tops and drizzle peppers with remaining 2 tbsp (30 mL) of oil. Bake in preheated oven until peppers are tender and slightly charred, about 30 minutes.

Parsley, lemon and potato risotto

Serves 4 to 6

This risotto is a quick and easy variation from traditional risottos in that the rice is added to the broth all at once and simmered until done, no stirring. The light lovely flavor of parsley and lemon are the perfect complement.

✥ Immersion blender or potato masher

2 tbsp	olive oil	30 mL
3	stalks celery with leaves, chopped	3
1/2 cup	chopped onion	125 mL
6 cups	Vegetable Broth (page 31) or store-bought	1.5 L
2 1/2 cups	coarsely chopped Yukon gold potatoes	625 mL
1/4 tsp	freshly ground black pepper	1 mL
1 1/2 cups	white jasmine rice	375 mL
1/2 cup	white wine	125 mL
1/4 cup	freshly squeezed lemon juice	60 mL
1/2 cup	chopped fresh parsley	125 mL
	Salt	

1. Place a large stockpot over medium heat and let pan get hot. Add oil and tip pot to coat. Add celery and onion and cook, stirring, until softened, 2 to 3 minutes. Add broth, potatoes and pepper. Reduce heat and simmer until potatoes are tender, about 15 minutes.

2. Remove pan from heat and using immersion blender, blend until well combined. Return pan to heat. Add rice and simmer, covered, for 15 minutes. Remove pan from heat. Stir in wine, lemon juice and parsley. Taste and adjust seasoning, adding salt, if needed. Cover and set aside for 4 to 5 minutes before serving.

Sake, shiitake and sesame risotto

The sake and shiitakes add a mellow woodsy layer to this rich and creamy risotto. Think of it as Asian-style comfort food. Serve as a light yet very satisfying lunch or dinner entrée.

Wire-mesh strainer, lined with doubled cheesecloth

1½ oz	dried shiitake mushrooms	45 g
2 cups	hot water	500 mL
4½ cups	Vegetable Broth (page 31) or store-bought	1.125 L
1 tbsp	toasted sesame oil	15 mL
1 tbsp	canola oil	15 mL
½	onion, finely chopped	½
2	cloves garlic, minced	2
1½ cups	Arborio rice	375 mL
½ cup	sake	125 mL
¾ tsp	freshly ground black pepper	3 mL
½ tsp	salt	2 mL
1 tbsp	finely chopped fresh cilantro	15 mL
1	green onion, white and green parts, finely chopped	1
¼ cup	toasted sesame seeds	60 mL

1. Soak mushrooms in warm water for 30 minutes. Drain mushrooms through prepared strainer into a bowl to catch soaking liquid. Chop mushrooms and set aside.

2. In a saucepan, combine vegetable broth and mushroom soaking liquid and bring to a simmer over medium heat. Reduce heat to low and keep hot.

3. Place a large saucepan over medium–high and let pan get hot. Add sesame and canola oils and tip pan to coat. Add onion, garlic and mushrooms and cook, stirring, until softened and starting to brown, 6 to 8 minutes. Reduce heat to maintain a simmer. Add rice and stir well to coat grains. Add sake and stir constantly until rice has absorbed the liquid. Add 1 cup (250 mL) hot broth mixture, stirring constantly until liquid is absorbed. Continue adding broth, ½ cup (125 mL) at a time, stirring constantly with each addition until liquid is absorbed before adding more and adjusting heat as necessary to maintain a simmer, until rice is softened and creamy with a slightly firm center, 15 to 20 minutes. Add pepper, salt, cilantro, green onions and sesame seeds and serve.

Indonesian pineapple fried rice

Serves 4 to 6

A colorful and exotic combination is strewn with sweet and savory bits of flavor. Serve with Spicy Adzuki Futomaki with Avocado and Micro Greens (page 186) or Horseradish Mustard and Panko-Encrusted Tofu (page 210).

4 tbsp	peanut oil, divided	60 mL
2	shallots, finely diced	2
1	green bell pepper, chopped	1
1/2	red bell pepper, chopped	1/2
2	cloves garlic, chopped	2
1	piece (2 inches/5 cm) gingerroot, peeled and cut into matchsticks	1
1	serrano chile, seeded and minced	1
1/2	medium pineapple, cut into 1-inch (2.5 cm) cubes (about 2 1/2 cups/625 mL)	1/2
4 cups	cooked and chilled jasmine rice, grains separated	1 L
1 tbsp	freshly squeezed lime juice	15 mL
1 tbsp	tamari	15 mL
2 tsp	brown sugar	10 mL
1/4 cup	chopped fresh cilantro	60 mL

1. Place a large skillet over medium–high heat and let pan get hot. Add 2 tbsp (30 mL) of the oil and tip pan to coat. When hot, add shallots and green and red bell peppers and cook, stirring frequently, until softened, 3 to 5 minutes. Add garlic, ginger and serrano and cook, stirring frequently, until fragrant and softened, about 1 minute. Add pineapple and cook, stirring frequently, until heated through and slightly browned, 4 to 5 minutes. Transfer mixture to a bowl and set aside.

2. Return pan to stove top over medium–high heat and let pan get hot. Add 2 tbsp (30 mL) of oil and tip pan to coat. When hot, add rice and stir to coat.

3. In a small bowl, whisk together lime juice, tamari and brown sugar until sugar is dissolved. Stir into rice. Cook, stirring occasionally, until rice is hot, 2 to 3 minutes. Stir in pineapple mixture and cilantro, mixing well to combine and cook, stirring frequently, until vegetables are heated through. Serve hot.

Indian pilau with crispy shallots

Crispy shallots add a savory crunch to the aromatic rice cooked with Indian spices and coconut milk. Serve with Chana Masala (page 227) or your favorite curry.

✖ Tip

Using a smaller saucepan enables you to use less oil for deep frying because a smaller space creates a deeper frying area.

Crispy shallots

1 cup	canola oil	250 mL
3	shallots, thinly sliced	3
1 cup	basmati rice	250 mL
1 tbsp	coconut oil	15 mL
1 tsp	ground cardamom	5 mL
1 tsp	ground cumin	5 mL
1 tsp	ground turmeric	5 mL
1 cup	coconut milk	250 mL
3/4 cup	water	175 mL
1/2 cup	golden raisins	125 mL
1/4 cup	chopped roasted pistachios	60 mL

1. *Crispy Shallots:* In a small saucepan, heat oil over medium-high heat until very hot. Add shallots, in batches, and cook, stirring until crispy, 4 to 5 minutes. Adjust heat as necessary between batches to prevent burning. Using a slotted spoon, transfer shallots to a plate lined with paper towels to further crisp and cool.

2. Place rice in a bowl. Cover with water and rub to loosen starch. Let stand for 30 minutes. Then drain rice in a colander to dry, shaking occasionally, about 30 minutes.

3. Place a saucepan over medium heat and let pan get hot. Add coconut oil and tip pan to coat. Add cardamom, cumin and turmeric and cook, stirring constantly, until fragrant, about 10 seconds. Add rice and stir to coat. Stir in coconut milk, water, raisins and pistachios and bring to a boil. Reduce heat, cover and simmer until all liquid is absorbed, 15 to 20 minutes. During cooking, do not lift lid or stir. Remove from heat and let stand, covered, 5 to 10 minutes. Serve hot, topped with crispy shallots.

Soups, Chilis and Curries

❌—❌—❌—❌—❌—❌—❌—❌—❌—❌—❌—❌—❌

Baked farro and fennel soup

Even after hours of soaking and cooking, farro, high in fiber and protein, still holds its shape and adds tooth to this unusual baked dinner soup.

▓ Tip

Use the slicing disk in a food processor on the thinnest setting to quickly slice vegetables.

▓ Preheat oven to 350°F (180°C)
▓ Large baking dish or Dutch oven, lightly oiled

2 cups	farro berries, soaked overnight and drained	500 mL
1 lb	fennel bulb, trimmed and thinly sliced	500 g
2	onions, thinly sliced	2
3	small carrots, thinly sliced	3
4	stalks celery, thinly sliced	4
2 tbsp	chopped fresh parsley	30 mL
1 tbsp	fresh thyme leaves	15 mL
1 tsp	chopped fresh sage	5 mL
2	bay leaves	2
6 cups	Vegetable Broth (page 31) or store-bought	1.5 L
3	garlic cloves, minced	3
3 tbsp	olive oil	45 mL
2 tbsp	freshly squeezed lemon juice	30 mL
$\frac{1}{2}$ tsp	salt	2 mL
$\frac{1}{4}$ tsp	freshly ground black pepper	1 mL

1. In prepared baking dish, layer fennel, onions, carrots, celery, parsley, thyme, sage and bay leaves. Top with farro and add vegetable broth. Cover with foil and bake on lowest rack of oven for $1\frac{1}{2}$ hours.

2. In a small bowl, stir together garlic, olive oil, lemon juice, salt and pepper. When soup has baked for $1\frac{1}{2}$ hours, remove foil, add oil mixture and stir to incorporate. Remove bay leaves, return baking dish to oven and bake for 20 minutes more. Serve hot.

Miso, shiitake and tofu soup

This simple and nourishing soup is made with white miso, a deliciously sweet fermented soy food that can be found in most grocery stores. Its delicate flavor pairs nicely with shiitake mushrooms and tofu to make a hearty soup on its own or a great starter to an Asian-inspired meal.

✜ Tip

Kombu is a mild tasting dried edible Japanese seaweed also referred to as kelp.

✜ Variation

Add 2 cups (500 mL) fresh spinach or thinly sliced savoy cabbage to the bowl and scatter a few toasted nori strips on each bowl.

2	dried shiitake mushroom caps	2
	Hot water	
1 to 2 tbsp	toasted sesame oil	15 to 30 mL
1 cup	thinly sliced fresh shiitake mushroom caps	250 mL
5 cups	water	1.25 L
1	piece (6 inches/15 cm) dried kombu seaweed (see Tip, left)	1
1	piece ($\frac{1}{2}$ inch/1 cm) gingerroot, peeled and cut into about 4 thin slices	1
$\frac{1}{2}$ cup	white miso paste	125 mL
1 cup	cubed ($\frac{1}{2}$ inch/1 cm) firm or extra-firm silken tofu	250 mL
$\frac{1}{2}$ cup	minced green onions	125 mL

1. In a bowl, cover dried shiitake mushrooms with hot water and let soak until softened, 30 to 40 minutes. Drain and chop.

2. Place a large pot over medium heat and let pan get hot. Add oil and tip pan to coat. Add fresh shiitake mushrooms and cook, stirring, until slightly softened, about 3 minutes. Transfer to a bowl and set aside.

3. Add water to same pot and place over medium-low heat. Add kombu and soaked dried shiitake mushrooms and heat until almost boiling. Reduce heat to low and simmer for 10 minutes. Using a slotted spoon, remove kombu and discard. Add ginger to pot and let simmer for 10 minutes.

4. In a bowl, combine miso paste and 1 cup (250 mL) of the hot mushroom and kombu broth, whisking to combine into a smooth mixture. Add back to remaining broth in pot. Add reserved mushrooms and tofu and simmer until tofu is heated through. Take care not to let broth boil after addition of miso. Taste soup and adjust flavoring, adding additional miso if stronger flavor is desired.

5. To serve, ladle soup into bowls and garnish with green onions.

Roasted corn chowder

Serves 4 to 6

Rich and velvety, this soup uses every bit of the delicious corn. Even the cobs are roasted and simmered with the vegetable broth for added flavor, a trick I learned from a young man in Texas.

Tip

To make this soup year-round, use frozen corn on the cob. Thaw before cutting.

Variations

Add roasted poblano or green chiles, red bell pepper with chopped cilantro or add chopped parsley, lemon juice and lemon zest.

- **Preheat oven to 400°F (200°C)**
- **Baking sheet, lined with parchment paper**
- **Blender**

4	ears corn, husked	4
8 tsp	olive oil, divided	40 mL
6 cups	Vegetable Broth (page 31) or store-bought	1.5 L
1	onion, chopped	1
2	stalks celery with leaves, chopped	2
1	carrot, peeled and chopped	1
$\frac{1}{2}$	green bell pepper, chopped	$\frac{1}{2}$
2	russet (Idaho) potatoes, peeled and cut into 1-inch (2.5 cm) cubes	2
1 tbsp	chopped fresh thyme	15 mL
1	bay leaf	1
$\frac{3}{4}$ tsp	salt	3 mL
$\frac{3}{4}$ tsp	freshly ground black pepper	3 mL
6	chives, chopped	6

1. Cut corn from cobs and spread kernels on prepared baking sheet. Toss kernels with 2 tsp (10 mL) of the oil. Add cobs to baking sheet. Roast in preheated oven until kernels are golden brown, 8 to 10 minutes. Set aside.
2. Pour vegetable broth into a stockpot. Add roasted corn cobs and place over medium heat. Bring just to a boil, reduce heat and simmer, 20 to 25 minutes. Remove corn cobs and discard. Set broth aside.
3. Place a large heavy-bottomed saucepan or Dutch oven over medium heat and let pan get hot. Add 2 tbsp (30 mL) of oil and tip pan to coat. Add onion, celery, carrot and bell pepper. Reduce heat to low and sweat, stirring occasionally, until softened, 8 to 10 minutes. Add reserved vegetable broth, potatoes, roasted corn kernels, reserving $\frac{1}{4}$ cup (60 mL) of kernels, thyme, bay leaf, salt and black pepper and simmer until potatoes are tender, about 15 minutes.
4. Let cool slightly. Remove bay leaf and transfer two-thirds of soup to blender and process until just smooth. Return soup to saucepan, stirring to thoroughly combine. Taste and adjust seasonings. Turn heat to low and simmer until soup is heated through. Serve topped with a sprinkle of roasted corn kernels and chives.

Sopa de lima

Serves 4

Avocado, tortilla strips and cilantro garnish the top of this citrusy Mexican vegetable soup.

1/3 cup	canola oil, divided	75 mL
2	corn tortillas, sliced into 1/4-inch (0.5 cm) strips	2
1/2	onion, chopped	1/2
2	cloves garlic, chopped	2
1	large jalapeño, seeded and sliced, divided	1
4 cups	Vegetable Broth (page 31) or store-bought	1 L
1 1/2 cups	cubed potato	375 mL
1	zucchini, cut into 1/2-inch (1 cm) dice	1
1	tomato, seeded and chopped	1
1/2 cup	roasted red pepper, chopped	125 mL
1/2 cup	roasted corn kernels	125 mL
1/4 cup	chopped cilantro, divided	60 mL
3 tbsp	freshly squeezed lime juice (about 1 large lime)	45 mL
1/2 tsp	ground cumin	2 mL
1/2 tsp	dried oregano	2 mL
1/2 tsp	salt	2 mL
1/2 tsp	freshly ground black pepper	2 mL
1	avocado, chopped	1

1. Place a large heavy-bottomed saucepan over medium-high heat. Add 1/4 cup (60 mL) of the oil and when very hot, add tortilla strips and fry, in batches, until crisp, about 1 minute. Transfer to a plate lined with paper towels and set aside.

2. Let pan and oil cool. Pour out excess oil and wipe outside edge of pan. Place same pan over medium heat and let pan get hot. Add 1 tbsp (15 mL) of oil and tip to coat. Add onion, garlic and half of sliced jalapeño and cook, stirring occasionally, 3 to 5 minutes. Add vegetable broth and potato, increase heat and bring to a boil. Reduce heat and simmer until almost softened, 5 to 6 minutes.

3. Add zucchini, tomato, red pepper, corn, 2 tbsp (30 mL) of the cilantro, lime juice, cumin, oregano, salt, pepper and remaining jalapeño slices and cook, stirring occasionally, until vegetables are softened and flavors are combined, 12 to 15 minutes. Remove from heat and serve topped with avocado, tortilla strips and remaining 2 tbsp (30 mL) of chopped cilantro.

Tomato basil soup

Using canned tomatoes eliminates the need to skin and seed, and using jarred marinara sauce to thicken cuts time. Adding garden fresh basil brightens the soup with a minimum of effort.

✖ Food processor

2 tsp	olive oil	10 mL
½	onion, chopped	½
1	can (28 oz/796 mL) whole tomatoes with juice	1
2 cups	Vegetable Broth (page 31) or store-bought	500 mL
2 cups	tomato marinara sauce	500 mL
½ tsp	salt	2 mL
½ tsp	freshly ground black pepper	2 mL
½ cup	packed fresh basil leaves, divided	125 mL
¼ cup	toasted pine nuts	60 mL

1. Place a medium saucepan over medium heat and let pan get hot. Add oil and tip pan to coat. Add onion and cook, stirring occasionally, until softened but not browned, 3 to 4 minutes. Add tomatoes with juice, vegetable broth, marinara sauce, salt and pepper. Reduce heat to low and simmer, stirring occasionally and breaking up tomatoes with the back of a spoon, about 10 minutes. Stir in ¼ cup (60 mL) of the basil. Let cool.

2. Transfer soup to a food processor and blend until smooth, 20 to 30 seconds. Return soup to saucepan, taste and adjust seasonings. Turn heat to low and simmer until soup is hot throughout. Chiffonade remaining basil leaves. Serve soup hot, topped with a scattering of basil and a sprinkle of pine nuts.

Cream of broccoli soup

Every time you make this soup you will ask yourself why you don't do it more often. It is so easy to prepare and delicious served hot or cold; truly a year-round winner. Serve with wheat crackers.

✖ Variations

Add ⅛ tsp (0.5 mL) ground nutmeg or allspice or more to taste.

Refrigerate and serve soup chilled.

✖ Food processor

1 cup	raw cashews	250 mL
1 lb	broccoli	500 g
2 tsp	olive oil	10 mL
½	onion, chopped	½
5 cups	Vegetable Broth (page 31) or store-bought	1.25 L
1	russet (Idaho) potato, peeled and cut into 1-inch (2.5 cm) cubes	1
¼ tsp	freshly ground black pepper	1 mL
½ tsp	salt	2 mL

1. Place cashews in a bowl and add water to cover by 3 inches (7.5 cm). Cover bowl and let soak for at least 2 hours.

2. Cut broccoli into 2-inch (5 cm) florets. Peel stalk and cut in half lengthwise and then crosswise into 1-inch (2.5 cm) pieces. You should have about 8 cups (2 L) total. Set aside.

3. Place cashews and 2 tbsp (30 mL) of the soaking water into food processor and process to a semi-smooth paste. Leave in processor and set aside.

4. Place a large saucepan over medium heat and let pan get hot. Add oil and tip pan to coat. Add onion and cook, stirring occasionally, until softened, 3 to 4 minutes. Add vegetable broth and potato, increase heat to high and bring to a boil. Reduce heat and simmer until slightly softened, 5 to 6 minutes. Add broccoli and black pepper, increase heat to high and bring to a boil. Reduce heat and simmer until potatoes and broccoli are tender, 6 to 8 minutes.

5. Let cool slightly. Working in batches, ladle soup into food processor with cashews and blend until smooth. Return to pan. Stir in salt. Taste and adjust seasonings and heat over low heat, stirring often, until soup is heated through. Serve hot.

Winter minestrone soup

Nothing says wintertime like a hearty bowl of minestrone soup. Absolutely packed with winter vegetables, beans and pasta, it is just the thing to warm your bones. Serve with a loaf of crusty rustic Italian bread for sopping.

2 tbsp	olive oil	30 mL
1	onion, chopped	1
2	carrots, peeled and chopped	2
2	stalks celery with leaves, chopped	2
1	acorn squash, peeled and cubed	1
3	cloves garlic, chopped	3
1	can (28 oz/796 mL) whole peeled tomatoes with juice	1
8 cups	Vegetable Broth (page 31) or store-bought	2 L
1/2 cup	chopped Italian flat-leaf parsley	125 mL
2	bay leaves	2
1 tsp	salt	5 mL
1 tsp	freshly ground black pepper	5 mL
1/2 tsp	hot pepper flakes	2 mL
2 cups	cannellini beans	500 mL
2	zucchini, cut into 1-inch (2.5 cm) pieces	2
1 cup	ditalini (soup pasta)	250 mL
2 cups	packed baby spinach	500 mL
1 cup	packed fresh basil	250 mL

1. Place a Dutch oven over medium heat and let pan get hot. Add oil and tip pan to coat. Add onion, carrots, celery, squash and garlic and cook, stirring frequently, until fragrant, 4 to 5 minutes. Stir in tomatoes with juice, vegetable broth, parsley, bay leaves, salt, black pepper and hot pepper flakes, breaking up tomatoes with the back of a wooden spoon. Reduce heat to low and simmer until vegetables are tender, 15 to 20 minutes.

2. Add beans, zucchini and pasta and simmer until pasta is tender, 8 to 12 minutes. Stir in spinach and basil and simmer for 3 to 4 minutes. Taste and adjust seasonings. Serve hot.

✛ Variation

Omit acorn squash and add cubed potatoes.

Curried french green lentil soup

The great thing about lentils, beside the gorgeous flavor, of course, is the whim factor. Due to the short cooking time, it is possible with little or no preplanning to decide at lunch to make this stew for dinner.

1 tbsp	olive oil	15 mL
1	large onion, chopped	1
3	carrots, peeled and chopped	3
2	stalk celery with leaves, chopped	2
4	cloves garlic, minced	4
1 tbsp	Curry Powder (page 311) or store-bought	15 mL
10 cups	Vegetable Broth (page 31) or store-bought	2.5 L
1	can (28 oz/796 mL) diced tomatoes with juice	1
2 cups	French puy lentils, picked through and rinsed	500 mL
2	bay leaves	2
2 cups	cubed (1 inch/2.5 cm) red potatoes	500 mL
3/4 tsp	salt	3 mL
3/4 tsp	freshly ground black pepper	3 mL
2 tbsp	chopped fresh parsley	30 mL

1. Place a large saucepan over medium heat and let pan get hot. Add oil and tip pan to coat. Add onion, carrots, celery and garlic and cook, stirring occasionally, until softened, 8 to 10 minutes. Stir in curry, broth, tomatoes with juice, lentils and bay leaves and bring to a boil. Reduce heat, cover and simmer, for 35 minutes. Add potatoes and cook until potatoes and lentils are tender, 15 to 20 minutes.

2. Remove from heat. Stir in salt, pepper and parsley. Discard bay leaves and serve hot.

French onion soup with garlic croutons

Serves 6

The trick to making this delectable classic is golden brown caramelized onions. Rich flavor and creamy texture are created by lengthy cooking and deliciously accentuated by a thick and crisp garlic toast topping.

✖ Variation

Ladle soup into ovenproof bowls, top each bowl with garlic crouton and ¼ cup (60 mL) vegan cheese alternative (preferably one that melts). Bake in a 325°F (160°C) oven until cheese is melted, 8 to 10 minutes.

2 tbsp	olive oil	30 mL
2 tbsp	vegan hard margarine	30 mL
6	onions, sliced	6
½ tsp	granulated sugar	2 mL
3 tbsp	all-purpose flour	45 mL
8 cups	Vegetable Broth (page 31) or store-bought	2 L
1 cup	dry white wine	250 mL
1	bay leaf	1
½ tsp	dried sage	2 mL
¼ tsp	ground thyme	1 mL

Garlic Croutons

6	slices rustic Italian baguette, about 2 inches (5 cm) thick	6
2 tbsp	vegan hard margarine	30 mL
2	cloves garlic, minced	2
3 tbsp	Sprinkle (page 30), optional	45 mL

1. Place a large heavy-bottomed saucepan over medium heat and let pan get hot. Add oil and margarine and tip pan to coat. Add onions, stirring to coat. Reduce heat to low, cover and cook, stirring frequently, for 20 minutes. Add sugar, increase heat to medium-low and cook, uncovered, stirring occasionally, until onions are golden brown, 30 to 35 minutes.

2. Reduce heat to low, stir in flour and cook, stirring, until blended, about 2 minutes. Gradually stir in vegetable broth, wine, bay leaf, sage and thyme. Increase heat to medium and bring to a boil. Reduce heat and simmer for 30 minutes.

3. Meanwhile, preheat oven to 350°F (180°C).

4. *Garlic Croutons:* Place bread slices on a baking sheet and bake in preheated oven for 10 minutes. Remove from oven, turn bread and spread each slice with 1 tsp (5 mL) margarine. Top with garlic and Sprinkle, if using, and return to oven. Bake until bread is toasted and garlic is softened and slightly browned, 4 to 5 minutes.

5. To serve, ladle soup into bowls and top with garlic crouton. Serve immediately.

Soup au pistou

A quick, strictly summertime soup makes good use of the garden's bounty. Set a table outside if possible and enjoy this beautiful green, green soup among the greens. Serve with rolls and a good vegan margarine.

3 tbsp	olive oil	45 mL
2 tbsp	chopped onion	30 mL
2 cups	chopped ($1/2$-inch/1 cm pieces) zucchini	500 mL
1	clove garlic, minced	1
$1/4$ tsp	freshly ground black pepper	1 mL
3 tbsp	Classic Pesto Sauce (page 286) or store-bought vegan pesto	45 mL
6 cups	Vegetable Broth (page 31) or store-bought	1.5 L
1 cup	orecchiette pasta	250 mL
$1 1/2$ cups	chopped Roma (plum) tomatoes	375 mL
1 cup	fresh or frozen corn kernels	250 mL
$1/2$ cup	dry white wine	125 mL
	Salt	

1. Place a pot over medium-low heat and let pan get hot. Add oil and tip pan to coat. Add onion and cook, stirring occasionally, until soft, about 5 minutes. Add zucchini, garlic and pepper, increase heat to medium and cook, stirring often, for 5 minutes.

2. Add pesto sauce, vegetable broth and pasta and bring to a boil. Partially cover, reduce heat and simmer until pasta is almost tender, 10 to 12 minutes. Add tomatoes, corn and white wine and simmer for 4 minutes longer. Season with salt to taste. Serve immediately.

Chardonnay, pumpkin and parsnip soup

Serves 4	

Sweet pumpkins and spicy parsnips are roasted and blended with a good-quality Chardonnay into a rich buttery gorgeous soup.

✖ Preheat oven to 375°F (190°C)
✖ Baking sheet, lined with parchment paper
✖ Food processor

1 lb	pie pumpkin, peeled, seeded and cubed	500 g
1 lb	parsnips, peeled and cubed	500 g
1/2	onion, cut into thick slices	1/2
1 tbsp	olive oil	15 mL
1 tsp	salt	5 mL
1/2 tsp	freshly ground black pepper	2 mL
6 cups	Vegetable Broth (page 31) or store-bought, heated	1.5 L
1 cup	Chardonnay wine	250 mL
1 tbsp	pure maple syrup	15 mL
	Salt and freshly ground black pepper	
4 tsp	walnut oil, optional	20 mL
2 tsp	minced fresh sage	10 mL

1. Place pumpkin, parsnips and onion on prepared baking sheet. Toss with olive oil, salt and pepper and spread out on sheet. Bake in preheated oven until tender, 20 to 25 minutes. Let cool. When cool enough to handle, transfer to food processor and pulse until smooth.

2. In batches, as necessary, add heated vegetable broth to food processor and process until blended. Transfer to a saucepan over medium heat. Stir in wine and maple syrup. Reduce heat and simmer until flavors are fully combined, 5 to 8 minutes. Season with salt and pepper to taste. Serve soup topped with a drizzle of walnut oil and a sprinkle of minced sage.

Easy blender gazpacho

The refreshing chill of garden vegetables stands up to a bit of hot pepper sauce. There are many on the market and this delicious soup is a perfect laboratory for testing. This meal begs for crusty French bread and a small bowl of good olive oil with a balsamic drizzle for dipping.

✖ Tip

Most of the vegetables used in this recipe are available fresh and flavorful year-round. Because fresh tomatoes are only flavorful in the summer, this recipe calls for canned. To use fresh, substitute 2 lbs (1 kg) fresh tomatoes for 28 oz (796 mL) canned.

✖ Food processor or blender

1	can (28 oz/796 mL) tomatoes with juice (see Tip, left)	1
2	stalks celery with leaves, cut into 1-inch (2.5 cm) pieces	2
1	green bell pepper, seeded and quartered	1
1	cucumber, peeled, halved, seeded and cut into 2-inch (5 cm) pieces, divided	1
1	red onion, quartered, divided	1
2	cloves garlic, finely minced	2
1 cup	tomato juice	250 mL
1/4 cup	olive oil	60 mL
1 tbsp	balsamic vinegar	15 mL
1 tsp	ground cumin	5 mL
	Hot pepper sauce	
	Salt and freshly ground black pepper	
2	green onions, white and green parts, finely chopped	2
	Olive oil, optional	

1. In food processor, combine half each of the tomatoes with juice, celery, bell pepper, cucumber and red onion and pulse until coarsely chopped. Transfer to a large bowl and place remaining half of vegetables into food processor along with garlic, tomato juice, oil, vinegar, cumin, and hot pepper sauce to taste and process into a purée. Add purée to chopped vegetables, stirring to combine. Add salt and pepper to taste. Cover and refrigerate until well chilled, about 2 hours or for up to 24 hours.

2. Serve in bowls topped with chopped green onions and a drizzle of olive oil, if using.

Havana black bean soup

Serves 6 to 8

Sofrito is the Cuban mirepoix generally agreed to be onion, green bell pepper and garlic. Sometimes cumin and oregano are considered essential, especially when you have more than one cook in the kitchen.

✖ Tips

If a blender is unavailable, omit that step because the soup is delicious without blending.

Substitute 2 cans (14 to 19 oz/398 to 540 mL) black beans for fresh, rinsing and draining well before using.

✖ **Blender or food processor (see Tips, left)**

1 lb	dried black beans (see Beans, page 231) (see Tips, left)	500 g
2 tbsp	olive oil	30 mL
1	onion, finely chopped	1
1	green bell pepper, finely chopped	1
3	cloves garlic, chopped	3
2 tsp	hot pepper flakes	10 mL
2 tsp	ground cumin	10 mL
2 tsp	ground oregano	10 mL
1	bay leaf	1
1/2 tsp	freshly ground black pepper	2 mL
1/4 cup	dry sherry	60 mL
	Salt	
1/2 cup	Basic Sour Cream (page 21) or store-bought vegan alternative	125 mL
2	green onions, white and light green parts only, finely chopped	2
2 tbsp	Sprinkle (page 30), optional	30 mL

1. Place beans in a large bowl and cover with water by at least 1 inch (2.5 cm). Let soak overnight.

2. When you're ready to cook, place a large heavy-bottomed saucepan over medium heat and let pan get hot. Add oil and tip pan to coat. Add onion, bell pepper and garlic and cook, stirring occasionally, until softened, 6 to 8 minutes.

3. Add soaked black beans with their water, hot pepper flakes, cumin, oregano, bay leaf, black pepper and enough water to cover beans by 2 inches (5 cm). Bring to a boil over high heat. Reduce heat and simmer, partially covered, until beans are tender, adding more liquid if necessary, 2 1/2 to 3 hours, adding salt to taste about 5 minutes before done.

4. Let soup cool slightly and, in batches as necessary, transfer to a blender and purée until smooth. Stir in sherry and reheat soup over low heat, stirring often, until steaming. Serve hot with a dollop of sour cream, a spoonful of green onions and a sprinkle of Sprinkle, if using.

Roasted poblano potato soup

Serves 4 to 6

Roasted poblanos
and potatoes go
well together, giving
this scrumptious
stick-to-your-ribs
soup a mellow yet
tasty kick.

Preheat broiler
Food processor

4	poblano chiles	4
4	cloves garlic, unpeeled	4
2 tbsp	olive oil	30 mL
1	onion, chopped	1
6	Yukon gold potatoes, peeled and cut into large cubes	6
3 cups	Vegetable Broth (page 31) or store-bought	750 mL
2 cups	Soy Milk (page 18) or hemp milk	500 mL
1/4 cup	chopped fresh cilantro	60 mL
1 1/2 tsp	salt	7 mL
	Heavy Cream (page 26) or store bought vegan non-dairy alternative, optional	

1. Place poblanos and garlic on a baking sheet and broil, turning poblanos frequently with tongs to char all sides, 10 to 15 minutes. Transfer charred poblanos to a dampened clean kitchen towel, wrapping to enclose, and steam for about 10 minutes to loosen skins. Peel poblanos, remove and discard stems and seeds. Chop and set aside. When garlic is cool enough to handle, squeeze pulp from their peels and set aside.

2. Place a large saucepan over medium-high heat and let pan get hot. Add oil and tip pan to coat. Add onion and cook, stirring occasionally, until softened, 3 to 4 minutes. Add potatoes, poblanos, garlic, vegetable broth and soy milk and bring to a boil. Reduce heat to medium-low and simmer until potatoes are fork-tender, about 10 minutes. Let cool.

3. Transfer to food processor. Add cilantro and salt and blend until smooth. Taste and adjust seasoning. Serve with a spoonful of heavy cream, if using.

Shallot saffron soup

This soup is light and delicious. The fennel and white wine provide a flavorful base for carrots, leeks, shallots and cauliflower. Saffron adds a lovely hue.

3 tbsp	olive oil, divided	45 mL
6	large shallots, thinly sliced	6
3	carrots, cut in half, lengthwise and thinly sliced	3
1	leek, trimmed and thinly sliced	1
1	small fennel bulb, thinly sliced	1
3 cups	cauliflower, trimmed into small florets (about 10 oz/300 g)	750 mL
4 cups	water	1 L
1 1/2 cups	dry white wine	375 mL
6 to 8	strands saffron, soaked in 1/4 cup (60 mL) water	6 to 8
2 tsp	Homemade Vegetable Bouillon (page 32) or store-bought	10 mL
1 1/2 tsp	salt	7 mL
1/2 tsp	freshly ground black pepper	2 mL
1/2 tsp	ground marjoram	2 mL

1. Place a large saucepan over medium–high heat and let pan get hot. Add 1 tbsp (15 mL) of the oil and tip pan to coat. Add shallots and cook, stirring frequently, until just softened, 1 to 2 minutes. Add remaining 2 tbsp (30 mL) of oil. Stir in carrots, leek and fennel and cook, stirring occasionally, until softened, 8 to 10 minutes.

2. Add cauliflower, water, wine, saffron, vegetable bouillon, salt, pepper and marjoram. Reduce heat to medium and cook, stirring occasionally, until vegetables are softened and flavors have combined, 10 to 15 minutes. Serve hot.

✖ Variation

Stir in 2 cups (500 mL) cooked chickpeas or artichoke hearts, if desired.

Mushroom and wild rice soup

In Minnesota when this creamy soup, loaded with sautéed mushrooms, hearty wild rice and a bit of brandy, pops up on local restaurant menus, it's a sure sign that fall has arrived. You don't have to travel to the Twin Cities to enjoy this autumn favorite.

✖ Tip

Wild rice is actually not rice but a grain. *To clean before cooking:* Place wild rice in a bowl, cover with water and let stand, stirring occasionally, for 2 to 3 minutes. Debris floats to the top. Pour off water, transfer rice to a strainer and rinse well.

3 cups	water	750 mL
⅔ cup	wild rice, rinsed (see Tip, left)	150 mL
¼ cup	olive oil, divided	60 mL
2 tbsp	vegan hard margarine	30 mL
18 oz	cremini mushrooms, sliced (about 7 cups/1.75 L)	540 g
1	onion, chopped	1
3	stalks celery with leaves, chopped	3
2 tsp	dried thyme	10 mL
3 tbsp	all-purpose flour	45 mL
2½ cups	Vegetable Broth (page 31) or store-bought	625 mL
2 cups	Soy Milk (page 18) or store-bought	500 mL
¼ cup	brandy, divided	60 mL
1½ tsp	salt	7 mL
½ tsp	freshly ground black pepper	2 mL
¾ to 1½ cups	Heavy Cream (page 26) or store-bought vegan alternative	175 to 375 mL

1. In a small saucepan bring water to a boil over medium–high heat. Add rice and return to a boil. Reduce heat to low, cover and simmer until rice has absorbed all liquid and is tender and puffed opened, 40 to 45 minutes. Set aside.

2. Place a large heavy-bottomed saucepan over medium–high heat and let pan get hot. Add 2 tbsp (30 mL) of the oil and margarine and when melted, tip pan to coat. Add mushrooms and cook, stirring occasionally, until wilted and juicy, about 6 minutes. Transfer cooked mushrooms with liquid to a bowl and set aside.

3. Return same pan to medium–high heat and let pan get hot. Add remaining 2 tbsp (30 mL) of oil and tip pan to coat. Add onion, celery and thyme and cook, stirring occasionally, until softened and slightly browned, 8 to 10 minutes. Stir in flour to coat vegetables. Gradually stir in broth and milk, scraping bottom. Bring to a low boil, stirring occasionally. Stir in reserved mushrooms, 3 tbsp (45 mL) of the brandy, salt and pepper. Reduce heat and simmer, stirring, until soup is thickened, 10 to 12 minutes. Stir in rice. Taste and adjust seasoning, adding additional brandy, if desired.

4. Serve soup hot with 2 to 3 tbsp (30 to 45 mL) heavy cream stirred into each bowl.

Black-eyed new year's chili for a crowd

Eating black-eyed peas on New Year's day is thought to bring prosperity. This black-eyed chili is so good you will want to eat it any day of the year!

✖ Tip

When preparing dry beans, it's best to add salt at the end of the cooking process to keep beans from becoming tough.

2 cups	dried black-eyed peas (see Beans, page 231)	500 mL
2 tbsp	olive oil	30 mL
1½ cups	chopped onions	375 mL
1½ cups	sliced celery	375 mL
1 cup	diced carrot	250 mL
1 cup	chopped green bell pepper	250 mL
2 tbsp	minced garlic	30 mL
1½ cups	canned tomato purée	375 mL
2 cups	canned tomatoes, chopped with liquid	500 mL
1½ cups	Vegetable Broth (page 31) or store-bought	375 mL
½ cup	chili powder	125 mL
1 tbsp	smoked paprika	15 mL
⅛ tsp	freshly ground black pepper	0.5 mL
1 tsp	salt	5 mL

1. Pick through black-eyed peas removing any grit. Place in a large bowl and cover with water. Soak overnight.

2. When ready to cook, place a large stockpot over medium heat and let pot get hot. Add oil and tip pot to coat. Add onions, celery, carrot, bell pepper and garlic and cook, stirring occasionally, until softened, 3 to 4 minutes. Add tomato purée, tomatoes, drained soaked peas, broth, chili powder, paprika and black pepper. Cook over low heat until chili is thick and peas are tender, about 1 hour, adding salt about 5 minutes before done. Add additional water as necessary to maintain desired consistency.

Boy howdy texas chili and beans

In Texas there is an ongoing spirited discussion over a true chili. Many feel the inclusion of beans in chili is blasphemy, negating any claim this concoction may have to the name. To play it safe I'm calling this hearty dish Chili and Beans.

✕ Tip

Refrigerate chili in an airtight container for up to 5 days.

10 oz	dried kidney beans (see Beans, page 231)	300 g
2 tbsp	olive oil	30 mL
1	large onion, chopped	1
1/2	red bell pepper, seeded and chopped	1/2
3	cloves garlic, chopped	3
1 tbsp	chili powder	15 mL
1 tsp	ground cumin	5 mL
1 tsp	dried oregano	5 mL
1	can (28 oz/796 mL) diced tomatoes with juice	1
2 cups	ground Old-School Seitan (page 28) or Quick Basic Seitan (page 29) or store-bought	500 mL
5 cups	Vegetable Broth (page 31) or store-bought	1.25 L
2 tbsp	tomato paste	30 mL
2 tbsp	liquid amino acids (see Tip, page 212)	30 mL
1/2 tsp	liquid smoke	2 mL
	Salt and freshly ground black pepper	

1. Pick through kidney beans and remove any grit. Place in a large bowl and cover with water. Let soak overnight.

2. When you're ready to cook, place a large heavy-bottomed stockpot over medium heat and let pan get hot. Add oil and tip pan to coat. Add onion and bell pepper and cook, stirring occasionally, until onion is translucent, 4 to 6 minutes. Add garlic, chili powder, cumin and oregano and cook, stirring, until garlic is softened, 1 to 2 minutes. Add tomatoes with juice, beans with their liquid, seitan, broth and enough water to cover all by 1 inch (2.5 cm). Stir in tomato paste, liquid amino acids and liquid smoke. Cover pan and bring to a boil. Reduce heat to low, partially cover, and simmer until beans are tender, 1 to 1 1/2 hours. About 10 minutes before beans are tender, season with salt and pepper to taste. Serve hot.

Smoky chipotle black bean chili

Chipotle peppers are smoked red jalapeño peppers packed in adobo, a sauce of vinegar, spices, tomato sauce and chiles. The heat is diminished, allowing the smoked earthy flavor of the chile to dominate. Add chipotles to stews, soups or purée to create a quick sauce.

✕ Tips

Substitute 3 cups (750 mL) drained canned black beans for dried, rinsing well before using.

Refrigerate chili in an airtight container for up to 1 week.

8 oz	dried black beans (see Tip, left)	250 g
1	can (7 oz/198 g) chipotle chiles in adobo sauce, drained, sauce reserved	1
½ cup	tomato juice	125 mL
1 cup	textured vegetable protein (TVP) flakes	250 mL
2 tbsp	olive oil	30 mL
1	onion, chopped	1
2	cloves garlic, chopped	2
½ tsp	ground cumin	2 mL
1	can (14 oz/398 mL) diced tomatoes with juice	1
1 tbsp	tomato paste	15 mL
¼ cup	chopped fresh cilantro	60 mL
	Salt and freshly ground black pepper	
	Vegan sour cream alternative, optional	
½ cup	chopped green onions, white and green parts	125 mL

1. Pick through black beans and remove any grit. Place in a large bowl and cover with water. Let soak overnight.

2. When you're ready to cook, remove chipotle chiles from sauce and set aside. In a small saucepan, combine tomato juice and adobo sauce and bring to a boil over medium-high heat. Remove from heat and stir in TVP, making sure to dampen all the flakes. Let stand until softened, about 5 minutes.

3. Place a large heavy-bottomed pot over medium heat and let pan get hot. Add olive oil and tip pan to coat. Add onion and cook, stirring occasionally, until onion is translucent, 4 to 6 minutes. Add garlic and cumin and cook, stirring, until garlic is softened, 1 to 2 minutes. Add reconstituted TVP mixture, tomatoes with juice, tomato paste, beans and enough water to cover all by 1 inch (2.5 cm). Roughly chop 3 to 4 chipotles to taste and stir into chili. Cover pot and bring to a boil. Reduce heat to low and simmer, stirring, until beans are tender, 1 to 1½ hours. About 10 minutes before beans are tender, stir in cilantro and salt and pepper to taste.

4. Serve bowls of chili topped with a dollop of sour cream alternative, if using, and a sprinkle of green onions.

Spinach and pumpkin curry

Make this soup in the fall when apples are plentiful and pumpkins dot the fields.

⠿ Variations

In place of a fresh pumpkin, you can use a 15-oz (425 mL) can, or 1¾ cups (425 mL) unsweetened pumpkin purée (not pie filling) and skip Step 1. Stir salt and pepper into purée and proceed with Step 2.

Add additional curry powder for a spicier soup.

⠿ Food processor
⠿ Steamer basket

1	pie pumpkin, halved and seeded	1
½ tsp	salt	2 mL
¼ tsp	freshly ground black pepper	1 mL
2 tbsp	olive oil	30 mL
2 tbsp	vegan hard margarine	30 mL
1	onion, chopped	1
2	carrots, peeled and chopped	2
1	green apple, chopped	1
1 tbsp	grated fresh gingerroot	15 mL
1½ tsp	Curry Powder (page 311) or store-bought	7 mL
2 cups	Vegetable Broth (page 31) or store-bought	500 mL
2 cups	plain hemp milk	500 mL
3 cups	packed spinach	750 mL
½ cup	Basic Sour Cream (page 21) or store-bought vegan alternative, optional	125 mL

1. Place steamer basket in a large saucepan and add water to about 1 inch (2.5 cm) below bottom of basket. Place pumpkin halves in basket, cover pan and turn heat to medium–high. When water boils, reduce heat to medium and cook until pumpkins are tender, 10 to 15 minutes, adding hot water, if necessary. Let cool. When cool enough to handle, scoop pulp from skins. Transfer to food processor, add salt and pepper and purée until almost smooth. Set aside.

2. Place a large heavy-bottomed saucepan over medium heat and let pan get hot. Add oil and margarine and when melted, tip pan to coat. Add onion, carrots, apple, ginger and curry powder and cook, stirring frequently, until softened, 6 to 8 minutes. Add pumpkin, vegetable broth, milk, and salt and pepper to taste, stirring well to thoroughly combine.

3. Reduce heat and simmer, stirring occasionally, until soup is slightly thickened, about 10 minutes. Stir in spinach. Taste and adjust seasonings and cook, stirring occasionally, until spinach is wilted, 4 minutes. Serve topped with a dollop of sour cream alternative, if using.

Taro and long bean green coconut curry

Taro grows underground and is similar to a potato with somewhat more fiber. The nutty, sweet and rich texture is delicious in this curry. Chinese long beans can grow up to a yard long but can become tough. Choose young tender beans 12 to 14 inches (30 to 35 cm) long.

1 tbsp	peanut oil	15 mL
1 lb	taro, peeled and cut into 2-inch (5 cm) cubes	500 g
1 lb	fresh Chinese long beans, trimmed and cut into 3-inch (7.5 cm) pieces	500 g
2 tbsp	green curry paste	30 mL
1 cup	Vegetable Broth (page 31) or store-bought	250 mL
2 cups	coconut milk	500 mL
3 tbsp	tamari	45 mL
2 tbsp	brown rice syrup	30 mL
¾ cup	fresh basil leaves	175 mL
4 to 6 cups	cooked rice	1 to 1.5 L

1. Place a large skillet over medium heat and let pan get hot. Add oil and tip pan to coat. Add taro and cook, stirring occasionally, for 8 minutes. Add long beans and cook until beans and taro are slightly browned, 4 to 6 minutes.

2. In a small bowl, thin curry paste with 1 tbsp (15 mL) vegetable broth and add to vegetables. Add remaining broth, coconut milk, tamari and brown rice syrup, stirring well to combine. Reduce heat to low. Stir in basil and simmer until slightly thickened, about 15 minutes. Serve in bowls with rice.

⠃ Variation

If Chinese long beans are unavailable, green beans are a great substitute.

Sauces, Dips and Spreads

✕—✕—✕—✕—✕—✕—✕—✕—✕—✕—✕—✕—✕

Asian pesto

This fresh and spicy
pesto is a simple way
to liven up grilled tofu
or vegetables. Add a
tablespoon to soups,
stews or a vegetable
smoothie.

⋇ Tip

Make a double batch and
freeze half in ice cube
trays. Spray trays with
vegetable oil and measure
1 to 2 tbsp (15 to 30 mL)
of pesto into each cube
slot. The cubes pop right
out after freezing and can
be stored in a resealable
freezer bag, ready when
you need them.

⋇ Food processor

2	cloves garlic, crushed (see Tip, page 285)	2
1 cup	packed fresh cilantro	250 mL
½ cup	packed fresh mint	125 mL
½ cup	packed fresh basil	125 mL
⅓ cup	roasted macadamia nuts	75 mL
1	can (4 oz/125 g) canned water chestnuts, drained	1
2 tbsp	freshly squeezed lime juice	30 mL
1 tbsp	grated gingerroot	15 mL
2 tsp	chopped Thai bird's-eye or serrano chile	10 mL
2 tsp	toasted sesame oil	10 mL
½ cup	sunflower oil	125 mL
Pinch	salt	Pinch

1. In food processor, with motor running, drop garlic
   through the feed tube and process until finely chopped.
   Scrape down sides, add cilantro, mint and basil and
   pulse until coarsely chopped, 10 to 15 times. Scrape
   sides, add macadamia nuts, water chestnuts, lime juice,
   ginger, chile and sesame oil and pulse to combine, 6 to
   8 times. Scrape sides. With motor running, slowly add
   sunflower oil through the feed tube and process until
   smooth, stopping to scrape sides as necessary. Season
   with salt. Use immediately or transfer to an airtight
   container and refrigerate for up to 1 week or freeze for
   up to 3 months.

Basil lemon gremolata pesto

**Makes about
1¾ cups (425 mL)**

A bright and fresh
mash up of gremolata
and pesto using lemon
peel and less oil is big
on flavor and low on
fat. Use a spoonful
in soups, stews,
smoothies, dressings,
dips or toss with hot
or cold pasta. For a
delicious sandwich
spread, mix with equal
parts of mayonnaise.

✻ Tip

When garlic is going into
a food processor, there
is no need to pre-chop,
however, crushing garlic
roughly once or twice
with the side of a knife
flattens the rounded sides
and garlic is then easily
incorporated into the
processing mixture.

✻ Food processor

1	lemon	1
2 cups	packed basil leaves	500 mL
2	cloves garlic, crushed (see Tip, left)	2
¼ tsp	salt	1 mL
¼ cup	olive oil	60 mL

1. Using a serrated knife, remove just the lemon peel in strips, avoiding the white pith. Reserve fruit for another use. Coarsely chop lemon peel.

2. In food processor, combine basil, lemon peel, garlic and salt and pulse until finely chopped. With motor running, slowly add oil through the feed tube and process until smooth or desired consistency is achieved. Use immediately or refrigerate in an airtight container for up to 5 days.

Classic pesto sauce

A classic pesto is
always so versatile and
should be prominently
included in everyone's
recipe repertoire. Add
a spoonful to soups,
stews, curries and
sauces or toss it with
steamed vegetables,
roasted potatoes and,
of course, pasta.

✖ Tip

Drizzling olive oil over top
of pesto during storage
helps prevent discoloration.

✖ Food processor or blender

6 cups	packed fresh basil leaves	1.5 L
1 tsp	salt	5 mL
½ tsp	freshly ground black pepper	2 mL
½ cup	olive oil	125 mL
¼ cup	pine nuts	60 mL

1. In food processor, combine basil, salt and pepper and
pulse until finely chopped, 3 to 4 times. With motor
running, slowly add oil through the feed tube and
process until just smooth, scraping down sides as
necessary. Add pine nuts and pulse to incorporate, 2 to
4 times. Use immediately or refrigerate in an airtight
container for up to 5 days.

Balsamic reduction sauce

So easy to make, this
versatile sauce will
add rich flavor to your
cooking. Use it in place
of straight vinegar
in salad dressings.
Luscious drizzled over
a fruit and nut platter.

1 cup	balsamic vinegar	250 mL
1 tbsp	granulated sugar	15 mL

1. In a small saucepan combine vinegar and sugar.
Bring to a boil over medium-high heat. Reduce heat
to medium-low, stirring occasionally, until vinegar
has reduced to ¼ to ⅓ cup (60 to 75 mL), 20 to
30 minutes. Remove from heat and let sauce thicken
as it cools. Use immediately or refrigerate in an airtight
container for up to 3 months.

Daikon dipping sauce

Makes about 1½ cups (375 mL)

White daikon radish is grated into a sweet and tangy combination to create a superb Asian dipping sauce. Delicious with vegetable tempura, spring rolls or drizzled over Light Savory Baked Tofu (page 26).

6 oz	daikon radish, shredded (about 1 cup/250 mL)	175 g
½ cup	tamari	125 mL
¼ cup	orange juice	60 mL
2 tbsp	freshly squeezed lemon juice	30 mL
2 tbsp	rice wine vinegar	30 mL
2 tbsp	water	30 mL

1. In a small bowl, combine radish, tamari, orange juice, lemon juice, vinegar and water. Sauce will be thick and may be thinned with additional water if desired. Cover and refrigerate before using for at least 2 hours. Refrigerate sauce in an airtight container for up to 2 days.

Fresh pomodoro sauce

Makes 7 cups (1.75 L)

Nothing tastes more of summertime than a simple blending of ripe Roma tomatoes, fresh and fragrant basil and good-quality extra virgin olive oil. Absolutely spectacular over pasta or ravioli topped with a few torn basil leaves. Amazing how something so simple can taste so good!

Tip

If tomatoes are out of season, substitute 2¼ cans (each 28 oz/796 mL) unsalted Roma tomatoes, drained.

½ cup	olive oil	125 mL
8 cups	chopped Roma (plum) tomatoes (about 4 lbs/2 kg) (see Tip, left)	2 L
2 cups	torn fresh basil leaves, divided	500 mL
1 tsp	salt	5 mL
½ tsp	freshly ground black pepper	2 mL

1. Heat a large skillet over medium-high heat. Add oil and tip pan to coat. Add tomatoes, 1½ cups (375 mL) of the basil, salt and pepper. Stir until tomatoes are just heated, 3 to 4 minutes. Taste and adjust seasoning. Serve topped with ½ cup (125 mL) of torn basil leaves.

Variation

Use this vibrant and flavorful sauce baked with stuffed shells, manicotti or lasagna.

Homemade barbecue sauce

An hour on the stove top reduces these ingredients into a tangy rich sauce. Make a double batch during the summer months to have on hand when you fire up the barbecue.

✖ Tip

If vegan Worcestershire sauce is unavailable, substitute 3 tbsp (45 mL) Henderson's Relish or tamari.

2 cups	water	500 mL
1 cup	tomato ketchup	250 mL
1	lemon, thinly sliced into circles	1
1/4 cup	packed brown sugar	60 mL
1/4 cup	apple cider vinegar	60 mL
1/4 cup	vegan Worcestershire sauce	60 mL
1 tbsp	tomato paste	15 mL
1 tbsp	All-Purpose Spicy Barbecue Dry Rub (page 308) or store-bought	15 mL
1 tsp	salt	5 mL
1 tsp	celery seeds	5 mL

1. In a heavy-bottomed saucepan over medium heat, combine water, ketchup, lemon, brown sugar, vinegar, Worcestershire sauce, tomato paste, barbecue rub, salt and celery seed, whisking well to incorporate. Reduce heat to medium-low and simmer until thick and saucy, 45 minutes to 1 hour. Use immediately or refrigerate in an airtight container for up to 2 weeks.

Pantry ponzu sauce

This is a versatile all-around dipping, marinating, roasting or drizzling sauce and is easily adapted to personal taste.

✖ Tip

For longer storing, omit herbs until just before use, and refrigerate for up to 2 weeks.

1/4 cup	tamari	60 mL
1/4 cup	freshly squeezed lime juice	60 mL
1/4 cup	orange juice	60 mL
3 tbsp	agave nectar	45 mL
2 tbsp	canola oil	30 mL
1 1/2 tbsp	minced gingerroot	22 mL
1 1/2 tsp	rice wine vinegar	7 mL
3	cloves garlic, minced	3
1 tsp	Asian chile sauce, such as sambal oelek	5 mL
1/2 tsp	toasted sesame oil	2 mL
1/4 cup	finely chopped fresh basil	60 mL
2 tbsp	chopped fresh cilantro	30 mL

1. In a glass jar, combine tamari, lime juice, orange juice, agave nectar, canola oil, ginger, vinegar, garlic, chile sauce, sesame oil, basil and cilantro and shake vigorously to combine. Use immediately or refrigerate in an airtight container for up to 4 days.

Lime sour cream dipping sauce

This cool and tangy dipping sauce is amazing with Chile-Dusted Chickpea Fries (page 42), blue corn chips or crudités.

1 cup	Basic Sour Cream (page 21) or store-bought	250 mL
½ tsp	grated lime zest	2 mL
2 tbsp	freshly squeezed lime juice	30 mL
2 tbsp	minced fresh cilantro	30 mL
¼ tsp	ground cumin	1 mL
¼ tsp	salt	1 mL
⅛ tsp	cayenne pepper, optional	0.5 mL

1. In a bowl, whisk together sour cream, lime zest, lime juice, cilantro, cumin, salt and cayenne until well combined. Let stand for 10 minutes to mingle flavors before using. Refrigerate in an airtight container for up to 4 days.

Roasted shallot yogurt sauce

This creamy sauce is great on grilled vegetables or tossed with hot or cold pasta.

❖ **Preheat oven to 375°F (190°C)**
❖ **Baking sheet, lined with parchment paper**
❖ **Food processor**

4	large shallots, unpeeled, ends cut off	4
4	cloves garlic, unpeeled	4
1 cup	plain soy yogurt	250 mL
5 tsp	freshly squeezed lemon juice	25 mL
1 tbsp	chopped fresh parsley	15 mL
¼ tsp	salt	1 mL
¼ tsp	ground lemon pepper or freshly ground black pepper	1 mL
Pinch	cayenne pepper	Pinch

1. Place shallots and garlic on prepared baking sheet and roast in preheated oven until tender, about 15 minutes. Let cool slightly.

2. In food processor, combine yogurt, shallots, garlic, lemon juice, parsley, salt, lemon pepper and cayenne and process until smooth. Taste and adjust seasoning, adding additional cayenne, if desired. Use immediately or refrigerate in an airtight container for up to 5 days.

Roasted tomatillo sauce

This rich and tasty sauce
is delicious when an
added kick of flavor
is desired. Spoon it
over grilled vegetables
or tofu, baked bean
burgers, roasted or
baked potatoes. Blend a
few tablespoons (30 mL)
with olive oil and toss
into chilled rice, potato
or pasta salad.

⠕ Tips

Roast extra poblano chiles,
cool and freeze unpeeled
as skins help retain flavor
while frozen. To use, thaw,
peel and remove seeds.

When processing herbs,
such as parsley or cilantro,
it is only necessary to
remove the large thick
bottom stems as upper
stems are more tender
and will be chopped finely
in the processor.

⠕ Preheat oven to 350°F (180°C)
⠕ Baking sheet, lined with parchment paper
⠕ Food processor

8	tomatillos, husked and washed	8
2	poblano chiles (see Tips, left)	2
2	tomatoes	2
1	small onion, quartered	1
3	cloves garlic, crushed (see Tip, page 285)	3
2 tbsp	freshly squeezed lime juice	30 mL
1/4 cup	lightly packed cilantro (large bottom stems removed) (see Tips, left)	60 mL
1/2 tsp	salt	2 mL
1/4 to 1/2 cup	water	60 to 125 mL

1. Halve tomatillos and arrange, cut side down, on prepared baking sheet along with whole poblanos and tomatoes. Broil until tomatillos and tomatoes are softened and skins are lightly blackened, 5 to 7 minutes. Transfer tomatillos and tomatoes to a food processor.

2. Continue to broil poblanos, turning frequently with tongs, until all sides are charred, 6 to 8 minutes. Transfer charred poblanos to a dampened clean kitchen towel, wrapping to enclose, and steam to loosen skins, about 10 minutes. Peel poblanos, remove stems and seeds and discard.

3. Add poblanos, onion, garlic, lime juice, cilantro and salt to food processor and process into a smooth sauce. Add water, a little at a time, until desired consistency.

Roasted vegetable sauce

Vegetable sauce on
vegetables is doubly
healthy and doubly
divine! The onion
adds a subtle base and
blends perfectly with
the roasted broccoli.
Scrumptious tossed
with pasta or on rice
or baked potatoes.

✖ Variation

Substitute cauliflower,
winter squash, carrots and
ginger or your favorite
vegetables.

✖ Preheat oven to 400°F (200°C)
✖ Baking sheet, lined with parchment paper
✖ Blender

4 cups	broccoli florets	1 L
1/2	onion, ends cut off, unpeeled, quartered	1/2
2	cloves garlic, unpeeled	2
2 tsp	olive oil	10 mL
1/2 cup	Vegetable Broth (page 31) or store-bought	125 mL
1/4 cup	plain hemp milk	60 mL
	Salt and freshly ground black pepper, optional	

1. Place broccoli, onion and garlic on prepared baking
   sheet. Drizzle and toss with oil. Bake in preheated oven
   until tender, 20 to 25 minutes. Let cool.

2. When cool, peel onion and garlic and transfer with
   broccoli to blender. Add broth and milk and blend until
   smooth. Taste and add salt and black pepper, if desired.
   Serve immediately or refrigerate in an airtight container
   for up to 2 days. Heat over low heat before using or
   serve chilled.

Avocado cilantro dip

A smooth and cool dip
for crudités or crunchy
tortilla and kettle chips.
Delicious with Roasted
Root Vegetable Chips
(page 56) or spooned
onto baked potatoes.

✖ Tip

Store dip with plastic wrap
gently pressed directly on
surface to prevent air from
discoloring dip.

✖ Food processor or blender

2	avocados, cut into large cubes	2
1/2 cup	Creamy Mayonnaise (page 19) or store-bought vegan alternative	125 mL
2 tbsp	finely chopped fresh cilantro	30 mL
1 tbsp	freshly squeezed lime juice	15 mL
1/2 tsp	onion powder	2 mL
1/4 tsp	garlic powder	1 mL
1/4 tsp	salt	1 mL
Pinch	cayenne pepper	Pinch

1. In food processor, combine avocado, mayonnaise,
   cilantro, lime juice, onion powder, garlic powder, salt
   and cayenne and pulse until smooth. Serve immediately
   or refrigerate in an airtight container for up to 1 day.

Roasted red pepper and chipotle dip

Makes 2 cups (500 mL)

This beautifully rich and spicy dip cuts the fat with a bean base. You will love it with crudités or fresh baked crisp pita chips.

✖ Tip

Substitute canned cannellini beans, taking care to rinse well and drain before adding.

✖ Preheat oven to broil
✖ Baking sheet, lined with parchment paper
✖ Blender

1	large red bell pepper, halved and seeded	1
1 cup	cooked cannellini beans (see Tip, left)	250 mL
1/2 cup	vegan cream cheese	125 mL
2 tbsp	Creamy Mayonnaise (page 19) or store-bought vegan alternative	30 mL
2	small chipotles, coarsely chopped	2
1	small shallot, finely chopped	1
2 tsp	adobo sauce from canned chipotle	10 mL
1/2 tsp	salt	2 mL
1 to 2 tbsp	white wine vinegar	15 to 30 mL

1. Place bell pepper, cut side down, on prepared baking sheet and broil until lightly charred, 6 to 10 minutes. Transfer pepper to a dampened clean kitchen towel, wrapping to enclose, and steam to loosen skins, about 10 minutes. Peel pepper, cut into large pieces and place in blender. Add beans, cream cheese, mayonnaise, chipotles, shallot, adobo sauce and salt and blend into a thick purée. If thinner consistency is desired, add white wine vinegar, 1 tsp (5 mL) at a time. Transfer to a serving bowl or refrigerate in an airtight container for up to 3 days.

Southwestern baba ghanouj

**Makes about
4 cups (1 L)**

Baba ghanouj is
traditionally served
with toasted pita
chips and with good
reason — it's delish!
For fun, try this spicy
and smoky version with
blue corn chips and a
bottle of cold Mexican
beer. For a great
homemade pita chips
recipe, see White Bean
Hummus with Spiced
Baked Pita Chips
(page 64).

✖ Preheat oven to 425°F (220°C)
✖ Food processor

2	medium eggplant	2
2	cloves garlic, crushed (see Tip, page 285)	2
1	can (4 oz/127 mL) roasted and diced New Mexican green chiles	1
1/4 cup	tahini paste	60 mL
2 tbsp	freshly squeezed lime juice	30 mL
3/4 tsp	salt	3 mL
1/8 tsp	ground cumin	0.5 mL
1/8 tsp	ground chipotle powder	0.5 mL

1. Place eggplant on prepared baking sheet and prick with
   a fork. Roast in preheated oven until collapsed and very
   tender, about 40 minutes. When cool, scoop out pulp
   and transfer to food processor. Add garlic, chiles, tahini,
   lime juice, salt, cumin and chipotle powder and process
   until smooth. Taste and adjust seasonings. Refrigerate in
   an airtight container for at least 2 hours before using or
   for up to 4 days.

Chipotle lime mayonnaise

**Makes about
1/2 cup (125 mL)**

Whip up this zesty
spread in just minutes
and slather on a huge
sandwich or juicy
vegan burger. Makes
a terrific dip for fries
or crudités.

1/2 cup	Creamy Mayonnaise (page 19) or store-bought vegan alternative	125 mL
1/2 tsp	grated lime zest	2 mL
1 tsp	freshly squeezed lime juice	5 mL
1/4 tsp	chipotle chile powder	1 mL
1/4 tsp	ground cumin	1 mL
Pinch	salt	Pinch

1. In a small bowl, whisk together mayonnaise, lime zest,
   lime juice, chipotle powder, cumin and salt until well
   blended. Serve immediately or refrigerate in an airtight
   container for up to 10 days.

> ✖ **Variation**
> Substitute 1 to 2 tsp (5 to 10 mL) minced chipotle
> for chipotle powder.

Apple Butter

Apples are cooked with
the skin to increase
flavor and nutrients,
so using scrubbed
organic apples is best.
The use of a food
mill is required for
this method. If you
preferred to skip that
step, see Variation.

✂ Tips

About 12 medium apples
will generally equal 4 lbs
(2 kg).

To sterilize canning jars,
immerse in a pot of
simmering, not boiling,
water for 10 minutes or
wash using the sterilizing
cycle in dishwasher. Keep
hot until filling.

✂ Food mill or small-holed colander

4 lbs	sweet, tart apples, such as Granny Smith, Cortland or Pippin, cored and quartered (see Tips, left)	2 kg
1¾ cups	apple cider or juice	425 mL
¾ cup	agave nectar	175 mL
2 tbsp	freshly squeezed lemon juice	30 mL
1½ tsp	ground cinnamon	7 mL
1 tsp	ground cardamom	5 mL

1. In a large heavy-bottomed saucepan over medium-high heat, bring apples and apple cider to a boil. Reduce heat and simmer, stirring occasionally, until very soft, 25 to 30 minutes. Let cool.

2. Press softened apples through a food mill or small-holed colander to remove skins.

3. Transfer apple purée to a clean large heavy-bottomed saucepan over medium-high heat. Stir in agave, lemon juice, cinnamon and cardamom and bring to a boil, stirring frequently. Reduce heat and simmer, stirring frequently to prevent any sticking and adjusting heat as necessary as mixture thickens, until mixture is very thick and mounds on a spoon, about 1½ hours.

4. Remove from heat and let cool. Spoon into sterilized canning jars (see Tips, left) or airtight containers and refrigerate for up to 1 month or freeze for up to 3 months.

✂ Variation

To avoid using a food mill to purée apples, peel, core and quarter apples and follow instructions through Step 1. Skip Step 2 and instead use a food processor to purée softened apples. Resume instructions at Step 3.

Chocolate hazelnut spread

**Makes about
1¾ cups (425 mL)**

This is a sublime
spread for sandwiches,
morning toast or
crêpes, a delectable dip
for fruits and a spot
of heaven spooned
into coffee or hot
milks. The possibilities
are endless. Terrific
thinned slightly and
drizzled on cakes,
frozen desserts and
waffles.

✂ Tip

*To toast and skin
hazelnuts:* Spread nuts in
a single layer on a baking
sheet. Toast in a 350°F
(180°C) oven, stirring
occasionally, until toasted,
8 to 10 minutes. Check
constantly because nuts
can burn quickly. Transfer
to a lightly dampened
clean kitchen towel, gather
up the sides and rub
briskly to dislodge majority
of skins.

✂ Food Processor

2 tbsp	soy powdered milk	30 mL
6 tbsp	plain soy milk (approx.)	90 mL
4 oz	vegan dark chocolate, chopped	125 g
1 cup	toasted hazelnuts, skins rubbed off (see Tip, left)	250 mL
¾ cup	Sweetened Condensed Milk (page 17) or store-bought vegan alternative	175 mL

1. In a small bowl, whisk powdered milk into soy milk. Set aside.

2. In a small microwave-safe bowl, microwave chopped chocolate on Medium (50%) power in 30-second increments until melted, stirring each time, about 2½ minutes.

3. In food processor, add hazelnuts and process into a smooth butter, 3 to 5 minutes. Add chocolate and condensed milk and process until combined into a thick paste. With machine running, add soy milk mixture through the feed tube, processing into a thick smooth but spreadable paste. If mixture is too thick, add soy milk, 1 tsp (5 mL) at a time.

4. Use immediately or transfer to airtight glass container and refrigerate for up to 1 week. Mixture thickens when chilled so remove 10 minute before using to soften.

Fresh pomegranate relish

Top grilled tempeh with this piquant sweet relish or tuck it into a luncheon wrap with baked tofu to add a fresh and vibrant twist.

✖ Tip

To remove seeds: Crack open pomegranate and submerge in a huge bowl of water. Gently urge seeds from skin with your fingers. Drain and sort out seeds. Brilliant!

1½ cups	pomegranate seeds (see Tip, left)	375 mL
½	small red onion, finely chopped (about ¼ cup/60 mL)	½
¼ cup	chopped fresh cilantro	60 mL
3 tsp	freshly squeezed lime juice	15 mL
	Salt and freshly ground black pepper	
1	avocado, chopped	1

1. In a bowl, combine pomegranate seeds, red onion, cilantro, lime juice, and salt and pepper to taste. Gently fold in avocado. Let stand at room temperature for 30 minutes before using. Taste and adjust seasoning, adding more lime juice, salt and pepper, if needed.

> ## ✖ Variation
> Swap out cilantro and lime with chopped parsley and lemon for a Middle Eastern flair.

Mango habanero chutney

It seems that new and hotter peppers are being discovered all the time, but as peppers go, habanero is one of the hottest. For this reason, wear gloves when handling.

✖ Tip

To make a tangy sauce or marinade, blend the chutney with additional liquid as necessary to achieve desired consistency.

½ cup	granulated sugar	125 mL
¼ cup	apple cider vinegar	60 mL
2	mangos, chopped	2
1	small habanero pepper, minced	1
1 tbsp	grated lime zest	15 mL
3 tbsp	freshly squeezed lime juice	45 mL
¼ cup	chopped onion	60 mL
3 tbsp	golden raisins	45 mL

1. In a saucepan over medium-high heat, stir together sugar and vinegar until sugar is melted. Add mangos, habanero, lime zest, lime juice, onion and raisins. Reduce heat to low and simmer, stirring occasionally, until slightly thickened, about 20 minutes. Let cool slightly and use immediately or transfer an airtight container and refrigerate for up to 1 week.

Maple rhubarb jam

Makes about 2 cups (500 mL)

This maple and vanilla–laced jam would be lovely spread on toast, as a tart filling, served with vanilla yogurt or eaten with a spoon. If you like tart and sweet you will love this treat.

Tip

Pack into decorative jars and give as a charming homemade hostess gift.

Preheat oven to 350°F (180°C)

1½ to 2 lbs	rhubarb stalks, cut into 1-inch (2.5 cm) pieces	750 g to 1 kg
½ cup	granulated sugar	125 mL
½ cup	pure maple syrup	125 mL
¼ cup	white wine, optional	60 mL
1 tbsp	freshly squeezed lemon juice	15 mL
1	vanilla bean, split	1

1. In a baking dish, stir together rhubarb, sugar, maple syrup, wine, if using, lemon juice and vanilla bean. Bake on lower rack in preheated oven, gently stirring once during cooking, until bubbly and thickened, about 1½ hours. Let cool, scrape vanilla bean into jam and discard bean. Stir to combine before serving. Refrigerate in an airtight container for up to 5 days.

Roasted roma tomato jam

Makes about 2½ cups (625 mL)

Served on crackers, over pasta or eaten with a spoon, this intensely sweet tomato jam will make your taste buds oh so happy.

Tip

Roma or plum tomatoes lend themselves beautifully to this recipe because they are less juicy than regular tomatoes, allowing less roasting time and netting a thicker jam.

Preheat oven to 400°F (200°C)
Rimmed baking sheet

8 cups	Roma (plum) tomatoes, halved lengthwise	2 L
⅓ cup	olive oil	75 mL
1 tsp	salt	5 mL
½ tsp	freshly ground black pepper	2 mL

1. In a large bowl, place tomatoes and toss with oil, salt and pepper. Spread evenly on baking sheet and roast on middle rack of preheated oven, stirring midway, until most of the liquid is evaporated, 20 to 30 minutes. Let cool until thickened. Transfer to an airtight container and refrigerate for up to 5 days.

Variation

For variety, add 2 cloves garlic, minced, and several torn fresh basil leaves to the tomatoes before roasting.

Raspberry curd

Makes 1½ cups (375 mL)

The pairing of scones or muffins with beautiful ruby-hued raspberry curd will make everyone a fan of the combination. It is also wonderful spooned over pudding or fruit; use anywhere a splash of berry goodness is needed.

Food processor

6 oz	fresh raspberries (about 1½ cups/375 mL)	175 g
¼ cup	light amber agave nectar	60 mL
4 oz	firm or extra-firm silken tofu	125 g
⅛ tsp	almond extract	0.5 mL

1. In food processor, purée raspberries until liquid. Pour purée through a fine mesh strainer into a bowl, pressing down hard with back of large spoon or spatula. Discard seeds. Stir in agave and set aside.

2. In clean food processor, add tofu and process until smooth, scraping down sides. Add raspberry purée and pulse to incorporate. Scrape down sides and process until mixture is a uniform ruby color. Add almond extract and pulse to combine. Refrigerate in an airtight container for at least 2 hours or for up to 1 week.

Salsa verde

Makes about 3 cups (750 mL)

Use a spoonful of this fresh and spicy salsa to perk up a morning scramble, add zip to luncheon tacos or dress up a dinnertime baked potato.

Tip

For milder salsa, remove seeds from chiles or omit chiles all together.

Food processor

3	cloves garlic, crushed (see Tip, page 285)	3
10	tomatillos, husked, washed and quartered	10
1	onion, cut into 2-inch (5 cm) pieces	1
1 cup	lightly packed cilantro (large bottom stems removed) (see Tips, page 290)	250 mL
2	small serrano chiles, halved and seeded (see Tip, left)	2
¼ cup	freshly squeezed lime juice	60 mL
2 tbsp	white wine vinegar	30 mL
1 tbsp	olive oil	15 mL
1 tsp	salt	5 mL

1. With motor running, drop garlic into food processor through the feed tube until finely chopped. Scrape sides and add tomatillos, onion, cilantro, chiles, lime juice, vinegar, oil and salt. Process into a thick chunky salsa. Taste and adjust seasoning, adding more lime juice, vinegar or salt, if needed. Let stand for 30 minutes. Refrigerate in an airtight container for up to 4 days.

Stone fruit salsa

Adding a sweet twist to this spicy dish creates a salsa that is hard to resist. Spoon fruit salsa into a decorative clear glass serving bowl set on a large platter. Surround the bowl with white and blue corn chips for a striking presentation.

✤ Tip

Stone fruits not only taste incredible but also are full of fiber and natural antioxidants.

✤ Food processor

1	serrano chile, halved and seeded	1
1/2	small red onion, quartered	1/2
4	green onions, white and light green parts only, trimmed into 2-inch (5 cm) pieces	4
4	Roma (plum) tomatoes, divided	4
1	roasted red bell pepper, coarsely chopped	1
2	nectarines, coarsely chopped	2
2	green plums, coarsely chopped	2
1	mango, coarsely chopped	1
2	cloves garlic, smashed	2
2 tbsp	freshly squeezed lime juice	30 mL
1 tsp	red wine vinegar	5 mL
2 tbsp	olive oil	30 mL
2 tbsp	chopped fresh cilantro	30 mL
2 tbsp	chopped fresh mint	30 mL
1 tsp	agave nectar	5 mL
1/2 tsp	ground cumin	2 mL
1/4 tsp	salt	1 mL
1/4 tsp	freshly ground black pepper	1 mL

1. In food processor, combine serrano chile, red onion and green onions and process until finely chopped. Transfer to a large serving bowl. Coarsely hand chop 2 tomatoes and add to serving bowl along with bell pepper, nectarines, plums and mango.

2. With motor running, drop garlic through the feed tube into food processor and process until finely chopped. Scrape sides. Coarsely chop 2 tomatoes and add to processor with lime juice, vinegar, oil, cilantro, mint, agave, cumin, salt and pepper and pulse into a rough purée.

3. Transfer to serving bowl and gently toss to combine. Refrigerate salsa for 30 minutes to 1 hour before serving. Taste and adjust seasoning before serving.

Year-round blender tomato salsa

You can't wreck this magic recipe that comes out perfect every time. It comes out different every time, but always perfect. Calling for canned tomatoes makes this a fabulous choice for a winter blues buster. Whip up a few mojitos, put out a bowl of chips and dig out that Gypsy Kings CD. You will be warm in no time.

✖ Tip

Nothing beats summer tomatoes picked at their flavor peak. This is why canned tomatoes rather than fresh should be used in recipes during winter months because tomatoes are picked and canned when ripe and flavorful. Rotel is a brand that includes spices and green chile peppers.

✖ Food processor or blender

2	cans (each 10 oz/284 mL) tomatoes with spices and green chile peppers (see Tip, left)	2
1	small onion, coarsely chopped	1
1	jalapeño, stem removed, coarsely chopped	1
1½ cups	lightly packed cilantro, large bottom stems removed (see Tips, page 290)	375 mL
	Juice of 1 lime	
½ tsp	salt	2 mL

1. In food processor, combine tomatoes, onion, jalapeño, cilantro, lime juice and salt and pulse into a thick salsa. Transfer to a serving bowl, cover and refrigerate for 30 minutes to 1 hour. Taste and adjust seasoning before serving. Salsa will keep refrigerated, in an airtight container, for up to 2 days.

Dressings and Spice Blends

Caper and pine nut vinaigrette

Warm or cool, this nutty vinaigrette is perfect tossed with Roasted Potatoes and Tofu (page 207) or as a dressing for mixed greens.

✖ Tip

Refrigerate in an airtight container for up to 5 days.

½ cup	olive oil	125 mL
¾ cup	chopped onion	175 mL
1 tbsp	minced garlic	15 mL
½ cup	chopped walnuts	125 mL
¼ cup	pine nuts	60 mL
½ cup	white wine vinegar	125 mL
3 tbsp	drained capers	45 mL
½ tsp	salt	2 mL
¼ tsp	freshly ground black pepper	1 mL

1. Place a medium skillet over medium–low heat and let pan get hot. Add oil and tip pan to coat. Add onion and garlic, stirring occasionally, until soft and translucent, 5 to 6 minutes. Add chopped walnuts and pine nuts and cook for 2 minutes. Add vinegar, capers, salt and pepper and cook for 1 minute to blend flavors. Use either warm or at room temperature. If using warm, toss immediately with warm vegetables to impart the best flavor.

Champagne vinaigrette

A glass jar with a tight-fitting lid does double duty here as a tool for blending and a container for storing.

✖ Tip

Store at room temperature for up to 3 weeks. Shake well to reblend before using.

✖ Glass jar with tight-fitting lid

½ cup	dry Champagne or Champagne vinegar	125 mL
½ cup	olive oil	125 mL
½ cup	agave nectar	125 mL
Pinch	salt and freshly ground black pepper	Pinch

1. In clean glass jar, combine Champagne, oil, agave, salt and pepper and shake vigorously until well blended. Taste and adjust seasoning, adding more salt and pepper, if needed.

✖ Variation

It is so easy to flavor this vinaigrette to your liking by adding chopped fresh herbs or smashed garlic cloves. If adding fresh herbs or garlic, refrigerate unused portions in a glass jar with tight-fitting lid. Let dressing come to room temperature before shaking to reblend.

Creamy tahini dressing

Makes about 2 cups (500 mL)

This dressing is easy to make and incredibly less expensive than store-bought, and you can create your own signature blend by adding herbs or substituting a favorite vinegar or citrus juice. Far beyond salads, try this on roasted vegetables, baked potatoes, crispy tofu or as a spread in your favorite wrap.

⅓ cup	tahini paste	75 mL
⅓ cup	apple cider vinegar	75 mL
3 tbsp	tamari	45 mL
2 tbsp	freshly squeezed lemon juice	30 mL
2	cloves garlic, minced	2
1 tbsp	finely chopped fresh parsley	15 mL
1 tbsp	finely chopped chives	15 mL
½ cup	sunflower oil	125 mL
¼ cup	water	60 mL
½ tsp	salt	2 mL

1. In a bowl, whisk together tahini, vinegar, tamari, lemon juice, garlic, parsley and chives until well combined. Add oil and whisk until incorporated. Add water, a little at a time to achieve desired consistency, making a thicker dressing if using as a sauce. Whisk in salt. Taste and adjust seasonings.

Italian herbed dressing

Makes about ⅔ cup (150 mL)

Easily doubled for a larger gathering, this dressing celebrates simple flavors. Toss with greens, mix into a pasta salad or drizzle over a baked potato.

✂ Tip

Use immediately or transfer to an airtight container and refrigerate for up to 3 days. Let dressing come to room temperature before using.

¼ cup	red wine vinegar	60 mL
1	clove garlic, smashed	1
½ tsp	chopped fresh basil	2 mL
½ tsp	chopped fresh thyme	2 mL
½ tsp	chopped fresh oregano	2 mL
¼ tsp	paprika	1 mL
Pinch	salt	Pinch
Pinch	freshly ground black pepper	Pinch
6 tbsp	extra virgin olive oil	90 mL

1. In a small deep bowl, whisk together vinegar, garlic, basil, thyme, oregano, paprika, salt and pepper. Drizzle in oil, whisking to thoroughly blend. Taste and adjust seasonings.

✂ Variation

Substitute herbs such as chives, parsley or chervil for the oregano.

Fresh raspberry mustard vinaigrette

Makes about ³/₄ cup (175 mL)

Splash on a dash of this delightfully different dressing when you are looking to liven up steamed vegetables, a tossed green salad or fruit bowl.

✖ Tip

Use immediately or transfer to an airtight container and refrigerate for up to 2 weeks. To serve, let vinaigrette set at room temperature for 15 to 20 minutes and shake vigorously to emulsify.

✖ Blender

½ cup	fresh or frozen raspberries	125 mL
⅓ cup	white balsamic vinegar	75 mL
1 tbsp	agave nectar	15 mL
1 tbsp	Dijon mustard	15 mL
½ cup	walnut oil	125 mL
Pinch	salt	Pinch
Pinch	freshly ground black pepper	Pinch

1. In blender, combine raspberries, vinegar, agave and mustard and purée until smooth. With blender running, slowly add oil through hole in lid until dressing is emulsified, about 30 seconds. Season with salt and pepper to taste and blend for 30 seconds.

> ## ✖ Variation
> If walnut oil is unavailable, a good olive oil is a nice substitute.

Mustard tarragon dressing

Makes about ⅔ cup (150 mL)

This tangy concoction adds a bright flavor to steamed vegetables and can give a nice little snap to cooked rice.

✖ Tips

Dressing can be stored at room temperature overnight or refrigerated for up to 3 days. If refrigerated, let dressing come to room temperature before using.

It is easy to make the dressing right in the same jar in which it will be stored. Simply add all ingredients and shake vigorously until well blended.

2 tbsp	white wine vinegar	30 mL
2 tsp	Dijon mustard	10 mL
1 tsp	freshly squeezed lemon juice	5 mL
1 tsp	chopped fresh tarragon	5 mL
Pinch	salt	Pinch
Pinch	freshly ground black pepper	Pinch
6 tbsp	olive oil	90 mL

1. In a small deep bowl, whisk together vinegar, mustard, lemon juice, tarragon, salt and pepper. Drizzle in oil, whisking to thoroughly blend. Taste and adjust seasonings. Transfer to a glass jar with a tight-fitting lid and use immediately.

✖ Variations

Substitute ¼ tsp (1 mL) dried tarragon for fresh.

To make a quick sauce for breaded cutlets, whisk in ¼ cup (60 mL) Creamy Mayonnaise (page 19) or store-bought vegan alternative.

Ranch dressing

**Homemade Ranch
Dressing is far superior
to store-bought.
Use it as a dip for
crudités or steamed
artichokes, tossed with
chilled potatoes and
vegetables or dolloped
on baked potatoes.**

❖ Tip

Use immediately or
refrigerate in an airtight
container for up to 10 days.

❖ Food processor

8 oz	firm or extra-firm silken tofu	250 g
2 tbsp	freshly squeezed lemon juice	30 mL
2 tbsp	white wine vinegar	30 mL
1 tbsp	sunflower oil	15 mL
1½ tsp	onion powder	7 mL
1 tsp	garlic powder	5 mL
Pinch	granulated sugar	Pinch
1 cup	Creamy Mayonnaise (page 19) or store-bought vegan alternative	250 mL
3 tbsp	minced fresh chives	45 mL
½ tsp	salt	2 mL
½ tsp	freshly ground black pepper	2 mL

1. In food processor, combine tofu, lemon juice, vinegar,
   oil, onion powder, garlic powder and sugar and process
   until very smooth. Add mayonnaise, chives, salt and
   pepper and process until thoroughly combined. Taste
   and adjust seasoning. If thinner dressing is desired add a
   little water, 1 tsp (5 mL) at a time, to thin.

❖ Variations

Think of this dressing as a base recipe to which
you can add fresh herbs, spices and flavors
to create your own signature Ranch Dressing.
Try adding 1 tbsp (30 mL) fresh parsley, dill,
marjoram, tarragon or cilantro; ¼ or ½ tsp
(1 to 2 mL) paprika, cracked peppercorns,
cayenne, dry mustard or Cajun seasoning; 1 to
2 tsp (5 to 10 mL) hot sauce, tamari, chopped
capers, sun-dried tomatoes or minced black
olives. You are only limited by your imagination.

Sesame citrus dressing

Makes about 2 cups (500 mL)

A sensational blending of sesame, orange and cayenne creates a zesty and zippy dressing to wake up any salad, chilled mixed grains, steamed vegetable or crispy tofu or tempeh dishes.

Tips

If Champagne vinegar is unavailable, substitute Champagne, even if it has lost its bubbles, white wine or white wine vinegar.

Use immediately or transfer to an airtight container and refrigerate dressing for up to 2 days. Let dressing come to room temperature before serving.

Blender

1/2 cup	orange juice	125 mL
1	clove garlic, finely minced	1
1 tbsp	Dijon mustard	15 mL
1/2 cup	Champagne vinegar (see Tips, left)	125 mL
1 tbsp	finely grated orange zest	15 mL
1 tsp	toasted sesame oil	5 mL
1 tsp	toasted sesame seeds	5 mL
1/4 tsp	salt	1 mL
1/4 tsp	freshly ground black pepper	1 mL
Pinch	cayenne pepper	Pinch
3/4 cup	olive oil	175 mL

1. Pour orange juice into a small saucepan over medium-high heat and bring to a boil. Reduce heat and add garlic and mustard and simmer until reduced by half, 6 to 8 minutes. Remove from heat, let cool and transfer to blender.
2. To blender, add vinegar, orange zest, sesame oil, sesame seeds, salt, pepper and cayenne and blend for 30 seconds to combine. With blender running, drizzle oil through hole in lid, blending until incorporated, about 20 seconds. Taste and adjust seasonings.

All-purpose spicy barbecue dry rub

Makes about 1 cup (250 mL)

A simple blend of ingredients you most likely have in your spice cupboard is great for tofu, tempeh and vegetables. Give an added kick to soups, marinades, dressings and sauces.

✖ Tips

Granulated dried onion and granulated dried garlic produce the same flavor as their powder versions, only the consistency differs. The larger grains of the granulated flavorings are a good texture to use in a rub. To substitute, use 1 tbsp (15 mL) powdered for each 2 tbsp (30 mL) granulated.

Use immediately or store in an airtight container for up to 3 months.

After making your first batch adjust flavors exactly to your liking, creating your very own signature rub. A half pint jar with a personalized label makes a great gift.

3 tbsp	brown sugar	45 mL
3 tbsp	salt	45 mL
2 tbsp	granulated dried onion (see Tips, left)	30 mL
2 tbsp	granulated dried garlic	30 mL
2 tbsp	smoky paprika	30 mL
2 tbsp	ground cumin	30 mL
2 tbsp	chile powder	30 mL
1 tsp	ground allspice	5 mL
1 tsp	dry mustard powder	5 mL
1 tsp	freshly ground black pepper	5 mL

1. In a bowl, combine brown sugar and salt, stirring until well combined. Add onion, garlic, paprika, cumin, chile powder, allspice, mustard powder and black pepper and stir until completely incorporated.

Autumn spice blend

Sold in grocery stores as pumpkin pie spice, it would be a shame to limit its use to sweet recipes. Add a spoonful to wake up baked or stir-fried vegetables, stove-top pasta and grains and oven-baked casseroles.

✖ Tip

Use immediately or store in a cool, dark place away from heat sources for up to 4 months.

2 tbsp	ground cinnamon	30 mL
4 tsp	ground ginger	20 mL
2 tsp	ground allspice	10 mL
2 tsp	freshly grated nutmeg	10 mL
1 tsp	ground cloves	5 mL
1/4 tsp	ground cardamom	1 mL

1. In an airtight container, combine cinnamon, ginger, allspice, nutmeg, cloves and cardamom.

✖ Variation

Add 1/2 tsp (2 mL) ground ginger or ground mace.

Bouquet garni

This classic blend is a reliable flavoring for soups and stews. Dried herbs are called for here. If you wish to use fresh herbs, bound them neatly in kitchen twine for a lovely bouquet.

✖ Tip

Recipe is easily doubled or tripled.

10	peppercorns	10
2	bay leaves	2
2 tbsp	dried parsley	30 mL
1 tbsp	dried thyme	15 mL
1 tbsp	dried rosemary	15 mL

1. In an airtight container, combine peppercorns, bay leaves, parsley, thyme and rosemary.

2. To use, spoon desired amount into a piece of cheesecloth. Secure the top with kitchen twine, leaving a nice long piece as a means of removal. Store bouquet garni in a cool, dark place away from heat sources for up to 4 months.

✖ Variation

Try adding fennel, lavender, savory, chervil or tarragon.

Cajun spice

This all-inclusive pungent spice adds heat and flavor to recipes beyond traditional Cajun dishes.

✖ Tip

Use immediately or store in a cool, dark place away from heat sources for up to 4 months.

2 tbsp	paprika	30 mL
5 tsp	salt	25 mL
1 tbsp	garlic powder	15 mL
1 tbsp	onion powder	15 mL
1 tbsp	dried oregano	15 mL
1 tbsp	dried thyme	15 mL
1 tbsp	freshly ground black pepper	15 mL
1 tbsp	cayenne pepper	15 mL
2 tsp	ground coriander	10 mL

1. In an airtight container, combine paprika, salt, garlic powder, onion powder, oregano, thyme, black pepper, cayenne pepper and coriander.

Caribbean seasoning

This general and aromatic combination of spices often found in Caribbean cuisine adds a distinctive gusto to most any dish.

✖ Tip

Use immediately or store in a cool, dark place away from heat sources for up to 4 months.

2 tbsp	dried onion flakes	30 mL
2 tsp	dried thyme	10 mL
2 tsp	ground allspice	10 mL
2 tsp	freshly ground black pepper	10 mL
1 tsp	granulated dried garlic (see Tips, page 308)	5 mL
½ tsp	ground cinnamon	2 mL
¼ tsp	hot pepper flakes	1 mL
¼ tsp	dry mustard powder	1 mL

1. In an airtight container, combine onion flakes, thyme, allspice, black pepper, garlic, cinnamon, hot pepper flakes and dry mustard powder.

✖ Variation

Create a tangy paste by adding olive, canola or grapeseed oil to desired consistency to rub on tofu, potatoes or vegetables before baking or grilling. Start with 1 tbsp (15 mL) oil to ¼ cup (60 mL) seasoning, adding more oil to achieve desired consistency.

Curry powder

A good all-around curry powder is a must to have in any pantry and just the thing to give a dish a good kick. Add to cold grain or pasta salads. Mix with nut smears or cream cheese to create dips, sprinkle on roasting vegetables or throw into a stir-fry.

✕ Tip

Use immediately or store in a cool, dark place away from heat sources for up to 4 months.

2 tbsp	ground cumin	30 mL
2 tbsp	ground coriander	30 mL
2 tbsp	ground turmeric	30 mL
1 tbsp	ground cardamom	15 mL
1 tbsp	ground fenugreek seeds	15 mL
1 tsp	freshly ground black pepper	5 mL
1 tsp	dry mustard powder	5 mL
1 tsp	cayenne pepper	5 mL

1. In an airtight container, combine cumin, coriander, turmeric, cardamom, fenugreek, black pepper, mustard powder and cayenne pepper.

> ## ✕ Variation
> Add 1 tsp (5 mL) each ground clove, ground cinnamon, ground nutmeg and ground ginger.

Easy chinese six-spice powder

Even better than the classic Chinese five-spice, this blend adds zip to any dish.

✕ Tip

Use immediately or store in a cool, dark place away from heat sources for up to 4 months.

2 tbsp	ground anise	30 mL
1 tbsp	ground fennel	15 mL
2 1/2 tsp	ground cinnamon	12 mL
2 tsp	freshly ground black pepper	10 mL
1/2 tsp	ground cloves	2 mL
1/2 tsp	ground ginger	2 mL

1. In an airtight container, combine anise, fennel, cinnamon, black pepper, cloves and ginger.

Fines herbes

Makes 1/4 cup (60 mL)

This delightful and somewhat delicate blend is best added toward the end of cooking. Try this sprinkled into scrambled tofu, over steamed vegetables or in soups.

Tips

Use immediately or store in a cool, dark place away from heat sources for up to 3 months.

Try this same combination with fresh herbs.

1 tbsp	dried tarragon	15 mL
1 tbsp	dried parsley	15 mL
1 tbsp	dried chives	15 mL
1 tbsp	dried chervil	15 mL
1 tbsp	dried marjoram	15 mL

1. In an airtight container, combine tarragon, parsley, chives, chervil and marjoram.

Herbes de provence

Makes about 1/2 cup (125 mL)

Lovely and aromatic herbs are delicious used in soups, sauces and vegetable dishes.

Tip

Use immediately or store in a cool, dark place away from heat sources for up to 4 months.

2 tbsp	dried marjoram	30 mL
2 tbsp	dried thyme	30 mL
2 tbsp	dried savory	30 mL
1 tbsp	dried lavender	15 mL
1 tsp	dried basil	5 mL
1 tsp	dried rosemary	5 mL
1 tsp	dried tarragon	5 mL

1. In an airtight container, combine marjoram, thyme, savory, lavender, basil, rosemary and tarragon.

Mediterranean seasoning

Flavors that are often found in Greek, Italian and Turkish recipes come together in a handy blend. Add lemon zest for a fresh change.

✜ Tip

Use immediately or store in a cool, dark place away from heat sources for up to 4 months.

1 tbsp	dried oregano	15 mL
2 tsp	dried parsley	10 mL
2 tsp	dried marjoram	10 mL
2 tsp	dried mint	10 mL
2 tsp	dried thyme	10 mL
1 tsp	dried onion flakes	5 mL
1 tsp	dried minced garlic	5 mL

1. In an airtight container, combine oregano, parsley, marjoram, mint, thyme, onion flakes and garlic.

✜ Variations

Add 1 tsp (5 mL) dried dill or add ½ tsp (2 mL) each ground cinnamon and nutmeg.

Nori sesame salt

Add this Asian-inspired salt to a marinade, dressing, broth or stir-fry to delight your taste buds.

✜ Tip

To toast nori sheets: Cut each sheet in half, then in half again. Using metal tongs, toast nori about 4 inches (10 cm) over medium-high heat until darkened and crisp, 3 to 5 seconds per side. Change the placement of the tongs so all of the nori sheet is toasted.

✜ Mini food processor or spice grinder

2	sushi nori sheets, toasted (see Tip, left)	2
¼ cup	sesame seeds	60 mL
1 cup	sea salt	250 mL

1. Crumble cooled nori sheets and transfer to a mini food processor.

2. Place a skillet over medium–high heat. Add sesame seeds and toast until fragrant while keeping the pan moving, 2 to 3 minutes. Let cool and transfer to mini food processor.

3. Add salt to mini food processor and pulse until nori is chopped to the size of sesame seeds and evenly incorporated. Use immediately or store in an airtight container for up to 3 months.

Sage seasoning blend

This is the seasoning that is generally associated with Thanksgiving and used in most all savory dishes served on that day. It is a delightful yet savory blend that works well in a dish requiring a lighter touch. New name, same traditional seasoning.

✖ Tips

Use immediately or transfer to an airtight container and store in a cool, dry dark place for up to 3 months.

Spices hold up well but do lose fragrance as they lose potency. Shake the jar and if fragrance is waning, use more spice than is called for, tasting as you go.

✖ Spice or coffee grinder

¼ cup	dried sage	60 mL
3 tbsp	dried marjoram leaves	45 mL
4 tsp	dried thyme leaves	20 mL
1½ tsp	celery seeds	7 mL
⅛ tsp	salt	0.5 mL

1. In a spice grinder, combine sage, marjoram, thyme, celery seeds and salt and pulse into a ground powder, 10 to 15 times.

Cocktails, Drinks and Smoothies

❌—❌—❌—❌—❌—❌—❌—❌—❌—❌—❌—❌—❌

Coco framboise

Definitely double trouble, this is a rich milkshake with a serious kick.

✖ Tip
For a festive flair, serve in a milkshake glass with a straw.

✖ Blender
✖ 2 tall glasses

1 cup	frozen raspberries	250 mL
2 cups	nondairy frozen chocolate dessert	500 mL
1/2 cup	crushed ice cubes (see page 317)	125 mL
1/4 cup	sparkling water	60 mL
4 oz	Crème de Framboise, divided	125 mL

1. In blender, combine raspberries, frozen dessert, ice and water and blend until smooth. Add 3 oz (90 mL) of the Crème de Framboise and pulse 3 to 4 times to blend. Divide between glasses. Drizzle each with 1/2 oz (15 mL) of Crème de Framboise and serve immediately.

> ## ✖ Variation
> Use raspberry or vanilla bean frozen dessert.

Sweet ride mudslide

Just like your favorite milkshake, this creamy cocktail is so scrumptious you will have to remind yourself not to drink it too fast. It's not the brain freeze that will get you!

✖ Blender
✖ 2 tall glasses, chilled

2 cups	crushed ice cubes (see page 317)	500 mL
2 oz	coffee liqueur, such as Kahlúa, divided (approx.)	60 mL
2 oz	McGillicuddy's Irish Cream (page 317)	60 mL
2 oz	vodka	60 mL
2 cups	Almond Milk (page 19) or store-bought	500 mL
2 tbsp	vegan whipped cream	30 mL

1. In blender, combine ice, Kahlúa, Irish Cream, vodka and almond milk and blend until smooth. Pour into prepared glasses. Spoon 1 tbsp (15 mL) whipped cream over top and top each with a drizzle of Kahlúa.

> ## ✖ Variation
> Replace Irish Cream with 2 tbsp (30 mL) Divine Chocolate Sauce (page 22) or store-bought vegan alternative, 1 tsp (5 mL) instant coffee granules and 2 oz (60 mL) vodka.

McGillicuddy's irish cream

Makes about 2¼ cups (550 mL)

This decadent vegan Irish Cream will put a twinkle in your eye and a bounce in your jig. As luscious as the original, it is an absolute must for the holidays. Double the batch to ensure you have enough on hand for when friends, or Santa, stops by for a visit.

✖ Tips

Refrigerate in an airtight glass container for up to 1 month. Shake well just before using.

If a blender is unavailable, place all ingredients in a quart jar and shake vigorously.

✖ Blender (see Tips, left)

¾ cup	Irish whiskey	175 mL
1 cup	Sweetened Condensed Milk (page 17) or store-bought vegan alternative	250 mL
½ cup	Heavy Cream (page 26) or store-bought vegan alternative	125 mL
1 tsp	espresso powder	5 mL
1 tbsp	Divine Chocolate Sauce (page 22) or store-bought vegan alternative	15 mL
1 tsp	vanilla extract	5 mL

1. In blender, combine whiskey, sweetened condensed milk, heavy cream, espresso powder, chocolate sauce and vanilla and blend until well combined, 30 to 45 seconds. Serve over ice or straight.

✖ Ice Cubes

Use filtered water in ice cube trays for clean-tasting cubes.

Always use large ice cubes because smaller cubes melt and dilute.

For crushed ice cubes, wrap ice in a clean kitchen towel, set on a solid work surface and pound with a rolling pin or side of a flattening mallet.

To make blending easier on your machine, place large ice cubes in a plastic resealable bag and crush with the bottom of a heavy pot before adding to blender.

Sake martini with fresh pomegranate and ginger

Serves 2

Crisp and fresh, this jewel of a cocktail goes down smooth. The pomegranate is balanced perfectly with the very dry sake with just a hint of ginger — yum.

✖ Tip

Thin-skinned gingerroot, such as Hawaiian ginger, is best to produce a good quality of juice and works well in the recipe.

✖ Fine-mesh tea-strainer
✖ Cocktail shaker with strainer
✖ 2 large martini glasses, well chilled

3 tbsp	grated gingerroot (see Tip, left)	45 mL
1 cup	cracked ice	250 mL
1 cup	dry sake, chilled	250 mL
1 cup	pomegranate juice, chilled	250 mL
2 tbsp	pure maple syrup	30 mL
2	pieces slit crystallized gingerroot, optional	2

1. Place grated ginger in tea-strainer set over a small bowl and press firmly with back of a spoon to release juice.

2. In cocktail shaker, combine ice, sake, pomegranate juice, maple syrup and ginger juice and shake vigorously to combine and chill.

3. Pour cocktail through strainer into prepared glasses and garnish rim with a piece of crystallized ginger, if using.

Amaretto joe

Serves 2

A true oxymoron, this creamy coffee drink, shaken and served over ice, is a relaxing pick-me-up.

✖ Cocktail shaker or 1-quart (1 L) jar with tight-fitting lid
✖ 2 tall clear glass mugs

1½ cups	brewed dark coffee, chilled	375 mL
2 oz	coffee liqueur, such as Kahlúa	60 mL
4 oz	Amaretto	125 mL
1 cup	vanilla almond milk	250 mL
10 to 12	ice cubes	10 to 12

1. In cocktail shaker, combine coffee, Kahlúa, Amaretto and almond milk and shake until blended. Place 5 to 6 ice cubes in each mug and divide shaken drink between them and serve.

George of the jungle

Serves 2

The party will be swinging in paradise when you serve your guests this luscious tropical cocktail.

✖ Blender
✖ 2 tall glasses, chilled

1 cup	crushed ice cubes (see page 317)	250 mL
1	banana	1
1/2 cup	coarsely chopped pineapple chunks	125 mL
1/2 cup	coarsely chopped mango	125 mL
6 oz	rum	175 mL
1 cup	coconut milk	250 mL
2	pineapple slices, optional	2

1. In blender, combine ice cubes, banana, pineapple, mango, rum and coconut milk and blend until smooth. Pour into prepared glasses and garnish with pineapple slices, if using.

> ✖ **Variation**
> Fresh fruit is always the first choice, but if it's unavailable, you can substitute frozen or canned.

Chocolate java rum frappé

Serves 2

Beware, these babies go down easy. Leave out the rum for a cool summer morning jolt. Or not.

✖ Blender
✖ 2 tall glass, chilled

1 1/4 cups	brewed strong black coffee, chilled	300 mL
1 cup	vanilla almond milk	250 mL
1/4 cup	Caramel Sauce (page 23) or store-bought vegan alternative	60 mL
1/4 cup	Divine Chocolate Sauce (page 22) or store-bought vegan alternative	60 mL
4 oz	dark rum	125 mL
2 cups	crushed ice cubes (see page 317)	500 mL
2 tbsp	vegan whipped cream	30 mL

1. In blender, combine coffee, almond milk, caramel sauce, chocolate sauce, rum and ice cubes and blend until a smooth slush. Pour into prepared glasses and top each with a dollop of whipped cream.

Apple dumpling

When Jack Frost comes nipping at your door, nip back with an Apple Dumpling.

✖ Tip

Substitute ground nutmeg for freshly grated.

✖ Blender
✖ 2 tall clear glass mugs, chilled

2 cups	nondairy vanilla bean frozen dessert	500 mL
1 cup	crushed ice cubes (see page 317)	250 mL
2 tbsp	pure maple syrup	30 mL
1 tsp	vanilla extract	5 mL
1/2 tsp	ground cinnamon	2 mL
1/4 tsp	freshly grated nutmeg	1 mL
4 oz	Calvados	125 mL
2 tbsp	vegan whipped cream	30 mL
2 pinches	freshly grated nutmeg	2 pinches

1. In blender, combine frozen dessert, ice cubes, maple syrup, vanilla, cinnamon, nutmeg and brandy and blend until smooth. Pour into prepared glasses and garnish with whipped cream and a pinch of nutmeg.

Golden autumn holiday

Cinnamon schnapps dancing with flecks of gold mimic falling amber leaves. Relax and shake up this tasty treat after a long day of raking.

✖ Tip

As alcohol does not freeze, store vodka in the freezer to ensure chilled vodka at a moment's notice.

✖ Cocktail shaker or 1-quart (1 L) jar with tight-fitting lid
✖ 2 martini glasses, chilled

2 tbsp	maple or Demerara sugar	30 mL
6 1/2 tsp	pure maple syrup, divided	32 mL
2 oz	vodka	60 mL
2 oz	Goldschlager Cinnamon Schnapps	60 mL
1 cup	ice cubes	250 mL
1/4 cup	sparkling water	60 mL

1. Pour sugar into a shallow saucer. Moisten rim of each chilled glass with about 1/4 tsp (1 mL) of the maple syrup and dip glass rims into sugar. Set aside.

2. In cocktail shaker, combine vodka, schnapps and remaining 6 tsp (30 mL) of maple syrup and shake a few times to blend. Add ice cubes and shake to chill mixture.

3. Pour shaken martini into prepared glasses, add a splash of sparkling water and serve immediately.

Cozy celtic

Serves 1

Curl up with a good book and a mug of this delightful drink for a truly relaxing evening.

✖ Tip
To pre-warm mug, fill with water and microwave for 1 minute. Discard water.

✖ Warmed mug (see Tip, left)

1 cup	plain hemp milk	250 mL
2 oz	Irish whiskey	60 mL
2 tsp	agave nectar	10 mL

1. In a small saucepan, heat milk over medium heat. Pour whiskey into prepared mug, add heated milk and stir in agave.

> ## ✖ Variation
> Substitute brown rice syrup or maple syrup for agave.

Holiday nut nog

Serves 4 to 8

This very traditional Yule punch starts showing up with the chill of winter and sets a festive tone through the holiday season. This makes a great party drink as well as a nice treat when you put your feet up after a long days work.

✖ Tip
Nog will keep refrigerated in an airtight container for up to 1 week.

✖ Blender

2 cups	unsweetened vanilla coconut milk	500 mL
2	packages (each 12.3 oz/350 g) firm or extra-firm silken tofu	2
1 cup	brandy	250 mL
1 cup	confectioner's (icing) sugar	250 mL
2 tsp	vanilla extract	10 mL
$\frac{1}{2}$ tsp	ground ginger	2 mL
$\frac{1}{4}$ tsp	freshly grated nutmeg, divided	1 mL

1. In blender, combine milk, tofu, brandy, confectioner's sugar, vanilla, ginger and $\frac{1}{8}$ tsp (0.5 mL) of the nutmeg and blend until smooth. Taste and adjust flavorings, adding additional brandy, sugar, nutmeg or ginger, if desired. Refrigerate until well chilled, for at least 2 hours. Serve chilled with a sprinkle of remaining nutmeg.

Piña colada

Who doesn't like Piña Coladas and takin' walks in the rain — well maybe walks on the beach.

✖ Tips

A Collins glass is a tall narrow glass typically holding about 14 oz (435 mL).

Coconut cream is very similar to coconut milk in taste but is very thick with a butter-like consistency. It is delicious with a mild taste and many times is used as a substitute for heavy cream in cooking.

✖ Blender
✖ 2 Collins glasses, chilled (see Tips, left)

2 cups	crushed ice cubes (see page 317)	500 mL
4 oz	light rum	125 mL
2 oz	dark rum	60 mL
1 cup	pineapple juice	250 mL
1/3 cup	coconut cream (see Tips, left)	75 mL
2 tbsp	freshly squeezed lime juice	30 mL
2	pineapple spears, optional	2

1. In blender, combine ice, light and dark rums, pineapple juice, coconut cream and lime juice and blend until smooth. Pour into prepared glasses and garnish with pineapple spears, if using.

✖ Variation
If coconut cream is not available, refrigerate a can of full fat coconut milk and scoop the cream off the top.

Oolong toddy

Enjoy a relaxing Scottish bedtime toddy — traditionally served to chase away the cold.

✖ Warmed glass mug

1 oz	whiskey	30 mL
1 tbsp	agave nectar	15 mL
1 tbsp	freshly squeezed lemon juice	15 mL
2	whole cloves	2
1 cup	prepared hot oolong tea	250 mL
1	piece (4 inch/10 cm) cinnamon stick	1

1. In warmed glass mug, combine whiskey, agave, lemon juice and cloves. Pour in hot tea and stir with cinnamon stick. Brew for 2 minutes. Enjoy while hot.

✖ Variation
Omit whiskey and substitute chamomile tea for oolong.

Blazing mary

After a blazing night on the town, this cocktail is a favorite at any proper brunch gathering. Fresh horseradish and celery seeds add zest and a savory flavor to this famous adult beverage.

✖ Cocktail shaker or 1-quart (1 L) jar with tight-fitting lid
✖ 2 Collins glasses (see Tips, page 322)

1½ cups	tomato juice	375 mL
4 oz	vodka	125 mL
2 tsp	freshly squeezed lemon juice	10 mL
1 tsp	prepared horseradish	5 mL
1 tsp	vegan Worcestershire sauce	5 mL
½ tsp	celery seeds	2 mL
½ tsp	freshly ground black pepper	2 mL
2 dashes	hot pepper sauce	2 dashes
½ tsp	salt	2 mL
3 cups	ice cubes (15 to 18 cubes)	750 mL
2	inside stalks celery with leaves	2

1. In cocktail shaker, combine tomato juice, vodka, lemon juice, horseradish, Worcestershire sauce, celery seeds, black pepper, hot pepper sauce and salt and shake until blended. Add 1 cup (250 mL) ice cubes and shake to chill mixture. Place 5 to 6 ice cubes in each glass. Pour drink over ice cubes, add celery stalk and serve.

> ✖ **Variation**
> If vegan Worcestershire sauce is unavailable, either omit or substitute liquid aminos or soy sauce.

Swiss alp

St. Germain liqueur is crafted from handpicked elderflowers found only in the foothills of the Swiss Alps a few weeks each year. The tiny annual harvest is handcrafted into an enchanting liqueur.

✖ 2 old-fashioned glasses, chilled

10 to 12	ice cubes	10 to 12
3 oz	vanilla vodka	90 mL
2 oz	St. Germain Elderflower liqueur	60 mL
6 tbsp	vanilla almond milk	90 mL

1. Place 5 to 6 ice cubes in each glass. Pour vodka over ice and top with St. Germain. Add almond milk and stir well to combine. Serve immediately.

The famous and fabulous st. germain cocktail

Serves 2

The signature drink using elderflower liqueur from the Swiss Alps is just too darn good to leave out of any beverage chapter.

⚒ 2 Collins glasses, chilled

8 to 10	ice cubes	8 to 10
4 oz	Brut Champagne	125 mL
3 oz	St. Germain Elderflower liqueur	90 mL
½ cup	sparkling water	125 mL
2	lemon twists	2

1. Place 4 to 5 ice cubes in each glass. Pour champagne into glasses over ice. Pour in St. Germain liqueur and add sparkling water. Stir to blend. Squeeze lemon peel over cocktail and drop twist into glass.

> ### ⚒ Variation
> Substitute your favorite fruit juice for St. Germain liqueur.

Frangelico chocolate almond brownie

Serves 2

This very chocolaty treat will satisfy even the most discerning sweet tooth. Is it dessert or is it a cocktail? Perhaps both.

⚒ 2 old fashioned glasses, chilled

10 to 12	ice cubes	10 to 12
1¼ cups	chocolate almond milk	300 mL
2 tbsp	Divine Chocolate Sauce (page 22) or store-bought vegan alternative	30 mL
4 oz	Frangelico liqueur	125 mL

1. Place 5 to 6 ice cubes in each glass. In a small pitcher, combine almond milk and chocolate sauce, stirring well to blend. Pour mixture over ice and top with Frangelico. Serve immediately.

> ### ⚒ Variation
> In a blender, combine ice, almond milk, chocolate sauce and Frangelico and blend until slushy smooth. Divide between 2 glasses and top with vegan whipped cream and chocolate shavings. Serve immediately.

Smith and kerns

Serves 2

Rumor has it this cocktail was created in North Dakota during an oil boom in the 1950s. Named after a couple of oilmen, Smith and Curran, the name was blurred with time, or was that slurred, but the drink remains a favorite.

- **2 old fashioned glasses, chilled**

10 to 12	ice cubes	10 to 12
4 oz	coffee liqueur, such as Kahlúa	125 mL
1/2 cup	plain hemp milk	125 mL
	Sparkling water	

1. Place 5 to 6 ice cubes in each glass. Pour Kahlúa and milk over ice cubes and fill glass with sparkling water. Serve immediately.

Variation

Add vodka and vegan-friendly cola to create a Smith and Wesson.

Blended top-shelf margarita

Serves 4

No alterations needed here to make this classic worldwide favorite. Use premium liquor for a true top-shelf cocktail.

- **Blender**
- **4 margarita glasses**

1/2 cup	coarse salt	125 mL
4	lime wedges	4
1 1/2 cups	best-quality tequila	375 mL
4 oz	triple sec	125 mL
2 oz	Cointreau	60 mL
1 cup	freshly squeezed lime juice	250 mL
4 cups	crushed ice cubes (see page 317)	1 L

1. Pour salt into a shallow saucer, moisten rim of each margarita glass with a lime wedge and dip rim into salt.
2. In blender, combine tequila, triple sec, Cointreau, lime juice and ice and blend until smooth. Pour into prepared glasses and serve immediately.

Mexican velvet elvis

Serves 4

Smooth as velvet but packing a punch just like the King himself. With this smoky, sultry cocktail you'll be singing "Love Me Tender" all the way back to the blender.

✂ Blender
✂ 4 margarita glasses, chilled

2 tbsp	salt	30 mL
1¼ tsp	ground New Mexico red chile powder, divided	6 mL
1 tsp	granulated sugar	5 mL
6 oz	good-quality gold tequila	175 mL
2 cups	chocolate soy milk	500 mL
1	package (12.3 oz/350 g) firm or extra-firm silken tofu	1
2 tbsp	Divine Chocolate Sauce (page 22) or store-bought vegan alternative	30 mL
2 tsp	vanilla extract	10 mL
1 tsp	ground cinnamon	5 mL
2 cups	crushed ice cubes (see page 317)	500 mL

1. In a shallow dish, combine salt, 1 tsp (5 mL) of the chile powder and sugar. Moisten rim of glasses with a little tequila and dip rims into chile salt.

2. In blender, combine soy milk, tofu, tequila, chocolate sauce, vanilla, cinnamon, ¼ tsp (1 mL) of chile powder and ice and blend until smooth. Pour blended mixture into prepared glasses and serve immediately.

Coconut russian

Serves 2

If a bartender from Moscow opened a little place in Bali, he would surely serve this popular cocktail, island-style.

✂ Cocktail shaker
✂ 2 old fashioned glasses, chilled

1½ to 2 cups	crushed ice cubes (see page 317)	375 to 500 mL
4 oz	vodka	125 mL
4 oz	coffee liqueur, such as Kahlúa	125 mL
¼ cup	coconut milk	60 mL
10 to 12	ice cubes	10 to 12

1. Fill cocktail shaker about two-thirds full with crushed ice. Add vodka, Kahlúa and coconut milk and shake until blended, 20 or 30 seconds. Place 5 to 6 ice cubes in each glass, strain cocktail into prepared glasses and serve.

Tropical breeze

Serves 2

Using frozen mango and banana make it possible to whip up a blender full of this tropical delight whenever the mood hits. Not to mention it is a great way to use up bananas that are thinking about going south.

✖ Tip

A hurricane glass is a footed 10- to 12-oz (300 to 375 mL) glass that is shaped like a vintage hurricane lamp. It is typically used for frozen, blended and tropical cocktails.

✖ Blender
✖ 2 hurricane glasses (see Tip, left)

1 cup	cracked ice	250 mL
1 cup	frozen mango pieces	250 mL
1	frozen banana, chopped	1
1 cup	guava nectar	250 mL
1/2 cup	coconut rum	125 mL
1/4 cup	orange juice	60 mL
2	orange slices, optional	2

1. In blender, combine ice, mango, banana, guava nectar, rum and orange juice and blend until very smooth. Pour into prepared glasses and garnish with orange slices, if using.

> ## ✖ Variation
> Use golden rum and substitute coconut milk for orange juice.

Green hornet

Serves 2

Loaded with vitamins and minerals, this smoothie will transform you into a superhero, or at least help you to feel like one.

✖ Blender

3 cups	packed kale leaves	750 mL
1 cup	chopped kiwi	250 mL
1 1/2 cups	apple juice	750 mL
1 tbsp	flax seed oil	15 mL
1 tbsp	wheat grass powder	15 mL

1. In blender, combine kale, kiwi, apple juice, oil and wheat grass powder and blend until smooth. Divide between 2 glasses and serve.

> ## ✖ Variations
> Try Swiss chard or spinach instead of kale.
>
> If you want a sweeter drink add 1 to 2 tbsp (15 to 30 mL) brown rice syrup.

Watermelon limeade

Always a hit, this summer thirst quencher is surprisingly easy to make. A great way to use up those last few pieces of that giant watermelon you bought for the family picnic.

✖ Tip

Because the watermelon seeds fall to the bottom of the blender, it is not necessary to use seedless watermelon, which often has less flavor.

✖ Blender

5 cups	chunked watermelon pieces	1.25 L
3 tbsp	agave nectar	45 mL
2 tbsp	freshly squeezed lime juice	30 mL

1. In blender, purée watermelon into a liquid. Strain watermelon through a wire mesh strainer into a measuring cup then pour into a pitcher. Stir in agave and lime juice, mixing well to blend. Taste and add more agave or lime juice, if desired.

✖ Variation

Watermelon Limeade Sparkler: Pour 1/4 to 1/2 cup (60 to 125 mL) Watermelon Limeade into a glass filled with ice. Fill with sparkling water and serve immediately.

Fresh ginger lemonade

This tangy crowd pleaser is great on its own or as a base for a refreshing cocktail.

4 cups	water	1 L
1/3 cup	shredded gingerroot	75 mL
1 cup	freshly squeezed lemon juice (6 to 8 lemons)	250 mL
1/4 to 1/2 cup	agave nectar	60 to 125 mL
4	sprigs mint	4

1. In a saucepan over medium heat, bring water to a boil. Reduce heat, add ginger and gently simmer for 5 minutes. Cover pan, remove from heat and let steep for 2 hours.

2. Strain gingered water and lemon juice through a wire mesh strainer into a glass pitcher. Stir in agave, starting with 1/4 cup (60 mL), mixing well to combine. Taste and adjust flavors, adding lemon juice and/or agave to taste. Cover pitcher and refrigerate for at least 1 hour to chill before serving. Serve over ice with a garnish of mint.

> ## ✖ Variations
> Add a splash of pomegranate or pineapple juice or a shot of vodka or tequila.

Sweet tart smoothie

Jump-start the day with a unique blending of sweet cherries, tart lime and a smooth banana.

✖ Tip
When bananas start to become over-ripe, place in the freezer for use in your morning smoothie.

✖ Blender

1 1/2 cups	pitted frozen cherries	375 mL
1	frozen banana, cut into 6 pieces	1
2 cups	vanilla soy yogurt	500 mL
3 tbsp	agave nectar	45 mL
2 tbsp	freshly squeezed lime juice	30 mL

1. In blender, combine cherries, banana, yogurt, agave and lime juice and blend until smooth. Divide between 2 glasses and serve.

Berry berry ginger smoothie

Sweet berries and tangy ginger with the added boost of protein powder start the morning right. Because all berries are delicious in this smoothie, use the freshest seasonal berries available.

✖ Tip

Plant protein powder, a fantastic protein supplemental option for anyone with a soy allergy, contains protein strictly from plant sources. Use it as you would use a soy protein powder in smoothies or blended with liquid such as almond milk.

✖ Blender

½ cup	fresh blueberries	125 mL
½ cup	fresh blackberries	125 mL
½ cup	frozen strawberries	125 mL
1	scoop plant protein powder (see Tip, left)	1
1 cup	cranberry juice	250 mL
1 tsp	grated gingerroot	5 mL
1 cup	crushed ice cubes (see page 317)	250 mL

1. In blender, combine blueberries, blackberries, strawberries, protein powder, cranberry juice, ginger and ice cubes and blend until smooth. Divide between 2 glasses and serve immediately.

✖ Variation

For added flavor include 1 banana.

Vermont maple morning smoothie

Serves 2

No time for a proper sit-down breakfast? Start the day in style with this guiltless gourmet treat.

✖ Tip

If smoothie is too thick, add additional almond milk.

✖ Blender

2 cups	vanilla soy yogurt	500 mL
1/2 cup	vanilla almond milk	125 mL
1	apple, cored, peeled and chopped	1
1 cup	maple almond granola	250 mL
1/4 cup	maple syrup	60 mL
1/2 tsp	vanilla extract	2 mL
1/2 tsp	ground cinnamon	2 mL

1. In blender, combine yogurt, milk, apple, granola, maple syrup, vanilla and cinnamon and blend until smooth. Divide between 2 glasses and serve.

Pomegranate ice smoothie

Serves 2

A beautiful jewel-toned drink packed with antioxidants is a great afternoon refresher.

✖ Blender

1 cup	fresh strawberries	250 mL
1 cup	frozen mixed berries	250 mL
1/2 cup	pomegranate juice	125 mL
1/2 cup	orange juice	125 mL
2 cups	crushed ice cubes (see page 317)	500 mL

1. In blender, combine strawberries, mixed berries, pomegranate juice, orange juice and ice and blend until smooth. Divide between 2 glasses and serve.

Desert sunrise

Bounty from the desert blends to create a healthy smoothie that tastes as good as it looks.

Blender

1	large fresh peach, peeled and quartered (about 1¼ cups/300 mL)	1
3	large pitted dates, coarsely chopped (about ¼ cup/60 mL)	3
½ cup	aloe vera juice	125 mL
1 cup	crushed ice cubes (see page 317)	250 mL
1 cup	sparkling water	250 mL
½ cup	pomegranate juice	125 mL

1. In blender, combine peach, dates, aloe vera, ice and sparkling water and blend until smooth. Divide between 2 glasses, top each with ¼ cup (60 mL) pomegranate juice and serve.

✖ Variation

If fresh peaches are unavailable, use frozen, decreasing ice to ½ cup (125 mL) and increasing sparkling water to 1¼ cups (300 mL).

Sweets

Jade green tea pound cake

This beautifully light green, delicate cake sets the perfect tone for a special spring occasion such as Mother's Day or a birthday tea party.

✖ Tip

Stir together egg replacer just before using as it loses its leavening power over time.

✖ Preheat oven to 350°F (180°C)
✖ Stand mixer with wire whisk attachment
✖ 10-inch (25 cm) Bundt pan, oiled and floured

Cake

4	green tea bags	4
1½ cups	boiling water	375 mL
3 cups	all-purpose flour	750 mL
⅓ cup	cornstarch	75 mL
1 tbsp	baking powder	15 mL
1 tsp	salt	5 mL
2 cups	granulated sugar	500 mL
¾ cup	coconut oil	175 mL
1 tsp	vanilla extract	5 mL
½ tsp	almond extract	2 mL
1 tbsp	powdered egg replacer (see Tip, left)	15 mL
¼ cup	warm water	60 mL

Glaze, optional

1 cup	confectioner's (icing) sugar	250 mL
4 to 5 tsp	freshly squeezed lemon juice	20 to 25 mL
	Edible flowers, such as daisies, pansies or small chrysanthemums, for garnish, optional	

1. *Cake:* In a measuring cup or heatproof bowl, steep tea bags in boiling water for 5 minutes. Discard tea bags squeezing gently and let tea cool in refrigerator for 20 minutes.

2. In a bowl, whisk together flour, cornstarch, baking powder and salt. Set aside. In bowl of stand mixer, stir together cooled tea, sugar, oil, vanilla and almond extracts. Set aside.

3. In a small bowl, thoroughly combine egg replacer and warm water. Add egg replacer mixture to wet ingredients in mixer bowl. Attach bowl to mixer and fit with wire whip attachment. Beat on low speed until blended. On low speed, gradually beat in dry ingredients until incorporated, scraping down sides of bowl as needed. Beat on medium speed for 2 minutes. Scrape batter into prepared pan, smoothing top.

4. Bake in preheated oven until tester inserted in the center comes out clean, 50 to 55 minutes. Let cool in pan on a wire rack for 15 minutes, then turn cake out onto rack and let cool completely.

5. *Glaze, if using:* In a small bowl, combine confectioner's sugar and enough lemon juice to make a thick yet spoonable consistency. Drizzle glaze over cake. Decorate with edible flowers, if desired.

⚏ Variation

Substitute white or Earl Grey tea in place of green tea.

Margarita icebox cake

Don't be hesitant to tackle this multi-step icebox cake. The steps can be done over the course of a few days and the cool tequila lime taste is really a showstopper for any summer gathering. Great on a scorching day.

✖ Tip
Either the cake or sorbet may be made and served independently of each other.

✖ Preheat oven to 350°F (180°C)
✖ 9- by 5-inch (23 by 12.5 cm) loaf pan, oiled and floured
✖ Ice cream maker

Cake

1½ cups	all-purpose flour	375 mL
1 cup	granulated sugar	250 mL
½ tsp	baking soda	2 mL
½ tsp	salt	2 mL
	Grated zest of 3 limes	
½ cup	freshly squeezed lime juice	125 mL
½ cup	water	125 mL
⅓ cup	vegetable oil	75 mL
½ tsp	vanilla extract	2 mL

Sorbet

¾ cup	granulated sugar	175 mL
1½ cups	water	375 mL
	Grated zest of 2 limes	
½ cup	freshly squeezed lime juice	125 mL
1 tbsp	tequila, preferably silver	15 mL
1 tbsp	orange-flavored liqueur	15 mL

Syrup

¾ cup	granulated sugar	175 mL
½ cup	freshly squeezed lime juice	125 mL
¼ cup	water	60 mL
2 tbsp	tequila, preferably silver	30 mL
1 tbsp	orange-flavored liqueur	15 mL
	Silken Crème Fraîche (page 16) or store-bought vegan alternative, optional	

1. *Cake:* In a bowl, stir together flour, sugar, baking soda and salt. Set aside. In a large bowl, whisk together lime zest, lime juice, water, oil and vanilla. Gradually whisk in dry ingredients, just until smooth. Scrape into prepared pan.

2. Bake in preheated oven until tester inserted in the center comes out clean, 35 to 40 minutes. Let cool in pan on a wire rack for 10 minutes, then turn out of pan onto rack and let cool completely. At this stage, cake can be frozen, well wrapped, for up to 1 week.

3. *Sorbet:* In a small saucepan, stir together sugar and water. Bring to a boil over medium heat, stirring until sugar is dissolved. Remove from heat and let cool. Transfer to an airtight container and refrigerate for at least 8 hours. Add lime zest, lime juice, tequila and orange liqueur, stirring to combine. Freeze in ice cream maker according to manufacturer's directions. Transfer to an airtight container and freeze for 1 hour, until firm, or for up to 1 week.

4. *Syrup:* In a small saucepan, stir together sugar, lime juice and water. Bring to a boil over medium-high heat, stirring until sugar is dissolved. Remove from heat and stir in tequila and orange liqueur. Let cool to room temperature. Syrup can be stored in airtight container in the refrigerator for up to 1 month.

5. *To assemble cake:* Using same loaf pan used to bake cake, line with plastic wrap, allowing several inches to hang over edges. Slice cake horizontally into 3 layers. Fit bottom layer into bottom of lined pan. Brush liberally with syrup. Stir sorbet to a spreadable consistency. Spread cake layer with about half of the sorbet. Add middle cake layer, brush with syrup and spread with remaining sorbet. Add top cake layer and brush with syrup. Fold hanging plastic wrap over top of cake and freeze for 2 hours, until firm, or for up to 1 week.

6. Lift cake out of pan using plastic wrap and transfer to a cutting board. Peel off wrap and cut into thick slices and serve with crème fraîche, if using, and drizzle with additional syrup, if desired.

Chocolate cake

Serves 8 to 10

No cookbook worth its salt is complete without the Holy Grail recipe: the best chocolate cake in the world, which just happens to be vegan!

✂ Tip

Serve with Divine Chocolate Sauce (page 22) or store-bought vegan chocolate sauce.

✂ Preheat oven to 350°F (180°C)
✂ 9-inch (23 cm) square metal baking pan, oiled and floured

1 cup + 2 tbsp	all-purpose flour	280 mL
1¼ cups	granulated sugar	300 mL
¼ cup	unsweetened cocoa powder	60 mL
1 tsp	baking soda	5 mL
½ tsp	salt	2 mL
¾ cup	brewed coffee or warm water	175 mL
¼ cup	vegetable oil	60 mL
1 tsp	vanilla extract	5 mL
1 tsp	apple cider vinegar	5 mL

1. In a large bowl, sift together flour, sugar, cocoa, baking soda and salt. Whisk to combine thoroughly.

2. In a 2-cup (500 mL) glass measuring cup or small bowl, whisk together coffee, oil, vanilla and vinegar. Pour into dry ingredients and whisk until smooth. Pour into prepared pan.

3. Bake in preheated oven until tester inserted in the center comes out clean, 25 to 30 minutes. Let cool in pan on a wire rack for 10 minutes. Serve warm or at room temperature.

Cranberry walnut cake with caramel sauce

Serves 8 to 12

This tart and sweet cake is sure to become your go-to dessert when having last-minute guests over. It is quick, easy and quite impressive topped with caramel sauce.

✖ Tips

If using frozen cranberries, there's no need to thaw them. Just pick through fresh or frozen cranberries to remove moldy or wrinkled produce, rinse and use as directed.

If you have a food processor, you can make quick work of mixing the flour, sugar, baking powder and margarine with a few pulses. Be sure to transfer to a bowl before stirring in cranberries, walnuts and milk.

✖ Preheat oven to 350°F (180°C)
✖ 10-inch (25 cm) pie plate, oiled and floured

2 cups	all-purpose flour	500 mL
1$\frac{1}{2}$ cups	granulated sugar	375 mL
2 tsp	baking powder	10 mL
$\frac{1}{4}$ cup	vegan hard margarine	60 mL
2 cups	fresh or frozen cranberries (see Tips, left)	500 mL
$\frac{1}{2}$ cup	walnuts, chopped	125 mL
1 cup	Almond Milk (page 19) or store-bought	250 mL
1 cup	Caramel Sauce (page 23) or vegan store-bought	250 mL

1. In a large bowl, stir together flour, sugar and baking powder. Add margarine and using a pastry blender or two knives, cut in margarine until mixture resembles coarse meal. Add cranberries, walnuts and milk and stir with a fork until flour is moistened. Pour batter into pie plate, spreading evenly.

2. Bake in preheated oven until golden brown and tester inserted in the center comes out clean, about 45 minutes. Let cool completely in plate on a wire rack. Cut into pie-shaped wedges and serve drizzled with caramel sauce.

Upside-down berry cornmeal cake

This golden cake makes the most of fresh berries in season while delivering big benefits: antioxidants, fiber and vitamin C.

✖ Tips

Using frozen berries is fine, just remember to thaw and drain well before using.

Store cake wrapped in plastic at room temperature and serve within 2 days.

✖ Preheat oven to 350°F (180°C)
✖ 8-inch (20 cm) round metal cake pan, oiled and bottom lined with oiled parchment paper

2 tbsp	ground flax seeds	30 mL
5 tbsp	water	75 mL
2 cups	fresh or frozen mixed blackberries, blueberries and raspberries (see Tips, left)	500 mL
1 cup	all-purpose flour	250 mL
1/2 cup	cornmeal	125 mL
1/3 cup	whole wheat flour	75 mL
2 tsp	baking powder	10 mL
1/4 tsp	salt	1 mL
1/2 cup	granulated sugar	125 mL
2/3 cup	Almond Milk (page 19) or Soy Milk (page 18) or store-bought	150 mL
1/3 cup	canola oil	75 mL

1. In small bowl, stir together ground flax and water and let stand for 10 minutes.

2. Place berries in prepared pan and set aside. In a large bowl, stir together all-purpose flour, cornmeal, whole wheat flour, baking powder and salt. Set aside. In another bowl, whisk together sugar, almond milk and oil. Stir in flax mixture. Add wet ingredients to dry ingredients and mix well.

3. Pour batter over berries in prepared pan. Bake in preheated oven until tester inserted in the center comes out clean, 40 to 45 minutes.

4. Let cool in pan on a wire rack for 5 minutes. Loosen sides by running a table knife around edge of pan. Invert a serving plate on top of pan, quickly invert onto plate and remove parchment. Let cool for 15 to 20 minutes before serving warm.

Caramelized bananas with rum sauce

Serves 4

Here's a quick dessert made from staples usually at hand. Something delicious happens when brown sugar, bananas and rum heat up together — absolute magic!

Tip

To toast coconut: Preheat oven to 325°F (160°C). Spread a thick layer of shredded coconut on a baking sheet and bake, stirring often, until golden, 8 to 10 minutes. Coconut burns quickly so don't walk away from the oven.

Long-handled igniter

3	bananas	3
1 tsp	freshly squeezed lime juice	5 mL
3 tbsp	vegan hard margarine	45 mL
6 tbsp	packed brown sugar	90 mL
1/3 cup	spiced, amber or dark rum	75 mL
1/4 tsp	freshly grated nutmeg	1 mL
2 tbsp	toasted sweetened shredded coconut, optional (see Tip, left)	30 mL

1. Peel bananas and slice in half lengthwise, then cut each half crosswise into 4 pieces. Place in a bowl and sprinkle with lime juice. Set aside.
2. Place a large heavy-bottomed skillet over medium heat and let pan get hot. Add margarine and let it melt. Add bananas, cut side down, and cook until browned, 3 to 5 minutes. Sprinkle brown sugar over bananas and, cook, shaking pan frequently until sugar melts. Turn bananas over and cook, until caramelized, about 3 minutes.
3. Remove pan from heat and add rum. Carefully ignite with long-handled igniter. Allow flames to burn off naturally.
4. Plate each serving with 3 banana sections, a few dribbles of sauce, nutmeg, and toasted coconut, if using. Serve immediately.

Variation

Use only 2 bananas and add 2 small, peeled, halved peaches to skillet or substitute fresh pineapple spears for bananas.

Mocha cupcakes with almond icing

Makes about 12

One of the great things about these cupcakes is that most of the ingredients are pantry staples. Yes, I think coffee liqueur is a staple! But even better is the taste. Moist chocolate cake with the coffee liqueur baked right in and gooey almond icing: need I say more?

❖ Tip

Store un-iced cupcakes in refrigerator, covered, for up to 3 days.

❖ Preheat oven to 350°F (180°C)
❖ 12-cup muffin pan, oiled

Cupcakes

1 cup + 2 tbsp	all-purpose flour	280 mL
¾ cup	granulated sugar	175 mL
¼ cup	unsweetened cocoa powder	60 mL
½ tsp	baking soda	2 mL
¼ tsp	salt	1 mL
½ cup	warm brewed coffee	125 mL
¼ cup	coffee liqueur, such as Kahlúa	60 mL
¼ cup	canola oil	60 mL
1 tsp	vanilla extract	5 mL
1 tsp	white vinegar	5 mL

Almond Icing

1½ cups	confectioner's (icing) sugar, sifted	375 mL
3 tbsp	vegan hard margarine, melted	45 mL
1½ tbsp	plain almond or soy milk	22 mL
½ tsp	vanilla extract	2 mL
¼ tsp	almond extract	1 mL
¼ cup	sliced almonds, optional	60 mL

1. *Cupcakes:* In a large bowl, sift together flour, sugar, cocoa, baking soda and salt. Stir to combine and set aside.

2. In small bowl, stir together coffee, liqueur, oil, vanilla and vinegar. Add to dry ingredients and stir briskly until batter is smooth. Divide among prepared muffin cups, filling half full. Any cups not filled with batter, fill half full with water.

3. Bake in preheated oven until tester inserted in the center of cupcake comes out clean, 15 to 20 minutes (cupcakes will be flat on top and moist). Let cool in pan on a wire rack for 10 minutes. Run a small knife around each cupcake to loosen. Invert rack on top of muffin pan and flip over together to invert cupcakes onto rack. Remove pan and let cupcakes cool completely on rack. (Cupcakes will be served upside down.)

4. *Almond Icing:* In small bowl, stir together confectioner's sugar and melted margarine, adding almond milk a little at a time to help blend until smooth. Stir in vanilla and almond extracts. Pour a heaping tablespoon (15 mL) on each cupcake, letting icing run down sides. Sprinkle with a few sliced almonds, if using. Serve immediately.

> ### ❖ Variation
>
> For an even more decadent, all-chocolate experience, omit almond icing. Sprinkle additional liqueur over each cupcake then cover with Divine Chocolate Sauce (page 22).

Chocolate espresso cowgirl cookies

Makes about 2 dozen cookies

Toasting the oatmeal and pecans lends these complex cookies an earthy and slightly smoky taste that is enhanced by the coffee and cinnamon. Lucky cowgirls can just close their eyes and imagine eating these gems by the campfire, without the bother of being out on the range!

✖ Tips

You may replace the instant espresso with ground coffee. Measure 2 tbsp (30 mL) ground coffee into coffee grinder and grind to a very fine powder, 20 to 30 seconds. Add to dry ingredients.

Allow baking sheet to cool between batches to prevent dough from spreading on hot pan. At Step 4, drop dough by rounded tablespoons (15 mL) onto a baking sheet and freeze. Transfer dough balls to a freezer bag and freeze for up to 1 month. Bake cookie dough directly from the freezer.

✖ Preheat oven to 350°F (180°C)
✖ Baking sheet, lined with parchment paper

1½ cups	large-flake (old-fashioned) rolled oats	375 mL
2 tbsp	ground flax seeds	30 mL
¼ cup	water	60 mL
2 cups	all-purpose flour	500 mL
1 tbsp	instant espresso powder (see Tips, left)	15 mL
1 tsp	baking soda	5 mL
½ tsp	ground cinnamon	2 mL
½ tsp	salt	2 mL
1 cup	vegan hard margarine, softened	250 mL
1 cup	packed light brown sugar	250 mL
½ cup	granulated sugar	125 mL
2 tsp	vanilla extract	10 mL
6 oz	semisweet chocolate chunks (1 cup/250 mL)	175 g
1 cup	chopped toasted pecans	250 mL

1. Place a large skillet over medium heat and let pan get hot. Add rolled oats and toast, shaking pan frequently, until fragrant and lightly browned, 5 to 7 minutes. Transfer to a bowl and let cool.

2. In small bowl, stir together ground flax and water and let stand for 10 minutes.

3. In another bowl, stir together flour, espresso powder, baking soda, cinnamon and salt. Set aside.

4. In a large bowl, using an electric mixer, beat together margarine, brown sugar, granulated sugar and vanilla just until smooth, about 1 minute. Using a wooden spoon, stir in flax mixture. Stir in dry ingredients until combined. Add cooled toasted oats, chocolate chunks and pecans. Stir just until combined.

5. Drop dough by rounded tablespoons (15 mL) on prepared baking sheet, at least 2 inches (5 cm) apart. Bake in preheated oven until edges are lightly browned, 10 to 12 minutes (do not over bake). Let cool on pan on a wire rack for 2 minutes, then transfer to rack and let cool completely. Store in an airtight container at room temperature for up to 3 days.

Chocolate macadamia drop cookies

Makes about 3 dozen

The rich crunch of macadamia nuts and a subtle hint of orange combine with chocolate to create a very special scrumptious treat. They make a beautiful gift, if you are able to bring yourself to give them away.

✖ Tip

Store cookies in airtight container at room temperature for up to 1 week or freeze for up to 1 month.

✖ Preheat oven to 350°F (180°C)
✖ Baking sheets, lined with parchment

2½ cups	all-purpose flour	625 mL
⅓ cup	unsweetened cocoa powder, sifted	75 mL
1 tbsp	baking powder	15 mL
1 tsp	grated orange zest	5 mL
½ tsp	salt	2 mL
¾ cup	vegan hard margarine, softened	175 mL
1½ cups	granulated sugar	375 mL
1 tsp	vanilla extract	5 mL
1 tbsp	powdered egg replacer	15 mL
¼ cup	warm water	60 mL
1 cup	chopped macadamia nuts	250 mL

1. In a bowl, stir together flour, cocoa, baking powder, orange zest and salt. Set aside.

2. In a large bowl using a stand or electric mixer, beat margarine and sugar until fluffy, about 1 minute. Beat in vanilla.

3. In a small bowl, stir together egg replacer and warm water. On low speed, alternately beat egg replacer and dry ingredients into margarine mixture, making two additions of egg replacer and three of dry ingredients. Stir in macadamia nuts.

4. Drop dough by rounded tablespoonfuls (15 mL) on prepared baking sheets, at least 2 inches (5 cm) apart. Bake, one sheet at a time, in preheated oven for 7 minutes. Then rotate pan from back to front and bake until edges are just beginning to turn golden and tops look dry, about 5 minutes. Let cool on pan on a wire rack for 5 minutes, then transfer to rack and let cool completely.

Crystallized ginger cookies

Makes about 2 dozen

These big cookies are for the ginger lovers among us. A pretty cookie topped with sparkling raw sugar, they look and taste like the gems they are.

✛ Tips

If a cookie scoop is unavailable, measure dough by the heaping tablespoon (15 mL).

Store in an airtight container at room temperature for up to 1 week.

✛ Preheat oven to 350°F (180°C)
✛ 2 baking sheets, lined with parchment paper
✛ 1½ tbsp (22 mL) cookie scoop (see Tips, left)

1 tbsp	ground flax seeds	15 mL
2 tbsp	water	30 mL
1¾ cups	all-purpose flour	425 mL
½ cup	whole wheat flour	125 mL
1 tbsp	ground ginger	15 mL
1 tsp	baking soda	5 mL
¼ tsp	salt	1 mL
1 cup	packed dark brown sugar	250 mL
¼ cup	canola oil	60 mL
⅓ cup	light (fancy) molasses	75 mL
1 tsp	vanilla extract	5 mL
1 cup	chopped crystallized ginger	250 mL
¼ to ½ cup	raw sugar crystals	60 to 125 mL

1. In a small bowl, mix together ground flax and water and let stand for 10 minutes.

2. In a large bowl, stir together all-purpose flour, whole wheat flour, ground ginger, baking soda and salt. Set aside.

3. In a bowl, using an electric mixer or a stand mixer fitted with paddle attachment, beat together brown sugar, oil, molasses and vanilla on medium speed. Beat in flax mixture. On low speed, gradually beat in flour mixture, just until combined. Using a wooden spoon, stir in crystallized ginger.

4. Scoop dough by 1½ tablespoons (22 mL) and roll into balls. Roll in raw sugar to coat then place on prepared baking sheets, at least 2 inches (5 cm) apart, and flatten lightly with palm of your hand.

5. Bake in preheated oven, one sheet at a time, rotating pans from back to front halfway through, until tops look dry, 15 to 18 minutes. Let cool on pan on a wire rack for 5 minutes, then transfer to rack and let cool completely.

Pistachio biscotti

Makes about 3 dozen

The crunch of the pistachios and almonds and the subtle hint of the lemon and orange peel make these biscotti almost addictive. Luckily they freeze beautifully so a stash can be as near as the freezer.

✖ Tip

Store biscotti in an airtight container at room temperature for up to 1 week or freeze for up to 1 month.

✖ Preheat oven to 350°F (180°C)

2 1/2 cups	all-purpose flour	625 mL
2 tsp	baking powder	10 mL
1/2 tsp	salt	2 mL
1 tsp	grated lemon zest	5 mL
1 tsp	grated orange zest	5 mL
1/2 cup	vegan hard margarine, softened	125 mL
1 1/4 cups	granulated sugar	300 mL
1 tsp	vanilla extract	5 mL
1 1/2 tsp	powdered egg replacer	7 mL
2 tbsp	warm water	30 mL
3/4 cup	pistachios	175 mL
3/4 cup	whole almonds	175 mL

1. In a bowl, stir together flour, baking powder, salt, lemon zest and orange zest. Set aside.

2. In a large bowl, using an electric mixer, beat margarine and sugar until fluffy, about 1 minute. Beat in vanilla.

3. In a small bowl, stir together egg replacer and water. On low speed, alternately beat egg replacer and dry ingredients into margarine mixture, making two additions of egg replacer and three of dry ingredients. Using a wooden spoon, stir in pistachios and almonds.

4. Divide dough in half. On baking sheet, shape each half into a log, about 16- by 2-inches (40 by 5 cm), placing logs at least 3 inches (7.5 cm) apart. Bake in preheated oven just until logs are beginning to brown and are firm to the touch, 20 to 25 minutes. Let cool on pan on a wire rack for 10 minutes.

5. Transfer logs to a cutting board and, using a serrated knife, cut into 1/2-inch (1 cm) slices on a diagonal. Return to baking sheets, turning each slice cut side down. Bake for 7 minutes, flip slices and bake for 5 minutes more. With biscotti still in oven, turn oven off, leave oven door ajar and let biscotti stand for 15 minutes. Transfer biscotti to a wire rack and let cool completely.

Figgy pudding with brandy hard sauce

Serves 8 to 10

How many desserts have their own song? The name is fun to say and the spicy, moist cake is definitely fun to eat. Add to the general festiveness by sprinkling with additional brandy and setting aflame!

Tip

To store pudding and hard sauce: Sprinkle pudding with brandy, wrap in foil and refrigerate in an airtight container for up to 1 month. If pudding becomes dry, sprinkle with additional brandy, if desired. Hard sauce may be refrigerated in an airtight container for up to 1 month.

- **8-cup (2 L) pudding mold or deep heatproof bowl**
- **Stockpot with lid, large enough to hold pudding mold**
- **Rack to fit inside stockpot**
- **Kitchen string**
- **Long-handled match or fireplace lighter**

Hard Sauce

1/2 cup	vegan hard margarine, softened	125 mL
1 1/2 cups	confectioner's (icing) sugar, sifted	375 mL
1/2 cup	brandy, divided	125 mL

Figgy Pudding

4 tbsp	vegan hard margarine, divided	60 mL
1 cup	all-purpose flour	250 mL
3/4 cup	whole wheat flour	175 mL
1/2 tsp	baking soda	2 mL
1/2 tsp	ground cinnamon	2 mL
1/2 tsp	ground nutmeg	2 mL
1/4 tsp	salt	1 mL
3/4 cup	unsweetened applesauce	175 mL
3/4 cup	packed brown sugar	175 mL
1/4 cup	plain almond milk	60 mL
1 1/2 cups	chopped dried figs, stems removed	375 mL

1. *Hard sauce:* In a large bowl, using an electric mixer, beat margarine until creamy. On low speed, gradually beat in confectioner's sugar and 2 tbsp (30 mL) of the brandy, until smooth. Transfer to an airtight container and refrigerate.
2. *Figgy pudding:* Using 1 tbsp (15 mL) of the margarine, heavily grease inside of pudding mold and one side of a piece of foil or parchment paper to fit over top of mold. Set aside.
3. Place rack in bottom of stockpot and add water to fill about one-quarter full. Bring to a boil over high heat.
4. In a bowl, stir together all-purpose flour, whole wheat flour, baking soda, cinnamon, nutmeg and salt. Set aside.

5. Melt remaining 3 tbsp (45 mL) of margarine in the microwave or in a small saucepan and place in a large bowl. Stir in applesauce, brown sugar and almond milk. Add dry ingredients and stir vigorously until smooth. Stir in figs. Pour batter into prepared mold and smooth top. Cover tightly with foil, coated side down. If needed, tie down foil with kitchen string.

6. Place mold on rack in stockpot. Boiling water should be a third of the way up the side of the mold. Add additional boiling water as needed. Cover stockpot tightly with lid. Reduce heat to medium–low and steam pudding until top springs back when lightly touched and tester inserted in the center comes out clean, $2\frac{1}{4}$ to $2\frac{1}{2}$ hours. Molds with center tubes (like a Bundt pan) will cook 10 to 15 minutes faster. Add additional boiling water to pot if level gets low. Remove mold from stockpot and let cool on a wire rack for 10 minutes. Unmold onto serving platter and cover to keep warm. Set aside.

7. Place remaining brandy in a small saucepan over low heat until warmed, about 3 minutes. Pour brandy over pudding and with a long-handled match or fireplace lighter, ignite brandy at base of pudding, dimming lights for best presentation. Serve each slice of pudding topped with a spoonful of hard sauce, which will melt slightly.

Coconut panna cotta with mango ginger sauce

This elegant panna cotta will impress and delight your vegan friends who have forgone this Italian classic usually made with heavy cream. Here we use coconut milk for a tropical twist.

✖ Tip

Arrange prepared ramekins on a tray before filling for easy transport to the refrigerator once filled.

✖ Variation

I think it's just right but the texture of panna cotta is up to you, controlled by the amount of agar powder used. Less will produce a softer panna cotta, while more will give you a firmer dessert.

✖ Food processor or blender

✖ Six ½-cup (125 mL) ramekins, lightly oiled with coconut oil (see Tip, left)

Coconut Panna Cotta

1²/₃ cups	coconut milk	400 mL
6 tbsp	natural cane sugar	90 mL
½ tsp	agar powder	2 mL
1 tsp	vanilla extract	5 mL
1	package (12.3 oz /340 g) firm or extra-firm silken tofu	1

Mango Ginger Sauce

1	mango	1
2 tbsp	agave nectar	30 mL
	Grated zest of 1 lime zest	
2 tbsp	freshly squeezed lime juice	30 mL
1 tsp	grated fresh gingerroot	5 mL

1. *Coconut Panna Cotta:* In a saucepan, whisk together coconut milk, sugar, agar powder and vanilla. Bring to a simmer over medium heat and cook, stirring constantly, until mixture thickens, 3 to 4 minutes. Remove from heat and let cool for 15 minutes.

2. In food processor or blender, combine tofu and coconut milk mixture and blend until smooth. Spoon mixture into prepared ramekins, cover with plastic wrap and refrigerate until firmly set, at least 2 hours or overnight.

3. *Mango Ginger Sauce:* In clean food processor or blender, combine mango, agave, lime zest, lime juice and ginger and process until smooth. Transfer to a bowl, cover and refrigerate until ready to serve.

4. To serve, place bottom of ramekins in hot water for a few seconds. Run a knife around the inside edge. Invert a serving plate on top of ramekin and while holding both the plate and the ramekin quickly invert. Gently shake the ramekin to loosen the panna cotta onto the plate. Top panna cotta with a spoonful of sauce and serve immediately.

Maple pecan bread pudding

The ultimate in comfort food, this bread pudding conjures up visions of evening gatherings around a crackling fire and snowflakes dancing at the windowpane. This is the perfect make-ahead dessert because it needs to be refrigerated for several hours before serving.

❌ Tips

No stale bread? Simply tear up a loaf of French bread, place it on a baking sheet and leave in a warm 200°F (100°C) oven for a few hours.

Instead of heating the entire dish in Step 3, individual servings may be microwaved on High for about 30 seconds each then topped with caramel sauce.

❌ Variation

In place of French bread, use 1 lb (500 g) torn up day-old Giant Cinnamon Rolls (page 72) or store-bought vegan cinnamon rolls.

❌ Preheat oven to 350°F (180°C)
❌ 13- by 9-inch (33 by 23 cm) glass baking dish, oiled

Pudding

3 cups	Soy Milk (page 18) or Almond Milk (page 19) or store-bought	750 mL
1 tbsp	all-purpose flour	15 mL
3/4 cup	unsweetened applesauce	175 mL
1/2 cup	pure maple syrup	125 mL
1 tbsp	vanilla extract	15 mL
1/2 tsp	ground cinnamon	2 mL
1 lb	day-old vegan French bread, torn into 1-inch (2.5 cm) pieces (see Tips, left)	500 g
1/2 cup	chopped toasted pecans	125 mL
1/2 cup	raisins	125 mL

Caramel Sauce (page 23) or vegan store-bought, optional

1. *Pudding:* In a large bowl, whisk together soy milk and flour until smooth. Stir in applesauce, maple syrup, vanilla and cinnamon. Gently mix in bread pieces and let stand for 15 minutes. Place in prepared baking dish. Sprinkle pecans and raisins over top, pressing down gently to submerge.

2. Bake in preheated oven until top is golden brown and edges are pulling away from sides of pan, 45 to 50 minutes. (A knife inserted in center will not come out clean.) Let cool slightly, then cover and refrigerate for at least 4 hours or for up to 2 days.

3. Preheat oven to 300°F (150°C) and heat pudding until hot, about 15 minutes. Serve with a generous helping of caramel sauce.

Mexican chocolate pudding

Serves 4

Ready to eat in a little over an hour, this smooth and chocolaty pudding tastes of almond and cinnamon, reminiscent of Mexican hot chocolate.

Tip

Refrigerate any leftover pudding in an airtight container for up to 2 days.

Blender or food processor

1	package (12.3 oz/350 g) firm or extra-firm silken tofu	1
4 oz	vegan semisweet chocolate, melted	125 g
1/4 cup	agave nectar	60 mL
1/4 tsp	ground cinnamon	1 mL
1/2 tsp	vanilla extract	2 mL
1/4 tsp	almond extract	1 mL
1 cup	Almond Crème Fraîche (page 16), optional	250 mL

1. In blender or food processor, combine tofu, melted chocolate, agave nectar, cinnamon and vanilla and almond extracts and purée, scraping down sides as needed, until mixture is thick and smooth.
2. Transfer mixture to a bowl, cover and refrigerate for 1 hour. Spoon into serving bowls and serve with a dollop of Almond Crème Fraîche, if using.

Variation

For a real Mexican kick, add 1/8 tsp (0.5 mL) ancho chile powder.

Cinnamon-almond rice pudding

Serves 4

Comfort in a bowl, this stove-top rice pudding is creamy and barely sweet. Perfect to cook on a cold day, when standing next to a warm stove, stirring, is restorative.

4 cups	Almond Milk (page 19) or store-bought	1 L
1 tsp	almond or canola oil	5 mL
1 cup	Arborio rice	250 mL
1/4 cup	packed brown sugar	60 mL
1 tsp	vanilla extract	5 mL
1/2 tsp	ground cinnamon	2 mL

1. In a saucepan, heat almond milk over medium heat to just under a simmer, then cover to keep warm.
2. Place a heavy-bottomed saucepan over medium heat and let pan get hot. Add oil and tip pan to coat. Add rice and cook, stirring frequently, until rice begins to color, 4 to 5 minutes. Add 1/2 cup (125 mL) warm almond milk, stirring constantly. Add brown sugar. Cook, stirring, until most of liquid is absorbed then add another 1/2 cup (125 mL) almond milk. Continue cooking, stirring and adding liquid until rice is thick and creamy, 40 to 45 minutes in total, adjusting heat as necessary to maintain a simmer. Stir in vanilla and cinnamon.
3. Serve warm or refrigerate in an airtight container for up to 2 days. To serve refrigerated pudding, reheat on the stove top over medium heat or in the microwave with additional almond milk.

Variation

Stir in grated zest of 1 orange and 1/3 cup (75 mL) golden raisins when adding vanilla.

Almond and cardamom spiced tapioca

Sweetly spiced and velvety smooth, this pudding is sure to become a family favorite. Lovely for dessert or a creamy snack.

⚙ Tips

Look for small pearl tapioca in natural food stores or Asian markets.

Pudding keeps, covered and refrigerated, for up to 1 week.

1/3 cup	small pearl tapioca (see Tips, left)	75 mL
1 cup	water	250 mL
2 1/4 cups	Almond Milk (page 19) or store-bought	550 mL
1/8 tsp	salt	0.5 mL
1/2 cup	granulated sugar	125 mL
1/4 cup	cornstarch	60 mL
1 tsp	vanilla extract	5 mL
1/2 tsp	rose water	2 mL
1/2 tsp	ground cardamom	2 mL
2 tbsp	slivered almonds	30 mL

1. In a bowl, combine tapioca and water. Cover and let soak at room temperature for 1 hour.

2. Drain pearls, discarding soaking water. Place tapioca pearls in a heavy-bottomed saucepan. Add 2 cups (500 mL) of the almond milk and salt. Bring to a gentle boil over medium heat, stirring constantly. Reduce heat to medium-low and cook, stirring constantly, until pearls become translucent, about 5 minutes. Remove from heat.

3. In a small bowl, stir together remaining almond milk, sugar and cornstarch, mixing until smooth. Add sugar mixture to tapioca and return to medium-low heat. Cook, stirring constantly, until tapioca thickens and becomes glossy, 1 to 2 minutes. Remove from heat.

4. Stir in vanilla, rose water and cardamom. Pour into a serving dish and refrigerate for at least 2 hours. Stir just before serving and scatter top with slivered almonds.

⚙ Variations

Omit rose water, if desired, and increase vanilla to 2 tsp (10 mL).

Orange flower water can be substituted for the rose water.

When tapioca is chilled, fold in 1 cup (250 mL) diced mango or peaches.

Oasis bars

Reminiscent of a
Fig Newton, these
nuggets are chock-full
of oasis fruits, such as
dates and figs, spiced
from the exotic east
and wrapped in a
sweetened delectable
crust.

✳ Tip

Store bars in an airtight
container at room
temperature for up to
1 week.

✳ Food processor
✳ 9-inch (23 cm) square metal baking pan, oiled

Filling

1 cup	dried figs	250 mL
1 cup	pitted dates	250 mL
¾ cup	mango nectar	175 mL
¼ cup	agave nectar	60 mL
½ tsp	ground cardamom	2 mL
½ tsp	ground ginger	2 mL

Crust and Crumble Topping

1½ cups	large-flake (old-fashioned) rolled oats, divided	375 mL
1 cup	whole wheat pastry flour	250 mL
1 tsp	baking powder	5 mL
¼ tsp	salt	1 mL
¼ cup	coconut milk	60 mL
2 tbsp	agave nectar	30 mL
2 tbsp	coconut oil	30 mL

1. *Filling:* In a saucepan, combine figs, dates, mango nectar, agave nectar, cardamom and ginger and bring to a boil over medium heat. Reduce heat and simmer, stirring occasionally, until liquid is syrupy, about 10 minutes. Remove from heat and let cool for 20 minutes.

2. Transfer to food processor and process until almost smooth. Transfer to a bowl and set aside.

3. *Crust and Crumble Topping:* Preheat oven to 350°F (180°C).

4. In clean food processor, process ½ cup (125 mL) of the oats until powdered. Add remaining oats, flour, baking powder and salt and pulse just to combine. Add coconut milk, agave nectar and coconut oil and pulse to just combine, 7 or 8 times. Scrape around blade and sides and pulse again 4 times.

5. Press two-thirds of the dough evenly into the bottom of prepared pan. Spread cooled fig filling over crust and crumble remaining oat mixture over top. Press down lightly.

6. Bake in preheated oven until firm, about 20 minutes. Let cool completely in pan on a wire rack before cutting into squares.

Northern oat shortbread

Makes 8 wedges

Oats add a charmingly rustic and chewy texture to this scrumptious shortbread. Though made in the traditional triangular shape, this is not as delicate but decidedly better for you.

Tip

Store shortbread in an airtight container at room temperature for up to 1 week.

- **Food processor**
- **8-inch (20 cm) round metal cake pan, oiled and lined with an oiled parchment paper**

1/2 cup	vegan hard margarine	125 mL
1/4 cup	packed light brown sugar	60 mL
1/2 tsp	vanilla extract	2 mL
1/2 cup	all-purpose flour	125 mL
1/4 tsp	baking soda	1 mL
1 cup	large-flake (old-fashioned) rolled oats	250 mL

1. In food processor, combine margarine, brown sugar and vanilla and process until smooth, scraping down sides as needed. Add flour and baking soda and pulse until smooth. Add oats and pulse 10 times. Scrape into prepared pan and smooth top. Cover with plastic wrap and refrigerate until chilled, for at least 30 minutes or for up to 24 hours.
2. Preheat oven to 350°F (180°C).
3. With tines of a fork, make indentations all round edge and prick the entire surface. Using the back of a knife, mark into eight equal wedges. Bake in preheated oven until golden brown, 20 to 25 minutes. Cut though marked sections and let cool completely in pan on a rack. Turn out of pan, peel off parchment, invert onto platter and serve in wedges.

Variation

Add up to 1/2 cup (125 mL) currants after adding the oats.

Apricot brownies

Makes 16 squares

A trip to the apricot farm inspired these moist and subtly fruity brownies.

✖ Tip

Brownies are best served the day they are made but may be frozen, well wrapped, for up to 1 month. Bring to room temperature before serving.

✖ Preheat oven to 350°F (180°C)

✖ 8-inch (20 cm) square metal baking pan, oiled and lined with parchment paper

½ cup	all-purpose flour	125 mL
¼ tsp	salt	1 mL
1 cup	granulated sugar	250 mL
¼ cup	vegan hard margarine, softened	60 mL
⅔ cup	unsweetened cocoa powder	150 mL
1 cup	puréed fresh or canned apricots	250 mL
1 tsp	vanilla extract	5 mL
½ cup	vegan chocolate chips	125 mL

1. In a small bowl, stir together flour and salt. Set aside. In another bowl, using a wooden spoon, cream sugar and margarine until fluffy. Beat in cocoa until smooth. Stir in puréed apricots and vanilla. Add flour mixture and stir just until combined. Fold in chocolate chips.

2. Pour batter into prepared pan, smoothing top. Bake in preheated oven until top looks dry and tester inserted in the center comes out with moist crumbs clinging to it, 20 to 25 minutes.

3. Let cool completely in pan on a rack. Remove from pan and peel off parchment paper. Transfer to a cutting board and cut into 16 squares.

Chocolate cherry brownies

Makes 25 small brownies

These sophisticated, brandy-accented brownies make an elegant and decadent ending to a dinner party.

✖ Tips

Brownies are best served the day they are made but may be frozen, well wrapped in foil, for up to 1 month. Bring to room temperature before serving.

For easiest cutting, when brownies are completely cool, refrigerate for 30 minutes.

✖ Preheat oven to 350°F (180°C)
✖ 8-inch (20 cm) square metal baking pan, oiled and lined with parchment paper or foil

½ cup	all-purpose flour	125 mL
¼ tsp	salt	1 mL
2 tbsp	ground flax seeds	30 mL
5 tbsp	water	75 mL
1 tbsp	brandy	15 mL
½ cup	dried cherries	125 mL
4 oz	vegan semisweet chocolate, chopped	125 g
2 oz	vegan unsweetened chocolate, chopped	60 g
¼ cup	vegan hard margarine	60 mL
1 cup	granulated sugar	250 mL
¼ cup	unsweetened cocoa powder	60 mL
½ cup	chopped walnuts	125 mL

1. In a small bowl, stir together flour and salt. Set aside. In another small bowl, mix together ground flax seeds and water and let stand for 10 minutes. In another small bowl, add brandy to cherries and let soak.

2. In a large microwave-safe bowl, microwave semisweet chocolate, unsweetened chocolate and margarine, on Medium, stirring every 30 seconds, until mostly melted, 1 to 2 minutes. Remove from microwave and stir until completely melted. Whisk in sugar, cocoa and flour mixture until smooth. Stir in flax mixture, cherry mixture and walnuts.

3. Pour batter into prepared pan, smoothing top. Bake in preheated oven until top looks dry and tester inserted in the center comes out with moist crumbs clinging to it, 20 to 25 minutes. Let cool completely in pan on a rack. Remove from pan and peel off parchment paper. Transfer to a cutting board and cut into 25 squares.

Pistachio brittle

Makes 1 lb (500 g)

This super easy microwave brittle takes all the guesswork out of creating candy. Kids will be wowed that fresh, homemade candy can be made in less than an hour, from ingredients likely found in your cupboard!

✳ Tips

I used a 700-watt microwave for this recipe. Generally, newer microwaves are likely to be 1000 watts. If your microwave is more powerful, use Medium (50%) power. The wattage is usually marked inside the door, on the back, or on the bottom of the microwave.

Do follow good safety precautions because boiling syrups are very hot. Make sure kids and pets are kept out of harm's way.

✳ Microwave-safe 2-quart (2 L) bowl
✳ Silicone spatula, oiled with almond oil
✳ Rimmed baking sheet, oiled with almond oil

1½ cups	shelled pistachios	375 mL
1 cup	granulated sugar	250 mL
½ cup	light (white or golden) corn syrup	125 mL
⅛ tsp	salt, optional	0.5 mL
1 tbsp	vegan hard margarine	15 mL
1 tsp	vanilla extract	5 mL

1. In microwave-safe bowl, combine pistachios, sugar, corn syrup and salt, if using. Stir gently until well combined.

2. Microwave on High until mixture is bubbly and nuts are starting to darken, 6 to 7 minutes (see Tips, left). Stir in margarine and vanilla and microwave until mixture is turning a pale golden color, 2 to 3 minutes.

3. Using oiled spatula, immediately spread onto prepared baking sheet. Let cool completely. Break into pieces and store in an airtight container at room temperature for up to 1 month.

> ## ✳ Variation
> Substitute almonds, walnuts, pecans, peanuts or a mixture of nuts for the pistachios.

Summer berry cobbler

Serves 6 to 8

Save the strawberries and raspberries for shortcakes. Bake up this easy cobbler highlighting the "cooking" berries. Blueberries and blackberries shine under a blanket of cakey batter. The perfect ending for cookouts and picnics.

✄ Preheat oven to 350°F (180°C)
✄ 8-inch (20 cm) square glass baking dish, oiled

Filling

6 cups	blackberries and/or blueberries	1.5 L
1/4 cup	granulated sugar	60 mL

Cobbler

1/2 cup + 2 tbsp	granulated sugar	155 mL
1/2 cup	whole wheat flour	125 mL
1/2 cup	all-purpose flour	125 mL
1 1/2 tsp	baking powder	7 mL
1/4 tsp	salt	1 mL
1/2 cup	Soy Milk (page 18) or Almond Milk (page 19) or store-bought	125 mL
1/3 cup	canola oil	75 mL

Topping

1 tbsp	granulated sugar	15 mL
1/2 tsp	ground cinnamon	2 mL

1. *Filling:* In prepared baking dish, gently mix berries and sugar. Set aside

2. *Cobbler:* In a large bowl, stir together sugar, whole wheat flour, all-purpose flour, baking powder and salt. Add soy milk and oil and stir vigorously until smooth. Dollop batter over top of berries, letting some berries show through.

3. *Topping:* In a small bowl, mix together sugar and cinnamon and sprinkle over cobbler.

4. Bake in preheated oven until berry filling is glossy and bubbly and a tester inserted in cake comes out with moist crumbs clinging to it, 50 to 55 minutes. If cobbler is browning too quickly, tent dish loosely with foil. Let cool in dish for 5 minutes and serve warm. Best eaten the day it is made but can be refrigerated overnight.

✄ Variation
Substitute sliced peaches or a combination of berries and peaches in the filling.

Apple brown betty

Serves 6 to 8

When the weather turns chilly, who doesn't love a warm apple dessert redolent of cinnamon and brown sugar? No one we know and it doesn't matter if you call it a crisp, a crumble, or a Betty — they're all good!

✖ Tip

Cover and refrigerate any leftovers for up to 3 days.

✖ Preheat oven to 350°F (180°C)
✖ 8-inch (20 cm) square glass baking dish, oiled

Topping

½ cup	large-flake (old-fashioned) rolled oats	125 mL
⅓ cup	packed brown sugar	75 mL
¼ cup	whole wheat flour	60 mL
¼ cup	all-purpose flour	60 mL
1 tsp	ground cinnamon	5 mL
Pinch	salt	Pinch
¼ cup	vegan hard margarine, melted	60 mL
¼ cup	finely chopped walnuts, pecans or almonds	60 mL

Filling

6 cups	sliced peeled apples, such as Granny Smith (about 6 medium)	1.5 L
1 tbsp	all-purpose flour	15 mL
1 tsp	ground cinnamon	5 mL
⅓ cup	pure maple syrup	75 mL

1. *Topping:* In a bowl, stir together oats, brown sugar, whole wheat flour, all-purpose flour, cinnamon and salt. Stir in margarine until combined. Add walnuts. Using your hands, squeeze handfuls of mixture into clumps then break up into smaller clumps. Set aside.

2. *Filling:* In prepared baking dish, toss apples with flour and cinnamon. Pour maple syrup over apples and toss to coat. Crumble topping mixture evenly over apples.

3. Bake in preheated oven until apples are tender and topping is browned, 40 to 45 minutes. Let cool for 5 minutes and serve warm.

> ## ✖ Variation
>
> Substitute other seasonal fruit for the apples. Plums, peaches, pears and apricots all make wonderful "Betties."

Chocolate lover's silk pie

Serves 12 to 16

This pie is all about chocolate: deep, dark, ultra-rich chocolate. Serve well-chilled, in very small slices, to chocoholics only.

✖ Food processor
✖ 9-inch (23 cm) glass pie plate
✖ Dried beans or pie weights

Crust

1 cup	all-purpose flour	250 mL
1/3 cup	unsweetened cocoa powder	75 mL
1/4 cup	granulated sugar	60 mL
7 tbsp	vegan hard margarine, chilled, cut into pieces	105 mL
2 tbsp	cold water	30 mL
1/2 tsp	vanilla extract	2 mL

Filling

12 oz	vegan semisweet chocolate chips	375 g
1	package (12.3 oz /350 g) firm or extra-firm silken tofu	1
1 tsp	vanilla extract	5 mL
2 cups	vegan whipped cream alternative, optional	500 mL

1. *Crust:* In food processor, combine flour, cocoa and sugar and pulse until uniformly mixed. Add margarine and pulse until mostly fine crumbs. With motor running, add cold water and vanilla through feed tube. Pulse just until mixture forms a loose ball. Press into a disk. Wrap in plastic wrap and refrigerate for 30 minutes.

2. Preheat oven to 400°F (200°C).

3. Place dough between two pieces of waxed paper or parchment paper and roll out to a 12-inch (30 cm) circle. Slide paper and dough onto a large baking sheet and refrigerate for 10 minutes. Remove top sheet of paper and invert into pie plate, gently drape to fit. Remove paper and trim dough to fit edges, crimping edge decoratively. Prick all over with fork. Refrigerate for 15 minutes. Line pie shell with foil or parchment paper and fill with dried beans.

4. Bake in preheated oven until edges look dry, 10 to 12 minutes. Remove dried beans and foil and bake for an additional 5 minutes. Let cool completely before filling.

5. *Filling:* In a microwave-safe bowl, melt chocolate chips on Medium, stirring every 30 seconds, for 1 to 2 minutes.

6. In food processor, purée tofu, melted chocolate and vanilla until smooth. Spoon into crust, smoothing top. Cover loosely and refrigerate until chilled and set, for at least 1 hour or for up to 24 hours. Serve small slices with a dollop of whipped cream alternative, if using.

⁑ Variation

Change the flavor by adding 1 tbsp (15 mL) orange-flavored liqueur and grated zest of 1 orange with the tofu, or 2 tbsp (30 mL) Kahlúa or other coffee-flavored liqueur for a coffee kick.

Key west pie

A perfect ending for a spicy tropical meal, this fresh key lime pie has a secret. The beautiful green hue and creamy richness comes from avocados! Not only do they provide good fats, fiber and vitamin C, avocados also pair with lime quite naturally. Key limes are very small and very juicy and sometimes come in a 1 lb (500 g) mesh bag in the produce section or at Latin grocery stores. Use any leftover limes for margaritas or limeade.

✖ Tips

If purchasing a prepared graham pie crust, be sure to avoid a honey graham crust (which is not vegan). You can find vegan prepared crusts at health food stores.

To make a crumb crust: Mix together 1½ cups (375 mL) vegan graham cracker or vegan gingersnap crumbs, ⅓ cup (75 mL) granulated sugar and 6 tbsp (90 mL) vegan hard margarine, melted. Press into an 8- or 9-inch (20 to 23 cm) pie plate and refrigerate for 1 hour.

Cover and refrigerate any leftovers and serve within 2 days.

✖ Food processor or blender

¼ tsp	agar powder	1 mL
⅓ cup	water	75 mL
½ cup	granulated sugar, divided	125 mL
	Grated zest of 4 key limes	
½ cup	freshly squeezed key lime juice (about 12 key limes)	125 mL
4	small avocados	4
1	8- or 9-inch (20 or 23 cm) prepared vegan graham cracker crust (see Tips, left)	1
2 cups	vegan whipped cream alternative, optional	500 mL
1	mango, sliced, optional	1

1. In a small saucepan, sprinkle agar over water and let stand for 5 minutes. Stir in ⅓ cup (75 mL) of sugar and heat over medium heat, stirring until sugar is dissolved. Boil, stirring occasionally, for 1 minute. Pour into a small bowl and let cool until mixture begins to gel, 25 to 30 minutes.

2. In food processor, purée lime zest, lime juice and avocados until very smooth. Add agar mixture and remaining sugar and pulse until incorporated and smooth. Pour into prepared crust, cover loosely and refrigerate until chilled and set, for at least 4 hours or overnight.

3. Serve pie topped with whipped cream and mango slices, if using.

Rustic open-faced peach pie

Serves 6 to 8

A blanket of sweet ground almonds surrounds plump peach halves in a flaky puffed crust. The easy glaze topping and a sprinkling of raw sugar finish it off beautifully.

❖ Preheat oven to 400°F (200°C)
❖ 10-inch (25 cm) glass pie plate
❖ Food processor

4 cups	peach halves in light syrup (one 28 oz/796 mL can)	1 L
8 oz	vegan frozen puff pastry, thawed (1 sheet)	250 g
1/3 cup	raw sugar, divided	75 mL
1 cup	chopped almonds	250 mL
2 tbsp	vegan hard margarine	30 mL
1 tbsp	vanilla bean paste	15 mL
1 tbsp	plain soy yogurt or other vegan yogurt	15 mL
1/4 tsp	ground nutmeg	1 mL
Pinch	salt	Pinch

1. Drain peaches, reserving 1/4 cup (60 mL) syrup. Pat peaches dry, lay on a kitchen towel and set aside

2. On floured work surface, roll out puff pastry to a 16-inch (40 cm) square. Fit into pie plate, letting pastry corners hang over edges. Refrigerate while preparing filling.

3. Set aside 1 tsp (5 mL) raw sugar for topping and place remainder in food processor. Add almonds, margarine, vanilla bean paste, soy yogurt, nutmeg and salt and process for 30 seconds. Scrape down sides and process until fairly smooth, for 30 seconds more.

4. Spread almond mixture in prepared crust, building up mixture a little higher around edges. Place peach halves, cut side down, on top of almond mixture. Press down lightly. Fold corners of pastry over top of peaches, scrunching square pastry to fit in round pan.

5. Bake in preheated oven until almond filling (showing around peaches) looks dry and peaches have a slightly golden color, 45 to 50 minutes. If pastry seems to be browning too rapidly, cover edges with strips of foil. Let cool on rack 10 minutes.

6. Meanwhile, place reserved peach syrup in a microwave-safe bowl and microwave on High until reduced by half, 3 to 4 minutes. Brush syrup over peaches and sprinkle with reserved sugar. Serve warm or at room temperature.

Plymouth rock pie

Serves 8 to 10

During the rushed, cool days of the winter holidays, it's good to take time to chop dried fruit, mix up the spices and fill the house with aromatic memories. This old-timey minced fruit and nut pie will put us in the proper frame of mind to count our blessings and rejoice in our abundance.

✖ Tips

It is useful to note that 1 medium apple weighs about 6 oz (175 g).

Pie will keep, covered at room temperature, for up to 3 days.

✖ **8- or 9-inch (20 or 23 cm) glass pie plate**

Filling

1/2	orange	1/2
2 lbs	apples, peeled, cored and chopped, such as Granny Smith (see Tips, left)	1 kg
3/4 cup	packed brown sugar	175 mL
1/2 cup	golden raisins	125 mL
1/2 cup	chopped dried figs, stems removed	125 mL
1/2 cup	chopped dried cranberries	125 mL
1/4 cup	apple cider vinegar	60 mL
1/4 cup	brandy	60 mL
1 tsp	ground cinnamon	5 mL
1/2 tsp	ground nutmeg	2 mL
1/2 tsp	Autumn Spice Blend (page 309) or store-bought pumpkin pie spice	2 mL
1/2 tsp	ground ginger	2 mL
1/4 tsp	salt	1 mL
1/2 cup	chopped walnuts or pecans	125 mL

Crust

2 1/4 cups	all-purpose flour	550 mL
1/2 tsp	salt	2 mL
3/4 cup	vegan vegetable shortening, chilled and cut into chunks	175 mL
6 tbsp	cold water (approx.)	90 mL

1. *Filling:* Zest 1/2 an orange, remove seeds and chop. In a large saucepan, combine apples, chopped orange and zest, brown sugar, raisins, figs, cranberries, vinegar, brandy, cinnamon, nutmeg, spice blend, ginger and salt and bring to a boil over medium–high heat. Reduce heat to medium–low, cover and boil gently, stirring frequently to prevent sticking, until apple pieces are somewhat tender, about 20 minutes. Uncover, stir in walnuts and simmer, stirring often, for 5 minutes. Mixture should be very thick and hold its shape when mounded on a spoon. If not, boil, uncovered, stirring, until thick. Transfer to a bowl, cover and refrigerate for at least 2 hours or for up to 1 month.

2. *Crust:* In a large bowl, stir together flour and salt. Add vegetable shortening and, using a pastry blender or two knives, cut in shortening until mixture resembles coarse meal. Add cold water and, using a sturdy fork, mix well until dough holds together. If dough seems too dry and will not hold together, add additional water, 1 tbsp (15 mL) at a time. Divide dough in half and gather dough into two balls, then press into disks. Wrap in plastic and refrigerate until chilled, for at least 30 minutes or for up to 24 hours.

3. Preheat oven to 450°F (230°C).

4. On floured work surface, roll one portion of dough into a circle slightly larger than the pie plate. Fit dough into pie plate and refrigerate. Repeat process to roll out remaining dough for top crust.

5. Pour cooled filling into pie shell. Fit top crust over filling, fold over bottom crust to seal and crimp edges decoratively. Cut vent holes in top crust.

6. Bake in preheated oven for 15 minutes. Reduce temperature to 350°F (180°C) and bake until crust is beginning to brown, 30 to 40 minutes. Let cool on a wire rack. Serve warm or at room temperature.

Just rhubarb pie

Serves 6 to 8

Forget the strawberry filler, especially those with all the scary additives, this all-rhubarb pie is a revelation. Beautifully pink and red inside, the balance of tart to sweet is just right.

✕ Tip

Keeps covered, at room temperature, for 1 to 2 days.

✕ Food processor
✕ 9-inch (23 cm) glass pie plate

Crust

2¼ cups	all-purpose flour	550 mL
½ tsp	salt	2 mL
¾ cup	vegan vegetable shortening, chilled and cut into chunks	175 mL
6 tbsp	cold water (approx.)	90 mL

Filling

1½ cups	granulated sugar	375 mL
⅓ cup	all-purpose flour	75 mL
⅛ tsp	salt	0.5 mL
2 lbs	rhubarb, sliced into ½-inch (1 cm) pieces (about 6 cups/1.5 L)	1 kg
2 tbsp	vegan hard margarine, cut into small pieces	30 mL

1. *Crust:* In food processor, combine flour and salt. Add vegetable shortening and pulse until mixture resembles coarse meal. With motor running, through feed tube, add cold water. Pulse until dough gathers into a ball. If dough seems too dry, add more water, 1 tbsp (15 mL) at a time. Divide dough in half and gather into two balls, then press into disks. Wrap in plastic and refrigerate until chilled, for at least 30 minutes or up to 24 hours.

2. Preheat oven to 450°F (230°C).

3. On floured work surface, roll one portion of dough into a circle slightly larger than pie plate. Fit dough into pie plate and refrigerate. Repeat process to roll out remaining dough for top crust.

4. *Filling:* In a large bowl, combine sugar, flour, salt and rhubarb and pour into pie shell. Dot with margarine. Fit top crust over filling, folding over bottom crust to seal and crimp edges decoratively. Cut vent holes in top crust.

5. Bake in preheated oven for 15 minutes. Reduce temperature to 350°F (180°C). Bake until juices bubbling from vent holes are thick and shiny and crust is golden, 30 to 40 minutes. Let cool on a wire rack. Serve warm or at room temperature.

Balsamic roasted figs in phyllo cups

A composed dessert to make when figs and blackberries are at their best, this is a celebration of the deep purple hues of summer. The stunning presentation makes this a great choice when entertaining.

✖ Tips

As balsamic vinegar ages it thickens and intensifies in flavor. A balsamic that is at least 7 years old provides a superior experience.

To make phyllo cups: Preheat oven to 375°F (190°C). Cut 3 sheets of thawed phyllo dough in half, making 6 sheets that measure 13 by 8.5-inches (33 by 21 cm). Layer all 6 sheets, each brushed with melted vegan margarine and sprinkled with granulated sugar, into a stack. Cut the stack into 4-inch (10 cm) squares and fit into oiled muffin tins. Discard extra phyllo or reserve for another use. Bake in preheated oven until crisp and golden, 10 to 15 minutes. Let cool in pan on a wire rack for 5 minutes, then transfer to rack to cool completely.

✖ Preheat oven to 375°F (190°C)
✖ Muffin pan, 4 cups oiled

½ cup	pure maple syrup or agave nectar	125 mL
1 tbsp	balsamic vinegar (see Tips, left)	15 mL
4	large figs	4
4	pre-baked phyllo cups, thawed (see Tips, left)	4
2 cups	fresh blackberries or raspberries	500 mL
4	sprigs mint	4

1. In a small nonstick skillet, heat maple syrup and balsamic vinegar over medium–low heat until just simmering. Add figs and roll gently in syrup until heated through, about 5 minutes. Remove from heat, leaving figs in syrup.

2. *To plate:* Spoon a 1½ tbsp (22 mL) pool of syrup in center of each dessert plate. Set a phyllo cup at edge of pool and drizzle a little syrup inside cup. Slice each fig in half lengthwise, almost, but not all the way through, and open slightly. Place a warm fig in phyllo cup and drizzle a little syrup inside fig. Scatter blackberries around plate and add one sprig of mint. Repeat with remaining portions and serve immediately.

✖ Variation

Lemon verbena is a lovely replacement for mint sprigs.

Decadent chocolate truffles

Really, must any more be said?!

✖ Variation

Omit unsweetened cocoa powder and roll truffles in finely chopped pistachios, almonds or macadamia nuts.

¼ cup	coconut milk	60 mL
3 tbsp	vegan hard margarine	45 mL
8 oz	vegan dark chocolate, chopped	250 g
¼ cup	unsweetened cocoa powder, sifted	60 mL

1. In a microwave-safe bowl, combine coconut milk and margarine and microwave on High until margarine is melted and mixture is very hot, 1 to 1½ minutes. Add chopped chocolate and stir until chocolate is melted. Refrigerate for 1 hour or until mixture is stiff enough to scoop.

2. Scoop by tablespoons (15 mL) and form into rough balls. Place on a plate and refrigerate for 10 minutes. Roll balls in cocoa. Store between layers of waxed paper or parchment and in an airtight container in refrigerator for up to 2 weeks or frozen for up to 1 month.

3. To serve, remove from refrigerator 20 minutes prior to serving. If frozen, thaw for 24 hours in refrigerator.

Blackberry mint sorbet

Makes 4 cups (1 L)

This is pure blackberry with a delicate mint infusion. The color is stunning and the flavor is absolute heaven! One taste will send you rushing to your secret berry patch hunting for more.

✖ Tip

Store frozen sorbet for up to 2 weeks.

✖ Variation

If fresh blackberries are unavailable, frozen whole berries are a fine substitute.

✖ Ice cream maker

1¼ cups	granulated sugar	300 mL
1¼ cups	water	300 mL
¾ cup	mint leaves	175 mL
2 cups	blackberries	500 mL

1. In a small saucepan, stir together sugar and water. Bring to a boil over medium-high heat, stirring constantly, until sugar is dissolved. Add mint, immediately remove pan from heat and let cool completely. Transfer to an airtight container and refrigerate for at least 8 hours or for up to 1 week.

2. Pour chilled syrup through a fine sieve into a large bowl and discard mint. In same bowl, using same sieve, mash blackberries discarding seeds. Whisk mixture to blend.

3. Freeze in ice cream maker according to manufacturer's instructions. Transfer sorbet to a chilled airtight container and freeze until firm, for at least 4 hours before serving.

Iced mocha granita

Granita is a fun and delightful frozen dessert that requires nothing more than a shallow pan and a freezer. Serve in chilled margarita glasses for a festive presentation.

✜ Tip

Refrigerate shallow baking dish ahead of time so it is cold when you start.

✜ **11- by 7-inch (28 by 18 cm) glass baking dish**

¼ cup	unsweetened cocoa powder	60 mL
¼ cup	agave nectar	60 mL
2 cups	cold strong-brewed dark-roast coffee	500 mL

1. In a bowl, whisk together cocoa powder and agave until smooth. Whisk in coffee, mixing thoroughly to blend. Pour mixture into baking dish, cover tightly and freeze until ice crystals begin to form, 30 to 45 minutes. Scrape ice crystals from sides of pan and stir into mixture. Repeat process every 30 minutes until mocha mixture is frozen into ice crystals but not frozen solid, 2 to 2½ hours depending on your freezer.

2. Use a large serving spoon to scrape and break up the crystals. If granita becomes to frozen use a food processor to process granita into frozen crumbs. Spoon granita into chilled margarita glasses or bowls. Serve immediately.

Banana chocolate chip frozen pops

Everyone loves frozen pops so fortunately they are super easy to make. The chips sink to the bottom, which when unmolded, becomes the top. How clever.

✜ **Blender**
✜ **Six ¼-cup (60 mL) frozen pop molds**

2	bananas, cut into large pieces	2
½ cup	coconut milk	125 mL
3 tbsp	agave nectar	45 mL
3 tbsp	vegan mini chocolate chips	45 mL

1. In blender, combine bananas, coconut milk and agave and purée until smooth. Divide among molds. Sprinkle 1½ tsp (7 mL) chocolate chips on top of banana mixture in each mold. Seal molds and freeze until solid, for at least 8 hours or for up to 2 weeks.

2. To serve, run mold under warm water for a few seconds then unmold pops. Serve immediately.

Chocolate coconut frozen pops

Makes 6

Super chocolaty, with rich strands of fresh shredded coconut to boot. What more could you ask for!

✖ Tip

Shredded fresh coconut is available in the refrigerated (or freezer) section of most Asian grocery stores and in some well-stocked supermarkets.

✖ **Six ¼-cup (60 mL) frozen pop molds**

1 cup	coconut yogurt	250 mL
¼ cup	chocolate-flavored hemp or soy milk	60 mL
¼ cup	Divine Chocolate Sauce (page 22) or vegan store-bought	60 mL
1 tbsp	shredded fresh coconut	15 mL

1. In a small bowl, whisk together yogurt, milk, chocolate sauce and coconut until well blended. Divide among molds. Seal molds and freeze until solid, for at least 8 hours or for up to 2 weeks.

2. To serve, run mold under warm water for a few seconds then unmold pops. Serve immediately.

Peaches and cream frozen pops

Makes 6

Just the thing for the long dog days of summer.

✖ **Blender**
✖ **Six ¼-cup (60 mL) frozen pop molds**

1 cup	frozen sliced peaches	250 mL
¾ cup	vanilla-flavored almond milk, divided	175 mL
3 tbsp	packed brown sugar	45 mL

1. In blender, combine peaches, ½ cup (125 mL) of the almond milk and brown sugar and purée until smooth. Add remaining almond milk and process to blend. Divide among molds. Seal molds and freeze until solid, for at least 8 hours or for up to 2 weeks.

2. To serve, run mold under warm water for a few seconds then unmold pops. Serve immediately.

Tomatillo-lime sorbet

Light, cool and unique, this refreshing and delightful sorbet is the perfect festive finale to a spicy, hearty Mexican dinner.

❖ Food processor or blender
❖ Freezer proof bowl
❖ Metal melon baller
❖ 4 margarita glasses, chilled

1 cup	chopped tomatillos (2 to 3 medium)	250 mL
1 to 2	serrano chile peppers, seeded and chopped	1 to 2
1/2 cup	water	125 mL
1/4 cup	granulated sugar	60 mL
1 tsp	grated lime zest	5 mL
1/2 cup	freshly squeezed lime juice	125 mL
4	sprigs mint, optional	4

1. In a small saucepan, combine tomatillos, chiles to taste, water and sugar and bring to a boil over medium heat, stirring occasionally. Reduce heat and simmer, stirring occasionally, until tomatillos are softened, 8 to 10 minutes. Transfer to food processor and purée until smooth.

2. Place a fine-mesh strainer over freezer proof bowl and pour in tomatillo mixture. Use back of a large spoon to press liquids through strainer into bowl. Discard solids. Stir lime zest and lime juice into liquid.

3. Cover tightly and freeze for 2 hours. Remove bowl from freezer and stir with a sturdy fork. Return bowl to freezer and freeze until firm, 4 hours or overnight.

4. When ready to serve, using melon baller, scoop sorbet balls into prepared glasses and garnish with mint, if using.

> ❖ **Variation**
> Add 1 oz (30 mL) good-quality tequila to create a frozen margarita you can eat with a spoon.

Tropical ice in fruit cups

A beautiful presentation is only the beginning of the delights in store with these mouthwatering frozen gems served right in the fruit. Equally at home dressed up for an elegant dinner party or enchanting a group of little ones for a healthy and fun treat.

✕ Tip

If baby pineapples are not available, substitute 1 large pineapple and serve tropical ice in bowls.

✕ **Food processor**
✕ **Shallow pan**

2	baby pineapples (see Tip, left)	2
1/4 cup	natural cane sugar	60 mL
1/2 cup	water	125 mL

1. Slice pineapples in half vertically, scoop out flesh and set aside, taking care to leave pineapple shells intact. Place pineapple shells onto a baking sheet and freeze until firm.

2. In a small saucepan, combine sugar and water and bring just to a boil over medium heat, stirring to dissolve sugar. Set aside and let cool. Cover and refrigerate until chilled, about 4 hours.

3. In food processor, combine reserved pineapple fruit and 1/4 cup (60 mL) cooled simple syrup and process to a smooth purée. Taste and add more simple syrup, if necessary. Pour mixture into shallow pan, cover with plastic wrap and place in freezer. Freeze until partially frozen, scraping ice crystals from sides and stirring them into mixture, about 1 hour. Return to freezer until mixture is mostly frozen but not solid, stirring occasionally to break up any large frozen pieces. Before mixture is completely frozen and still granular, scoop into frozen pineapple halves and freeze to desired consistency. Remove from the freezer a few minutes before serving.

Green tea and coconut rum ice cream

A beautiful pale ivory green combination of matcha green tea and coconut milk blend into a luscious frozen dessert.

✖ Tip

If 15-oz (425 mL) cans cream of coconut aren't available, buy two 8½-oz (241 mL) cans and measure 1¾ cups + 2 tbsp (455 mL), then transfer the extra to an airtight container and refrigerate for up to 2 weeks or freeze for up to 3 months.

✖ Ice cream maker

2	matcha green tea bags	2
1 cup	hot water	250 mL
1	can (15 oz/425 mL) cream of coconut, chilled (see Tip, left)	1
½ oz	rum	15 mL

1. In a bowl or teapot, combine tea bags and hot water and let steep for 5 to 6 minutes making a strong cup of tea. Squeeze and discard bags. Let tea cool completely and refrigerate for at least 2 hours.

2. In a bowl, whisk together green tea, coconut cream and rum. Freeze in ice cream maker according to manufacturer's instructions. Transfer ice cream to a chilled airtight container and freeze to desired consistency. Remove from freezer a few minutes before serving to allow ice cream to thaw slightly.

> ## ✖ Variation
>
> If an ice cream maker is unavailable, pour mixture into an 11- by 7-inch (28 by 18 cm) glass baking dish. Freeze until frozen, stirring every 30 minutes, until desired consistency is achieved.

Index

Library and Archives Canada Cataloguing in Publication

Roussou, Deb
    350 best vegan recipes / Deb Roussou.

Includes index.
ISBN 978-0-7788-0294-5

1. Vegan cooking. 2. Cookbooks. I. Title. II. Title: Three hundred fifty best vegan recipes.

TX837.R68 2012   641.5'636   C2011-907498-2